THE FAMILY IS THE PATIENT
an approach to behavioral pediatrics
for the clinician

THE FAMILY IS THE PATIENT
an approach to behavioral pediatrics
for the clinician

BAYARD W. ALLMOND, Jr., M.D.

Co-Director, Child Study Unit,
Associate Clinical Professor, Pediatrics,
University of California, San Francisco

WILMA BUCKMAN, M.A., M.S.W.

Associate Clinical Professor Emeritus, Pediatrics,
University of California, San Francisco

HELEN F. GOFMAN, M.D.

Co-Director, Child Study Unit,
Associate Professor, Pediatrics,
University of California, San Francisco

Illustrated

The C. V. Mosby Company

ST. LOUIS • TORONTO • LONDON   1979

Printed in the United States of America

The C. V. Mosby Company
11830 Westline Industrial Drive, St. Louis, Missouri 63141

Library of Congress Cataloging in Publication Data

Allmond, Bayard W
  The family is the patient.

  Bibliography: p.
  Includes index.
  1. Pediatrics — Psychological aspects.   2.   Sick
children — Psychology.   3.   Family — Health and hygiene.
4.   Parent and child.   I.   Buckman, Wilma, joint author.
II.   Gofman, Helen F., joint author.   III.   Title.
[DNLM: 1.   Behavioral sciences.   2.   Child development deviations.   3.   Family.   4.   Pediatrics.
5.   Social environment.   WS100.3 A439f]
R547.5.A43   618.9′2′00019   79-16622
ISBN 0-8016-0131-2

C/VH/VH   9   8   7   6   5   4   3   2   1   01/A/081

To

OUR TRAINEES—STUDENTS, INTERNS, RESIDENTS,

and FELLOWS

They have been our faithful teachers

Foreword

Family-focused pediatrics has been given considerable lip service as the desirable way to practice pediatrics. In fact, however, it has been little practiced. In spite of calls by eminent authorities over the past two decades and recent announcements by the Task Force on Pediatric Education, which strongly recommends education of pediatricians in the biosocial and family aspects of child health, to date there has been little practical education of pediatricians in the skills needed for providing family therapy. This text is one of the first written by, and for, pediatricians to help them learn the skills of family therapy.

Reading a book on family therapy can no more produce a skilled family therapist than reading a book on skiing can make one an accomplished skier. It can help, however, both before starting the experience and after one has made some first clumsy attempts. This book avoids the use of jargon and is heavily illustrated with case examples that all clinicians can recognize. Examples of common behavioral problems in physically well children, as well as behavioral aspects of chronic disease, hospitalized patients, and psychosomatic disorders, are presented. The case examples include the actual verbal dialogue between family members and pediatrician. As the authors comment, "verbal dialogue tends to lose something . . . the juices and the flavor . . ." when written down, but the presentation of the cases in this text comes as close to the real thing as the written word can. Behavioral pediatrics is now an "in" word to define the new pediatrics, but it has been hard to define or to point the interested clinician to references that would help. This book is such a help.

Clearly family therapy is not for every pediatrician. This text will help those who are on the fence decide whether they want to obtain the training to do it well. Doing it well requires considerable experience, training under supervision, and skill. We still do not have carefully controlled studies to demonstrate which patients are most likely to be helped nor how the long-term effects of such therapy compare with other methods of treatment. However, there is so much validity to the cases presented that most readers will find that the methods and results "ring true." For pediatricians who recognize that the family is *the* patient, this book will be a guide to an exciting new diagnostic and therapeutic skill.

Robert J. Haggerty, M.D.

Professor of Public Health and Pediatrics,
Harvard School of Public Health;
Visiting Professor of Pediatrics,
Harvard Medical School

Preface

We began writing this book regarding behavioral or biosocial issues in pediatrics in November 1977, nearly 30 years after the Child Study Unit first began teaching pediatricians how to deal effectively with the psychosocial aspects of children's health care. Our trainees (over 200 pediatric residents and 26 fellows) often stated that the training they received from us in this area was the most valuable of any obtained during their medical education. This fact was often made all the more surprising, they added, because of their preconceived conclusion that any rotation in behavioral pediatrics would probably be dull and a waste of time. We knew different, of course. The behavioral realm of pediatrics is both exciting and important, and its teaching can and should reflect that same excitement and importance.

Naturally our specific approaches in teaching pediatricians and working with children have changed and evolved with the years. But regardless of the strategies and techniques used, we have singlemindedly held to the view that pediatricians in training should have expertise in the management of those behavioral and psychosocial issues that appear along with the child himself in the practicing pediatrician's office. Attention to the psychosocial needs of children is as much the responsibility of a pediatrician as the traditional concern for their physical well-being. Both aspects, not just one or the other, exert exceedingly important influences on the health and growth of all children. Pediatricians should therefore have practical, working skills for the handling of both biological and psychological dilemmas in children.

We have attempted to impart to our trainees this practical, working skill regarding the management of children's biosocial needs. Their response to our efforts over the years has been gratifying and enthusiastic. It is increasingly apparent to us as well that the work in which we have been engaged is both unique and successful and that the time has come to share our approaches to children's health and behavior with a wider audience. This book is intended for pediatricians, family practice physicians, nurses, social workers, psychiatrists, psychologists, and family therapists—as well as teachers and students in all of these disciplines. Since much of our own teaching focuses currently on the utilization of a family approach to children and their problems, we have decided to address most specifically the use of family interviews and family therapy principles by a physician or other health professional engaged in the clinical practice of pediatrics.

To be sure, we are joined by many others in our view that behavioral pediatrics is important and necessary for the training of all pediatric clinicians. This was dramatically verified in a recent publication of the Task Force on Pediatric Education, titled *The Future of Pediatric Education.** The task force was formed because of a recognition that many of the important health needs of infants, children, and adolescents were not being met as effectively and fully as they should be. Members represented ten societies that shared a common concern for the welfare of children (the American Academy of Pediatrics, American Academy of Child Psychiatry, Ambulatory Pediatric Association, American Medical Association Residency Review Committee, and Society for Pediatric Research, among others). Their primary goal was to identify the unmet health needs of children and to point out the educational strategies that would be required to prepare the pediatricians of the future to meet them. The published report was in their words "a distillation of two years of thought, testimony, and research."†

Early in their report, the task force acknowledged the omnipresence of behavioral issues in clinical pediatrics: "During the course of discussion the following issues repeatedly emerged at the core of current problems in pediatric education. They can only be addressed by commitment of talent, space, and money. . . . Biosocial and developmental problems, such as early family adjustment difficulties and school failure, adversely affect the health of many children and adolescents. These problems are serious and very widespread. All pediatricians should have the skill to cope with them."‡ The group further stated that children's

---

*Report: The Task Force on Pediatric Education. The future of pediatric education, 1978, Evanston, Ill.
†Report: The Task Force on Pediatric Education. The future of pediatric education, 1978, Evanston, Ill., p. viii.
‡Report: The Task Force on Pediatric Education. The future of pediatric education, 1978, Evanston, Ill., p. ix.

health needs are changing such that pediatricians in the future "will be called upon *increasingly* to manage children with emotional disturbances, learning disabilities, chronic illnesses, and other problems of a developmental, psychological and social nature.*

Perhaps most importantly, the task force identified those categories of needs in children most often underemphasized in current pediatric education. Foremost among them were "the biosocial and developmental aspects of pediatrics (early adjustment problems and school failure as well as all those deriving from abnormal growth and development in the child who is chronically ill or is socially, mentally, or emotionally disturbed)."†

A section of the task force report devoted to discussion of biosocial and developmental aspects of pediatrics seemed so pertinent to our teaching and to the writing of this text that we decided to include here a lengthy quotation from that portion of the report:

> By biosocial problems the Task Force means those health problems which are socially induced or complicated by social and environmental factors. These problems are sometimes referred to as "psychosocial" or "behavioral," but the Task Force prefers the term "biosocial" because it indicates that these aspects of child health are as much a part of human biology as those to which the term "biomedical" is commonly applied. The developmental aspects of pediatrics often involve both biomedical and biosocial concerns.
>
> The roles of pediatricians in practice are changing and pediatricians are increasingly being consulted regarding problems of a biosocial and developmental nature. With increasing frequency, the practicing pediatrician is being called upon to aid parents and children in coping with the challenges of modern society. Finally, to be effective in the promotion of healthy lifestyles and in health education, the pediatrician will need to be competent in the biosocial aspects of the discipline.
>
> The increasing national emphasis on primary care and the increasing visibility of biosocial problems have brought about changes in the nature of pediatric practice. Parents report numerous biosocial and behavioral problems in their children, turn most often to pedia-

---

*Report: The Task Force on Pediatric Education. The future of pediatric education, 1978, Evanston, Ill., p. 13.
†Report: The Task Force on Pediatric Education. The future of pediatric education, 1978, Evanston, Ill., p. 1.

tricians for help, and express a willingness to pay for the extra amounts of the physician's time required for counseling in these areas. . . .

Practitioners are becoming involved in management of biosocial and developmental problems not only because of the great need, but also because the growth of group practices allows individual pediatricians to pursue areas of special interest. Among the areas of special interest most frequently selected by general pediatricians are those which require a commitment to biosocial and developmental concerns: i.e., behavioral and psychosocial pediatrics, adolescent medicine, the child with handicaps, child abuse and neglect, and community medicine.

About half (54 percent) of young pediatricians rated their residency as providing insufficient experience with psychosocial and behavioral problems; 36 percent rated training in the management of mental or emotional disorders as insufficient. It is understandable, therefore, that pediatricians are expressing a desire for additional training in the biosocial and developmental areas.

The content of experience in biosocial pediatrics should include normal and abnormal growth and development, basic behavioral science information, reactions of children of various ages to illness, education for healthy lifestyles, and the principal literature regarding child development. Residents should also learn about the nature of psychologic and achievement tests, the principal psychological therapies, the principles of psychopharmacology, and the techniques of family counseling. They should be familiar with the developmental characteristics of the parent-child interaction, child care practices, and dysfunctions in parenting.

Residents should learn to manage such family crises as death and bereavement, suicide attempts, sexual assault, accidents, child abuse, birth of a defective child, separation, divorce, abortion, and a wide range of common behavioral disorders. Furthermore, they should be able to work with the family to resolve problems in parenting, well child care, adoption/foster care, school adjustment, and learning. They should be familiar with the role of the pediatrician in the management of disease states in which psychological elements play an etiologic or contributory role. . . .

Residents need to acquire skills in interviewing and obtaining a history from parents, parent surrogates, children, and adolescents. The interview should create a positive relationship between physician and patient while eliciting data leading to the diagnosis of organic or psychosomatic disease. Residents must learn to hear what children are saying.

Another important skill is the systematic observation of behavior and personal interactions in settings in which children are nurtured, cared for, and educated. Behavioral observations often offer important diagnostic clues. Developmental and psychosocial evaluation . . . should be part of every thorough physical examination. The physical examination should be an emotionally therapeutic experience.

Empathy and the ability to use subjective personal reactions in the care of patients are additional important skills. The pediatrician's development of self-awareness, particularly of personal temperament and preferences in lifestyle, may enable him or her to become more aware and accepting of the patient's total life situation, respecting the autonomy, privacy, and value preferences of the families served. The pediatrician can often promote healing and prevent biosocial complications by personal concern and kindness.

Other skills include the ability to communicate with parents and the child in the ways which enable them to increase their confidence in themselves and to engage actively in their own health and sickness care.*

We hope that the reader — pediatrician, family physician, nurse, social worker, psychiatrist, psychologist, or family therapist — will find this text responsive to the preceding observations and recommendations, a useful tool for enhancing one's knowledge regarding the biosocial aspects of pediatrics, and a book that may be used for developing specific clinical skills in working effectively with children and their families.

We are very grateful for the unflagging support and professional comradeship offered by our colleagues in the Child Study Unit. Their ideas, skills, and yeoman work efforts have in large part made the writing of this text possible. To each we say thank you. The staff includes: Mary Crittenden, Ph.D., pediatric psychologist; Sarah Dean, M.A., pediatric psychologist; Richard Flower, Ph.D., speech, language, and hearing consultant; Donya Harvin, M.A., pediatric psychologist; Paula Johnson, M.S.N., N.P., clinical nurse specialist; Diana Kennedy, M.S., pediatric psychologist; Marc Lehrer, Ph.D., pediatric psychologist; Alan Leveton, M.D., consulting psychiatrist and family therapist; Jack Obedzinski, M.D., pediatrician and family therapist; Louise Taichert, M.D., pediatrician and family therapist; Alice Whitsell, B.S., educational specialist; and Leon Whitsell, M.D., consulting neurologist and psychiatrist. One other staff member in the Child Study Unit has literally

---

*Report: The Task Force on Pediatric Education. The future of pediatric education, 1978, Evanston, Ill., pp. 19-21.

made the writing of this volume possible. Our secretary, Nancy Colvin, has tirelessly and expertly nursed this manuscript through its typing and retyping periods, serving not only as typist but also as grammarian and informal reviewer. Her contribution is acknowledged and most appreciated.

Another informal reviewer deserves mention. Nancy Allmond, in the wings, has listened and listened. She has also provided ideas, encouragement, suggestions for revisions, and enthusiasm. Grateful acknowledgment is made of her contributions to the project.

The Child Study Unit has continued to receive considerable financial support over the years from the Division of Maternal and Child Health, Department of Health, Education and Welfare (Grant #MCT-002001-13-0). We are grateful for this steadfast support of our teaching and research efforts. Such funding has played no small part in the development and completion of this text.

Bayard W. Allmond, Jr.
Wilma Buckman
Helen F. Gofman

Contents

Introduction

This text describes a clinical approach that has been developed over the years within the Child Study Unit of the Department of Pediatrics at the University of California, San Francisco. A brief history of that unit will help the reader to glimpse the setting that has nurtured our ideas.

The unit began 30 years ago with two staff members and one trainee. It was established by the late Dr. George Schade, a pediatrician at the University of California, San Francisco; he was one of four pediatricians selected throughout the country in the 1930's to receive 2 years of training with Drs. Frederick Allen and Jessie Taft at the Philadelphia Child Guidance Clinic. Training for the four pediatricians, directed toward increasing their knowledge in the management of pediatric emotional and behavior problems, was supported by the Commonwealth Foundation. The organization hoped through this project to improve the training of many more pediatricians in the management of common emotional and behavioral problems in children. It was explicitly expected that the four pediatricians, following training, would return to their respective pediatric departments in university teaching hospitals and establish teaching programs devoted to this aspect of pediatrics. In 1948 Dr. Schade, with the aid of a small grant from the Commonwealth Foundation and subsequent support from the University of California and its Department of Pediatrics, fulfilled this expectation by formally opening the Pediatric Mental Health Unit. The staff consisted of Dr. Schade himself, a psychiatric social worker, and Dr. Helen Gofman, his first pediatric fellow.

From the beginning, the purpose of this unit was to provide opportunities for pediatricians "to become better pediatricians." Pediatric house officers were helped to understand and manage the behavior problems commonly seen in pediatric practice. Particular emphasis was

1

placed on understanding the normal development and developmental differences in children. Frederick Allen's view had been that a child's behavior was often a manifestation of his own "growth toward independence." This view, one of the early attempts to understand children utilizing a "growth" model rather than a "pathology" model, was incorporated into teaching efforts with pediatric trainees in the unit. Clinical approaches as taught by the staff, again largely influenced by Allen, were concerned most often with the present rather than with the past and with an emphasis on practical interventions and strategies, the latter especially appealing to pediatricians. The early work of the unit was greatly aided by the contributions of the late Dr. Olga Bridgman, a psychologist and psychiatrist who had long been associated with the Department of Pediatrics and also with the Department of Psychology at the University of California, Berkeley. Her main interest was in the développmental assessment and management of children with visual handicaps, hearing deficits, cerebral palsy, and/or mental retardation. Through her efforts pediatric psychologists with expertise in the developmental assessment of children were added early to the staff of the Pediatric Mental Health Unit, their number growing from one to the five now in the unit.

Mrs. Wilma Buckman joined the Pediatric Mental Health Unit 2 years after its inception in 1950 as a psychiatric social worker. Aside from her background in social work, she had also had experience as an elementary and nursery school teacher and director; she had received a masters degree in child growth and development and had operated several day care nursery schools for working mothers during World War II. She thus also stressed the unit's clinical emphasis on the developmental aspects of child growth and behavior. In the 1950's Mrs. Buckman and Dr. Gofman began working steadily on the development of a practical teaching program for pediatric house officers in interviewing and pediatric counseling.

Following the sudden death of Dr. Schade in 1961, Dr. Gofman assumed the directorship and began to concentrate her energies on another area of training: the evaluation of children with learning problems. As a result of this interest, she was gradually able to increase the size and diversity of the unit staff, adding a neurologist and educational consultant to the roster and forming a close alliance with the Department of Otolaryngology, Speech, and Audiology. As more and more children were referred to the unit for learning and developmental problems, in addition to those referred for behavioral complaints, a change in name seemed indicated. The title, Child Study Unit, was adopted in 1966.

By this time financial support had been obtained, first from the U.S. Children's Bureau and then from the Division of Maternal and Child Health, Department of Health, Education, and Welfare. The support allowed the addition of a psychiatrist and a second pediatrician to the staff. A third pediatrician, Dr. Bayard Allmond, joined the unit in 1969. During this period, in the middle and late 1960's, the members of the unit became interested in the newly developing field of family therapy and the possible application of family therapy approaches to pediatrics and to pediatric interviewing. As a result both Mrs. Buckman and the unit's consulting psychiatrist, Dr. Alan Leveton, received training directly from Virginia Satir in family therapy and Frederick Perls in Gestalt therapy. Returning to share their training experiences with the remainder of the Child Study Unit staff, these two individuals became largely responsible for the incorporation of family therapy and Gestalt therapy principles into the ongoing training program for pediatric residents. These new dimensions in interviewing, the subject of this book, were firmly established in the unit's pediatric training endeavors by the early 1970's, significantly altering the program in interviewing that had been offered to pediatricians-in-training.

In the mid 1970's another pediatrician and a pediatric nurse practitioner were added to the staff. Thus from two individuals, the staff has grown to fifteen professionals: four pediatricians, five pediatric psychologists, one psychiatrist, one neurologist, one pediatric nurse practitioner, one educational specialist, and two secretaries.

Just as the staff has grown and diversified over the years, so have the trainees. In the early years training was somewhat irregular, directed toward whoever was willing to be taught and/or "unlucky" enough to have been assigned a patient with a behavioral problem requiring assistance. Training became more formalized—and apparently quite successful—with time. By the early 1950's a pediatric resident could elect a specific 3-month rotation through the Pediatric Mental Health Unit. The rotation was always filled, and in 1969 the pediatric house officers themselves requested that the Child Study Unit be a required, rather than an elective, rotation for all pediatric residents. That situation has been the case ever since. Every PL-II trainee at the University of California, San Francisco, spends 2 months in the Child Study Unit.

In addition to pediatric residents, since 1965 the Child Study Unit has been training two postgraduate pediatric fellows per year in a 1- or 2-year fellowship in behavioral pediatrics. This aspect of the training has received continuing support from the Division of Maternal and Child Health, Department of Health, Education, and Welfare.

The Child Study Unit is also considered core curriculum for medical students at the University of California, San Francisco. Consequently the majority of third or fourth year medical students spend time with the staff of the Child Study Unit.

Other trainees have participated in Child Study Unit programs regarding behavioral pediatrics depending on their specific interests and time. These individuals have included nurses, physicians in primary care residencies, and genetics counselors. While the unit, its staff, and its trainees have grown and changed over the years, the main purpose remains the training of pediatricians in children's behavior and development. The setting previously described and the main purpose just stated form the basic professional underpinnings for the authors and for the text that follows.

FORMAT

Case illustrations using specific dialogue are used heavily throughout this book. We are aware that this style of writing has both advantages and disadvantages. On the negative side, accounts of a verbal dialogue tend to lose something once they are written. Many of the nuances of nonverbal behavior, setting, and mood are unavailable to the reader, and he must either imagine those aspects of the conversation or do without them. In any case the juices and flavor of the dialogue may suffer, rendering the interchange somewhat flat and one-dimensional. This limitation of the written word to describe events that are both visual and auditory is regrettable but unavoidable. As an additional disadvantage, lengthy sections of dialogue may make cumbersome reading, requiring a different set from that to which the reader is accustomed — in much the same way that reading drama differs from reading prose and necessitates a different approach by the reader. We have attempted to minimize the reader's possible struggle over dialogue by deleting obviously clumsy grammatical and syntactical constructions that are so much a part of literal verbal language (the hems and haws, repetitions, grunts and groans, and so on) when doing so would not change the flavor of the dialogue itself. In many of the situations presented, the dialogue has been "neatened up" to allow for less effort and difficulty in the reading process. The conversations themselves are actual, and beyond the editorial deletions, the gist of a person's speech has not been changed. However, to ensure the privacy of patients and their families we have freely changed names and sometimes sexes, geographic locations, ages, and occupations.

In spite of the drawbacks attendant upon the use of written dialogue for clinical illustration, we have chosen to use it, and to use it considerably, for very particular reasons. This text is concerned with demonstrating clinical approaches that are practical and specific. We have felt that our illustrations must share with the reader situations in which practical skills are being utilized, that is, clinical interviews with specific dialogues between physicians and families.

The text is also concerned very much with "how" questions, that is, *how* does a certain family member react to a given comment, *how* does a doctor handle this certain situation, *how* does one tell a mother this particular news, and so forth. Examples of clinical dialogue can effectively answer such "how" questions, perhaps more succinctly than any other written device, in a way that is often unlabored and to the point.

There is a third reason for our inclusion of so much illustrative dialogue. To be an effective teacher of behavioral pediatrics, one must be willing to risk exposing one's own interviewing style and clinical techniques with patients — for better or worse, through the successes and through the failures as well. Some of the cases that follow, particularly those in the first part of the book, sound very neat, easy, almost too successful. While we do not feel constrained to apologize for these successes — they did in fact occur — we have attempted to present also a few of our clinical failures and partial failures to balance the scale and to gently encourage others to risk themselves in like situations. We hope with our own risk-taking, demonstrated in the pages to follow, to invite that of the reader in his or her own clinical work with children and families. For risk-taking, as we all know, ultimately separates the successful from the unsuccessful learner.

Most often an interviewer in the examples presented is referred to as "the pediatrician" or "the doctor" or "the physician." These terms are meant to be generic and broad, standing for any health care worker who may be involved in the medical and psychological care of children: family physician, pediatrician, nurse, social worker, psychologist, psychiatrist, or family therapist. Each of these professionals may conduct family interviews, and the substance of this book is directed to them all. It would, however, have been awkward to list every one of those terms in the text whenever an interviewer is mentioned. We trust that readers, especially those who are not physicians but for whom our approach seems useful, will understand that a desire for simplicity in writing style rather than professional chauvinism motivated our choice of terms.

The text is divided into two major parts. The first part, "Principles," presents in four chapters the work of four theorists and clinicians who have strongly influenced not only the character of our clinical work with children and families, but also our teaching approaches with pediatric trainees. Our granting each of these individuals a separate, extensive discussion may be misleading for some readers. One could assume from this format that we see our clinical work as simplistically limited to a literal application of the ideas developed by each or all of the four theorists. This is not the case. We would find such a clinical approach to be constricting, unimaginative, and too artificially compartmentalized. We are indeed grateful for the ideas of Satir, Minuchin, Haley, and Perls, the four individuals reviewed in Part I. Their work is often at the heart of what we do clinically with families and trainees. However, we are also mindful of the writings of Sigmund Freud, Erik Erikson, Milton Erickson, Carl Jung, Frederick Allen, Murray Bowen, and many others.

To these innovators in the field of psychological thought, we have seen fit to add elements of our own choosing, our own style, our own creativity. It is this mix of (1) Satir, Minuchin, Haley, and Perls, (2) legendary others in the field, and (3) our own individuality—distilled into a clinical approach—that we have attempted to present through case illustrations in the nine chapters of Part II, titled "Clinical Application."

Some readers may prefer to begin with the second part of the text, learning something first of our specific clinical approaches and style and turning thereafter to Part I and our discussion of many of the principles that underlie our work. Since we suspect that many busy pediatricians will probably do this anyway, we would like to sanction such an approach to the reading of this text.

We insert one final balancing statement. This book is enthusiastic in its view that family therapy principles can be applied to pediatric practice for both the diagnosis and management of pediatric problems, particularly those in the behavioral and psychological realms. Our enthusiasm stems from the fact that we have found a family systems approach to be practical, effective, exciting, congruent with our ideas about children and their families, and thus comfortable for us to use. However, in sharing our approaches with the reader we are not suggesting the arrival of *truth,* nor in our enthusiasm do we seek to nullify other theoretical hypotheses and alternate clinical approaches to the same human problems as those we have encountered. Rather our work in this text is intended to introduce a method, a model, an approach that has worked well for us.

PART I

PRINCIPLES

The family as the treatment unit and the pediatric practitioner as the interviewer

THE LOCKSLEY FAMILY

Joan, age 7, sits quietly, very prettily, in her chair. She is swinging her legs to and fro as her grandmother explains to Dr. Henry Abbott, the pediatrician:

Grandmother: She's not sleeping, Doctor. And neither am I — none of us has had a good night's rest in 7 weeks or so. Even if I get her in bed by 8 P.M., usually about 11 she wakes up — terrified, screaming. Then I'm up all night with the poor child. And once she does settle down again, maybe 3 or 4 A.M., she still thrashes and screams out — in her sleep! Why, I've had to bring her in to the emergency room twice in the past 2 weeks . . . she just gets hysterical. The doctor who saw her said something about epilepsy.

Doctor: Well, Mrs. Locksley, I wonder if . . .

Grandmother: Screams bloody murder — it wakes the neighbors. We're all on pins and needles now at night. And look at the circles under her eyes . . . low blood, somebody told me . . .

Doctor: What I meant to say . . .

Grandmother: I've tried everything — night-light, waking her up, talking, taking her to the bathroom, stories, rocking, hot milk — my own mother used to do that. Could it be worms, Doctor?

Doctor: That's something to consider. Now back to . . .

Grandmother: What could cause a child to cry out in her sleep like that? Well, I don't know if she's asleep or not. But I do know she just won't stay in bed once the whole thing starts . . . oh, and

11

stomachaches—I almost forgot. She complains constantly about that—in bed 5 minutes and then "Gramma, my tummy hurts." Then I know we're in for it for the rest of the night. Makes no difference when she goes to bed, early or late, it's the same thing.

Doctor: When does she usually . . .

Grandmother: I think more of this child than myself, Doctor—I want you to know that. Why, I've raised her since she was 4 years old. We're never apart, isn't that right, honey?

Joan: (nods)

Doctor: Do the two of you live alone?

Grandmother: Well, we did, but no, my daughter, Joan's mother, she lives with us now. She was separated recently. And my other daughter, divorced too, she's moved back in with me. And she has her own little girl, Cheryl, just 6 months younger than Joan. The two kids get along really well. What's that? Yes, the house is crowded, but we're making do. But Joan's business has been getting to everybody. With the last episode 3 nights ago, we *all* came to the emergency room. She certainly needs some sort of checkup, don't you think? Can growing pains ever do this?

Doctor: Sometimes. The stomachaches you mentioned, just where does she complain of pain?

Grandmother: All over, isn't that right, Joan? Show him, sweetie . . . now don't be that way. The doctor is here to help us. Speak right up and talk to the nice man; he wants to know where you hurt. There's nothing to be afraid of . . . she doesn't like doctors. Doctor . . . you're not going to give her any shots are you, she hates that. Now Joan, sweetie, don't cry.

The culmination of this interview between a pediatrician, a patient, and her grandmother is maddeningly familiar. A history of sorts has been obtained, along with a physical examination. More than likely the youngster's sleep disorder and other assorted symptoms have remained intact, as have grandmother's notions about epilepsy, worms, growing pains, low blood—and physicians; she is communicating these notions to the child as well. Only the doctor is altered; he experiences a definite depletion of energy—his, which was to have carried him through his office day. This was the case with Joan, Mrs. Locksley, and her pediatrician. The situation, while not included as a laudatory example of fancy interviewing footwork, did occur, and it serves to introduce an initial tenet of the authors: in many clinical pediatric situations it is useful to raise one's sights above the child, focusing on the family constellation surrounding the child via a family interview. For Joan and others like her, the clinician would do well to enlarge his* vision to include *all* the family for the purpose of understanding the family's interaction and its relationship to the presenting problem. Having done so, one may then recognize that the focus for both diagnosis and treatment is no longer a single individual, nor, if the family includes others, is it limited to one parent and child; it is rather that group of relationships called "the family."

Focusing on the family constellation surrounding a child is hardly a new idea. It is a time-honored tradition in pediatrics to obtain a complete family history when undertaking the medical care of a child. Indeed, pediatricians seem to be particularly family-oriented in their views of children and children's health care. No pediatrician finishes training without the realization that he is almost always working with at least two patients simultaneously—a child and a parent. So in this sense pediatricians are already committed to the idea that working with children means working with others (usually the mother) in a child's family. Likewise family practitioners today need no convincing that treating children involves work with other family members. It goes with the territory, so to speak. Yet little is written in medical literature regarding the use of family interviewing or a family-oriented interviewing approach in pediatric or family practice.

We are suggesting something considerably more specific than a general consensus that families are important, something more direct than the compilation of a thorough family history obtained by talking with one parent. We are suggesting that, since pediatrics and family medicine are family-oriented disciplines and since children in most instances cannot be considered or treated apart from their family context, pediatric practitioners should consider the treatment unit quite often to be the family; the family becomes *the* patient. Most explicitly we are suggesting that physicians develop a specific skill for working with "patients," name-

---

*All three authors (two are women) recognize that pediatric practitioners and interviewers come in male and female varieties. It is cumbersome to use constructions such as he/she and so on repetitively in writing. Use of the masculine pronoun throughout the book was therefore chosen for convenience. Sexual inequity is acknowledged.

ly, the ability to conduct a family interview. It is a skill based on specific principles, as learnable as ausculation of the heart, and it may be equally useful in clinical pediatrics.

The specific principles to which we refer derive from a body of theoretical and clinical work developed over the past 30 years in psychiatry and social work. Family interviewing and family therapy began as a ground (or more correctly, an underground) swell, without credentials or acceptance, in the late 1940's. Haley, writing in 1962, stated:

> The treatment of an entire family, interviewed together regularly as a group, is a new procedure in psychiatry. Just when family therapy originated is difficult to estimate because the movement has been largely a secret one. Until recently, therapists who treat whole families have not published on their methods, and their papers are still quite rare, although we may soon expect a deluge. The secrecy about family therapy has two sources: those using this method have been too uncertain about their techniques and results to commit themselves to print (therapists of individuals have not let this dissuade them), and there has apparently been a fear of charges of heresy because the influence of family members has been considered irrelevant to the nature and cure of psychopathology in the patient. As a result, since the late 1940's, one could attend psychiatric meetings and hear nothing about family therapy unless, in a quiet hotel room, one happened to confess that he treated whole families. Then another therapist would put down his drink and reveal that he too had attempted this type of therapy. The furtive conversations ultimately led to an underground movement of therapists devoted to this most challenging of all types of psychotherapy and this movement is now appearing on the surface.*

Actually Freud himself gave a nod to the importance of family members in one of his most famous cases, "Little Hans."[5] In 1909 he undertook the treatment of that child's phobia by working exclusively with the father. Hans himself was not interviewed. It is a matter of record, however, that family therapy was not born of this case. Freud preferred to work with individuals apart from their families. And psychoanalysts eventually developed strong feelings against the inclusion of families in the treatment of individuals, stating as the major objection that transference between patient and therapist could never be satisfactorily established with intrusions by other family members.[4]

---

*Haley, J.: Whither family therapy, Family Process 1:69, 1962.

Certainly the work of Harry Stack Sullivan, with his stress on the interpersonal aspects of mental illness, was an important developmental step toward the inclusion of family members in a child's psychiatric treatment. For him the mother-child relationship was all important and became the focus of treatment. His ideas were thus one of the most important foundations of the child guidance movement, which in some ways forwarded the cause of family treatment but did so unfortunately at mothers' expense. One of the negative outgrowths of this view of treatment was a tendency to blame mothers for all the difficulties observed in a child. In the zeal to shift sights off the child and onto the mother-child relationship, all too often the sighting was overcorrected and focused squarely on the other individual in the relationship, Mom. The (then) truism, "There are no bad children, only bad mothers" was unfortunately a hallmark of many child guidance clinics of the 1930's and 1940's.

The structuring of such a clinic was often as follows: the child (helpless victim) was weekly whisked into the playroom to spend a secret hour of play with the child psychiatrist in "the corrective emotional experience." In the meantime Mama (the cause) would spend the hour talking with a psychiatric social worker. In the 1940's in many clinics the psychiatrist and social worker did not talk together; each viewed the other's work as contaminating his/her own therapeutic efforts and professional silence was rigorously observed. Needless to say, fathers were almost never included in the treatment; even if they were considered important, they were usually dismissed as "unavailable." Siblings were ignored. This format, incidentally, may still be found in some communities even in the 1970's.

The 1950's produced the next forward surge in the growth of family treatment. At the Mental Research Institute in Palo Alto, California, four co-workers, Gregory Bateson, Don Jackson, John Weakland, and Jay Haley, were formulating a hypothesis that would become a keystone of subsequent family theory. In their now classic paper[3] they suggested that the symptoms of schizophrenia could be produced by a family's placing one family member in something called the "double bind." This "double bind hypothesis" will be discussed in more detail in Chapter 2, "Communication and the Family." Suffice it to say that such a hypothesis implicated the family directly and explicitly in the development of an individual's psychiatric symptoms. This hypothesis logically suggested to some that the treatment should include the family.

Coincident with the publication of this hypothesis, one of the investigators, Don Jackson, introduced another term equally basic to the future development of family therapy, "family homeostasis."[6] He observed that families with a mentally ill member acted as a unit with all members in dynamic equilibrium; he perceived a balance in family relationships that was maintained by each family member in some way. Dr. Alan Leveton, our consulting psychiatrist, has pointed out the analogy with a mobile.[7] Visualize a mobile with four or five pieces suspended from the ceiling, gently moving in the air. The whole is in balance, steady yet moving. Some pieces are moving rapidly; others are almost stationary. Some are heavier and appear to carry more weight in the ultimate direction of the mobile's movement; others seem to go along for the ride. A breeze catching only one segment of the mobile immediately influences movement of every piece, some more than others, and the pace picks up with some pieces unbalancing themselves and moving chaotically about for a time. Gradually the whole exerts its influence in the errant part(s) and balance is reestablished but not before a decided change in direction of the whole may have taken place. You will also notice the changeability regarding closeness and distance among pieces, the impact of actual contact one with another, and the importance of vertical hierarchy. Coalitions of movement may be observed between two pieces. Or one piece may persistently appear isolated from the others; yet its position of isolation is essential to the balancing of the entire system. Virginia Satir (whose work is discussed extensively in succeeding chapters) also likens a family to a mobile:

> In a mobile all the pieces, no matter what size or shape, can be grouped together in balance by shortening or lengthening the strings attached, or rearranging the distance between the pieces. So it is with a family. None of the family members is identical to any other; they are all different and at different levels of growth. As in a mobile, you can't arrange one without thinking of the other.*

Jackson also acknowledged "so it is with a family"—the whole and its pieces. In his view family members were moving constantly and in such a way as to maintain a precarious balance in their individual relationships with one another. He concluded this after noting that in the individual treatment of a schizophrenic patient:

> Other family members interfered with, tried to become a part of, or sabotaged the individual treatment of the "sick" member, as though the

---

*Satir, V.: Peoplemaking, Palo Alto, Calif., 1972, Science and Behavior Books, Inc., p. 119.

family had a stake in his sickness. The hospitalized . . . patient often got worse or regressed after a visit from family members, as though family interaction had a direct bearing on his symptoms. Other family members got worse as the patient got better, as though sickness in one of the family members were essential to the family's way of operating.*

This notion of homeostasis also seemed to call for a treatment process that could include all parts of the mobile. It may have been that following the acceptance of this term "family homeostasis," clinical work including the entire family began in earnest.

In 1958 Nathan Ackerman in New York published the first full-length study combining theory and practice, in which he emphasized the importance of role relations within the family.[1] He was already an experienced family therapy clinician by this time, having independently moved from a theoretical set to one that utilized clinical intervention with the family unit. In 1964 Virginia Satir was on the family treatment scene with her famous text entitled, *Conjoint Family Therapy: A Guide to Theory and Technique.*[9] Hence by this time in the fields of psychiatry and social work, the technique of treating emotional disturbance by working with the family together had been aggressively and successfully launched. John Howells said:

> In family psychiatry a family is not regarded merely as a background to be modified to help the present patient alone. Family psychiatry accepts the family itself as the patient, the presenting member being viewed as a sign of family psychopathology.†

These words, written in 1963, had by the close of the decade become accepted enough to be read almost as a commonplace. Currently in psychiatry the family therapy field is a burgeoning and already mammoth subdiscipline. It is now struggling with the dubious trappings of professional respectability: formalized societies, organization, journals, licensure, and bickering among the differing schools of family therapy. Differing schools or not, family therapy in psychiatry is here to stay.

Pediatrics has not been particularly quick to enter the family interviewing and family therapy field. It is understandable. In spite of the often-cited need for increasing liaison between pediatricians and child psychiatrists (most recently addressed in an article by Anders entitled

*Satir, V.: Conjoint family therapy: a guide to theory and technique, Palo Alto, Calif., 1964, Science and Behavior Books, Inc., p. 2.
†Howells, J.: Family psychiatry, Springfield, Ill., 1963, Charles C Thomas, Publisher, pp. 4-5.

"Child Psychiatry and Pediatrics: The State of the Relationship,"[2] with a succeeding commentary by Rothenberg[8]), an almost palpable "something" remains that keeps the two disciplines separate and wary of one another. Psychiatric treatment is too often dismissed out of hand by pediatricians as "impractical, too time-consuming, not worth the effort, unlearnable, illogical, and/or not within the province of pediatrics." Indeed in many ways a psychiatric model of treatment does not translate well into a busy clinical pediatric setting. Few pediatricians would be eager to initiate weekly play therapy for 1, 2, or 3 years with an encopretic 7-year-old. For one thing it would be an affront to the pediatrician's (almost inborn, it seems) need for action and visible results over a short period of time. Second, of course, very few pediatricians within the structure of their practices would have time for such an extended course of therapy. Third and most important, most pediatricians wouldn't know how to go about it. Nor would very many want to learn how. This is all reasonable. But it is not reasonable to extrapolate from this illustration and conclude that all forms of psychotherapeutic intervention with children are beyond the pediatrician's interest, skill, and tolerance. One should not throw out the baby with the play therapy. In selected pediatric situations family interviewing and family therapy have proved to be practical, relatively timesaving, worth the effort, learnable, logical, and very definitely within the province of pediatrics. We should be clear: we are not recommending that pediatricians undertake the long-term care of a schizophrenic teenager through the use of conjoint family therapy. All the objections by pediatricians to other forms of psychotherapy, those raised previously, would surface within 30 minutes of the first interview. Rather we are suggesting that a variety of conditions appear in a pediatrician's office that, were the physician equipped with some knowledge of family theory, family intervention techniques, and a modicum of courage, would lend themselves to alleviation and resolution under care by that physician alone.

What pediatric conditions would so lend themselves? In our experience the following have been successfully managed by pediatricians utilizing a family orientation in their work:

School phobia
Eating disorders including anorexia nervosa
Enuresis
Encopresis
Sleep disorders

Behavioral aspects of psychosomatic conditions such as recurrent abdominal pain and headaches

Juvenile diabetes mellitus

Short stature

Acting-out behavior

Psychosocial complications of such chronic illnesses as asthma, seizure disorders, cystic fibrosis, hemophilia, and so on

Awesome psychosocial aspects of fatal diseases, for example, leukemia, solid tumors

Difficulties associated with a wide variety of developmental disorders, from specific learning disabilities to mental retardation

Coping problems accompanying physical handicaps

Multitudinous behavioral problems associated with no particular disease, for which anxious parents consult physicians regularly (in fact the physician is often the first professional to be consulted in such situations).

A review of the preceding list, which is in no way complete, will illustrate that we do not propose that physicians should expand their practices to include the treatment of serious mental illness. We are asking that they develop some additional skills for themselves to help the patients who are *already* sitting in their waiting rooms, patients whom they already know—Joan and her grandmother, for instance, the pair who introduced this chapter. These two would certainly not be out of place in a family physician's office, even though the doctor might like them to be.

The doctor who insists on an individual (versus a family) orientation to the situation that Joan presents may be headed for trouble. For doctor and patient are only a requisition away from an EEG, complete blood count, pinworm preparation, and maybe a barium swallow and upper gastrointestinal x-ray series. This could easily be followed by a chaser of Donnatal and/or Valium—and very likely a continuation of symptoms. We are not recommending such a course of treatment, but the reader must admit that the sequence is not unusual in current medical practice.

What if the physician were to utilize a family approach in this situation? In fact he did after the first encounter; all five females—the family—were seen together. In the initial family interview the following was disclosed: several years before Joan's mother had left the child in Grandmother's care to run off and remarry. She had recently returned, contrite, and desired very much to assume a responsible mothering role with Joan. Grandmother by now saw Joan as her own and resented the return of Joan's mother; the two quickly locked in a struggle over who would mother the child. To complicate matters, Grandmother's older daughter (with her own child) had returned to the family home to lick her wounds after a particularly bitter separation and divorce. These two joined forces with Grandmother against Joan's mother, and the battle was joined. Joan, squarely in the middle, was handling her situation by refusing to sleep, literally jumping from bed to bed at night, staying with whomever she could entice to comfort and hold her. Her sleep disturbance and psychosomatic symptoms were automatic triggering mechanisms for beginning the contest anew each night—who would mother.

What seemed called for then was not a diagnostic evaluation of Joan's gastrointestinal tract but a family cease-fire and a clarification of specific family rules. The physician facilitated this, and after three family sessions, Joan's (and the family's) difficulties with sleep disappeared permanently. Family counseling continued thereafter but around substantially different issues.

How to gather such diagnostic family information, how to use it, and how to facilitate a change in a family's behavior, all accomplished by the pediatrician just mentioned in three interviews—the hows—are really the subject of the remainder of this book.

REFERENCES

1. Ackerman, N.: Psychodynamics of family life, New York, 1958, Basic Books, Inc., Publishers.
2. Anders, T.: Child psychiatry and pediatrics: the state of the relationship, Pediatrics **60:**616, 1977.
3. Bateson, G., and others: Toward a theory of schizophrenia, Behav. Sci. **1:**251, 1956.
4. Foley, V.: An introduction to family therapy, New York, 1974, Grune and Stratton, Inc.
5. Freud, S.: Analysis of phobia in a five year old boy. In Strachey, F., editor: The complete works of Sigmund Freud, vol. 10, London, 1964, The Hogarth Press, Ltd., pp. 5-148.
6. Jackson, D.: The question of family homeostasis, Psychiatr. Q. Suppl. **31:**79, 1957.
7. Leveton, A.: Personal communication, 1969.
8. Rothenberg, M.: Child psychiatry and pediatrics, Pediatrics **60:**649, 1977.
9. Satir, V.: Conjoint family therapy: a guide to theory and technique, Palo Alto, Calif., 1964, Science and Behavior Books, Inc.

CHAPTER 2

Communication and the family

CONTENT AND PROCESS

Two pediatric residents, a man and a woman, have just arrived in the Child Study Unit for the beginning of their 2-month training period in behavioral pediatrics. It is their first afternoon in the unit and their first teaching session with one of the authors (B.A.). At the moment, both are silent and busily engaged in an assigned nonverbal task. A large sheet of butcher paper, perhaps 2 feet by 3 feet, has been spread on a table before them, a box of crayons has been provided, and with a minimum of explanation they have been asked to "work together on the piece of paper for 30 minutes, without talking to one another or to me." Their requests for clarification have been handled mostly by a shoulder shrug. Their very obvious uncertainty, discomfort, and anxiety have been met by as reassuring a tone of voice as the instructor can muster. Otherwise they are being left to struggle with the task themselves. Within 3 minutes they have begun working in earnest, relatively oblivious to the clock and the presence of the instructor, and they are not at the moment visibly concerned with the silliness of the task. In fact, they appear to be enjoying themselves.

While she is busy drawing a country scene with mountains and trees and he is occupied with a tall fence around a structure, let us explain. This technique, the conjoint drawing, is actually a device that is often used with families in the course of family therapy.[2] (See Chapter 6.) We are also using it as a teaching device with our trainees in family interviewing. It has proved an immediate and effective method for introducing them to a focus on communication. We find it useful and interesting to begin a study of communication by insisting on silence, so our residents can experience the communication of silence. Also many of our

21

residents arrive for their training immediately following an exhausting and intense 5-week rotation in the pediatric intensive care nursery. They are not only weary; they are understandably still immersed in the life and death issues of caring for a critically ill infant. The nursery rotation is a hard act to follow. How then can we introduce them to another very different facet of training so that they will find it stimulating and rewarding to include in their practice of pediatrics? We have found that some sort of experiential task is helpful is assisting residents to shift their orientation from blood gases and intubation to a study of the various communications that can be used either constructively or destructively in family interactions. The conjoint drawing often does just that; it definitely arouses curiosity and anxiety. In most instances the former prevails and permits the trainees to complete the task. In fact, no one has ever refused to participate. Most often, as with the pair described above, the drawing elicits enthusiasm and even playfulness.

Of more importance than its value as a device to catch the pediatrician's interest in working with families, however, is the opportunity it affords to focus on two elementary aspects of communication: content and process. With these two definitions we most often introduce trainees to a study of family communication patterns. The terms are not ours, not new; however, their definitions here may also serve the function of initiating our discussion of communication with the reader.

The content of a communication refers to the literal, denotative aspect of that verbal message; process refers to the way in which the content is expressed. Process therefore includes all aspects of a communication outside the words and the specific subject matter delivered. It encompasses the tone of voice, body language, facial expression, hidden meaning, general feeling tone, and so on—in short all that is *implicit* in a message. If content has to do with "words," process has to do with the "music" of a communication; if content is the "figure," process is the "background." Content includes the "what" of a message; process contains the "how." Content is verbal; process is largely nonverbal.

Much of this can be illustrated specifically in a conjoint drawing. The picture can easily be recognized as the content (the "what") of that particular communication, and thus identified it can be set aside for an unobstructed look at process. The process comprises the ways (the "how") in which that particular picture came to be developed and drawn by the individuals participating. We return to the two residents, now energetically engaged in their mutual project. Their completed drawing is shown below.

The content is clear. It consists of a landscape with mountains, sun, clouds, trees, a stream, pond, animals, and a fence-enclosed men's room. The description of "how" that drawing arrived on the paper is infinitely less static, much richer in detail and interest; it says much about how these two individuals were relating to one another during the interchange. In short it summarizes the process of their communication with one another during a communication task.

Initially they were not so pleasantly engaged. First there was an uncomfortable, strained silence, particularly after both participants realized they were being asked to perform the task on their own without assistance from the instructor. For a few seconds some mutual fiddling with the crayons occupied both of them. Within 1 minute, however, Dr. Joan Lyons stood up, leaned over the paper, and with a sweepingly broad stroke drew the horizon line of mountains that extended across the entire paper. She then rapidly added the large sun in the middle of the drawing. She sat back and glanced at her co-worker. Dr. Fred Ascot was sitting immobilized in his chair, nervously removing the wrapper from his black crayon. He had yet to put a mark on the paper. Joan re-

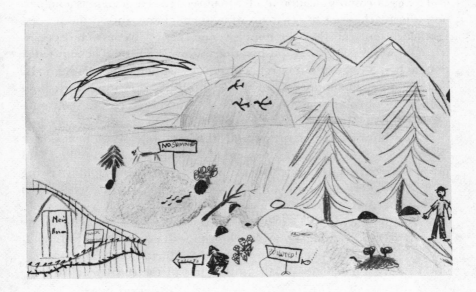

turned to her work and energetically began to fill in her landscape with trees and other objects. Periodically she would sense her partner's inactivity and draw the beginning of an object on the paper close to him. Fred was quickly losing available space by default, for Joan's drawing was taking up more and more territory. Reluctantly, it seemed, he began drawing, careful not to complete or adorn any of the items that Joan was offering as mutual projects. Instead he began to draw something of his own, a pond, very slowly and deliberately. This seemed to stimulate Joan's cooperative urge, and she offered him even more figures to which he might add his own touches. He did not. Undaunted, she then began to add to what he was drawing. When his pond was invaded by her trees, her rocks, he promptly put up a *NO SWIMMING* sign and moved on to build a house, deep in his territory. Joan returned to her side for a while but eventually returned to work on Fred's house. At this he labeled his structure "MEN'S ROOM." This time, when Joan moved back to her mountains and trees, Fred began construction of a wall surrounding his men's room, and on that project he continued diligently until the end of the task. Her final tour de force came when she added finials to his fence posts and thus completed the construction of a barrier obviously intended for her. It was a fascinating process to observe.

In discussing their experience, both residents were able to see parallels between their drawing behavior and some aspects of their more general styles of communication in life. Joan recognized herself as a helper, one who reaches out to others to draw them closer, and in the process she had often seen that her impulsiveness, aggressiveness, and persistence crowded people out, pushed them away. Fred could acknowledge that he had often lost out in relationships by withholding, waiting to be invited, and maintaining a loner stance. Both had unwittingly acted out these styles of communication and behavior in the process of their nonverbal content interchange on the paper.

However, a discussion of the individual and interactive behavior of these specific residents goes beyond our purpose here. Content and process are our focus, particularly as they apply in medical interviewing and/or the interview of a family. Physicians are beautifully schooled in the ways of content; as content gatherers they are probably without peer. The discipline and rigors of medical education have emphasized the importance of obtaining a complete history with no pertinent facts omitted. This is no more glaringly apparent than during students' introduction to clinical medicine, usually at the start of the third year. In their first experiences with "a new patient workup" they are very often over-whelmed, and they in turn often overwhelm patients and preceptors with elaborate medical histories that can read like the rough draft of a master's thesis. This variation of a "paper chase" and the pursuit of medical data is reinforced by the structure of medical teaching itself. Case presentations, rounds, clinical pathological presentations, and so on are often exercises in one-upmanship around content; expertise and competence of the student physician come to be judged by such things as the quantity and thoroughness of one's presentation, the intricacy and completeness of material placed on the blackboard for discussion, and an exceptional familiarity with the literature (it certainly doesn't hurt to have a neglected, obscure, yet pertinent reference in one's pocket). The more data and the more stunningly presented, the more favorably a physician-in-training is viewed by his peers and teachers. The ability to accumulate and organize content in this fashion is a skill with an extremely high priority in medical training. Content is a physician's friend.

Not so with process. Of course, there is a place in the traditional medical write-up for such items as "general behavior of patient," "mental status," and "reliability of informant." However, these are hardly given equal billing with "history of presenting illness," "review of organ systems," or a summary of "past medical history"—all primarily concerned again with content. The patient's communication process is rarely given mention in a formal medical history and physical examination write-up. As a result of such training, many physicians during their first conjoint family interview will naturally focus on the content of a particular interview, and within a short period of time they will admit to feeling hopelessly lost in a conversation with four or five family members, apparently having to do with who takes out the garbage on weeknights or what family rules obtain for watching nighttime television. And so, ensnared in those "problems" that the family brings into the interview situation, such an interviewer is diverted from paying attention to the process of the interview being played out before him. Yet the process is there, to be taken into consideration *even before* the family enters the office. For instance:

> Who initiates the referral? Who takes responsibility for seeking assistance from the doctor? How does that person sound on the telephone: desperate, angry, obsequious, suspicious?
> Who attends the first interview? Who is missing in spite of a specific

request from the physician that all family members attend? Who
seems to speak for the missing member?

Who determines when the interview will take place? Is it strictly on
the physician's terms or is it on the family's? ("Sorry, Jane has a
clarinet lesson that afternoon, Doctor. No, Thursday isn't good
either.")

The family continues to show their process once in the office:

How does the family enter the interview room? Who leads the way?
Who holds back? Do the parents seem to be in charge? Or are the
children controlling the situation by disruptive behavior or some
other tactic?

What is their seating arrangement? Does one family member sit apart
from the others? Do the parents sit together, or is the identified
patient (the reason for coming, Doctor) sandwiched between them?
Is one child sitting close to one parent and far from the other? Do
the children appear physically close or alienated from one another?

Who begins the interview? Again, who seems to be in charge of the
family? Do family members listen to one another? How are disruptions handled and by whom?

As the family's story is being told, what are their feelings? Are they
allowed into the telling and if so, by whom? Are changes in facial
expression and feeling tone noticed, acknowledged, accepted?
How do family members react when strong feelings are displayed,
that is, tears, anger, and so on? What is the family's general tone:
somber, angry, chaotic, anxious?

What is the family's general appearance and dress? Is that appearance consonant among all family members? What individual and
collective body language is displayed? Do closeness and even touching occur? How do family members handle themselves spatially in
the interview room?

All of these processes, and of course infinitely more, are occurring
simultaneously as one learns that Alfred, age 6, has been throwing up at
his desk at school for the past 3½ weeks. To focus on that fact to the exclusion of the preceding is to miss a wealth of useful information, information that discloses many significant aspects of that family's particular
structure—its mobile, its shifting balance of relationships, its family
homeostasis. In summary then, attention to a family's process is essential
in family interviewing, for a family reveals through its observable pro-

cess significant elements of its homeostatic pattern. A clear understanding of the homeostatic balance — the structure of the mobile — will form the basis for subsequent therapeutic interventions by the physician.

THE COMMUNICATION MODEL OF VIRGINIA SATIR

Simply understanding the difference between content and process is hardly enough to allow one to piece together a family's structure of relationships or its communication pattern. Such an understanding is important. It is a start, even though it may often require a conscious and disciplined shift away from content issues on the part of a physician who undertakes a family-oriented approach to interviewing. Even after having successfully done so, the physician will need other concepts to guide his observations of family function. Those presented in the work of Virginia Satir are quite useful. As mentioned earlier, this author contributed significantly to the growing family therapy field with the publication in 1964 of a textbook, *Conjoint Family Therapy*.[5] Largely as a result of this book, together with her subsequent writings and presentation of workshops, she is recognized today as a major force in the field of family therapy and is included among the three most important communication theorists in family work by one author.[4]

Her book begins (p. 1): "Family therapists deal with family pain. When one person in a family (the patient) has pain which shows up in symptoms, all family members are feeling this pain in some way."[5] In agreement with the basic notion of family homeostasis proposed by other communication theorists and mentioned earlier, she feels that the marital relationship is one of the major determining influences in a particular family's homeostatic balance, referring to the marital pair as the "architects" of a family. If there is pain in a marital relationship, then in her view dysfunctional parenting occurs, and very often the end result of dysfunctional parenting is a child with overt symptoms. Since Satir addresses herself almost exclusively to these interactional issues in the appearance of behavioral symptoms, one will find no references in her work to the role of traditionally recognized intrapsychic factors in symptom development. One could thus conclude from her 1964 writing alone that she proposes this path (pained marital relationship → dysfunctional parenting → child with symptoms) as the exclusive route for development of behavioral symptoms in children. However, in a subsequent book, *Peoplemaking*, published in 1972, Satir expands her view on the origins of behavior (p. xi): "Any piece of behavior at a moment in time is the outcome of the four-way interplay of the person's self-worth and his place in time and space and situation."[6] We, too, would agree that *all* behavioral difficulties in children cannot be attributed simply to dysfunctional parenting caused by a pained marital relationship. Many can be, and certainly if a pained marital relationship is present, dysfunctional parenting and symptomatology in a child are likely to follow. But, like Satir, we feel that much behavior, functional and dysfunctional, is multidetermined. An important determinant of behavior that we add to Satir's list is presented by the child himself in terms of his own individual temperament, behavioral individuality, and developmental pattern. These attributes the child brings to any situation himself. They are innately his and represent his contribution to a relationship with others, his parents included. He is not merely the passive recipient of parenting. His own temperament and developmental pattern (with or without developmental deviation) affect and often determine many aspects of the parenting that he receives, thus also determing many aspects of the parent-child relationship itself. Extensive work on the individual behavioral style and temperament of children can be found in the work of Chess and associates.[3] We feel a child's own temperament should be included as a variable in any hypothesis regarding the origin of behavioral difficulties and symptoms.

Returning to Satir's original 1964 model, which assumes that dysfunctional parenting is present in a given situation, we find no quarrel with the next step in her hypothesis; that is, that one member of the family, often a child, may be so significantly affected by the dysfunctional parenting that he develops symptoms. That child then becomes the "identified patient," and the symptoms are an "SOS" not just about the child but also about parental pain and family imbalance: the symptoms seem to be a message that the child is distorting his or her own emotional growth in an effort to alleviate and absorb the parents' pain.

Maturation: functional and dysfunctional communication

In Satir's book (p. 91), individuals are either functional or dysfunctional depending on their degree of maturation, "the most important concept in therapy."[5] She defines maturation as the state in which a human being is fully in charge of himself. A mature and therefore functional person is one who is able to make choices and decisions based on accurate perceptions about himself, others, and his context, acknowledging these choices and decisions as his own.

Such a functional person communicates clearly with others. He is in touch with and able to express what he feels; he can additionally accept responsibility for what he feels, thinks, hears, and sees, rather than denying or attributing to others. He views the presence of "differentness" between himself and others as an opportunity for learning, rather than one in which he feels threatened. He is able to negotiate, successfully checking out and clarifying communication between himself and others. A person who communicates in a functional manner therefore can:

1. Firmly state his case
2. At the same time clarify and qualify what he says
3. Ask for feedback
4. Be receptive to feedback when he gets it.

A dysfunctional person, on the other hand, is one who has not learned to communicate properly. This person:

1. Delivers unclear and perhaps conflicting messages
2. Is unable to check out meanings
3. Is unable to listen to feedback
4. Views differentness in others as a threat to himself and his integrity.

A dysfunctional communicator tends to overgeneralize and make false assumptions. There are many ways to do this. Satir includes among them:

False assumption 1: One instance is an example of all instances.
"Why don't you *ever*. . ."
"I *always* have to. . ."
"*Nobody* wears that!"

False assumption 2: Other people should share my feelings, thoughts, perceptions.
"I don't see how you can stand. . ."
"You should know how I feel about that."

False assumption 3: My perceptions are complete.
"Makes no difference what you tell me. I won't believe it."

False assumption 4: My perceptions won't change.
"That's the way he is. Period."
"Oh well, that's life."

False assumption 5: There are only two possible alternatives; things are or are not.
"If you cared for me, you wouldn't do that."
"You're either for me or against me."

False assumption 6: Characteristics of behavior define the person himself.

"She's a greedy person."
"He is an extremely hostile individual."
False assumption 7: I can get inside the skin of others.
"What she means to say is. . ."
"You don't really want that; what you want is. . ."
"I know what you're thinking."
False assumption 8: Others should be able to get inside my skin.
"You know what I mean."
"Why do I always have to tell you what I feel?"

A functional individual on the receiving end of any of these dysfunctional openers would ask for clarification and/or qualification rather than responding in kind. However, the original sender, if truly committed to a dysfunctional stance, would then handle such a request with an open rebuff, an unaltered restatement of his original case, an attack on the questioner, or simply evasion of the question, demonstrating an unwillingness to handle clarification, feedback, or difference. From there, of course, the interchange would go downhill, no matter how functional one member of the communication pair might be. For, Satir says (p. 70), "if verbal communication is to be reasonably clear, then both the sender and the recipient of a message must assume responsibility for making it so."[5]

For the reader who is suddenly awash in a flood of recognition at his/her own dysfunctional style of communicating, Satir does concede that we all generalize when we communicate and that anyone who perpetually clarifies and qualifies would seem just as dysfunctional as the person who rarely does so. A sender who too rigorously asks a receiver for feedback puts himself in the position of being inundated by it. Similarly, a receiver who continually asks for a sender to clarify would seem testy, uncooperative, and irritating. It is perhaps a matter of degree.

> Absolutely clear communication is impossible to achieve because communication is, by its very nature, incomplete. But there are degrees of incompleteness. The dysfunctional communicator leaves the receiver groping and guessing about what he has inside his head or heart. . .He behaves as though he is not aware of the fact that he generalizes or that he operates from assumptions.*

———

*Satir, V.: Conjoint family therapy: a guide to theory and technique, Palo Alto, Calif.,1964, Science and Behavior Books, Inc., pp. 71 and 73.

Self-esteem and parental validation

Observe the following interchange at a breakfast table:

She: I don't suppose you want another cup of coffee, George.
He: This stuff tastes like hot water!
She: You never have two cups.
He: Pass the sugar, Alice.
She: Anybody who likes sugar in coffee must be sick.

George and Alice, according to many of the characteristics cited, are having a dysfunctional interchange. Sidney, their 4-year-old son seated at the table, agrees. He may be on the way to dysfunctional interchanges of his own. This seems entirely possible if one agrees with Satir that the development of a dysfunctional communication style is connected to the particular family behavior in which one lives as a child. For one thing modeling behavior by parents is very influential. If their messages to one another and to their children are unclear and contradictory over time, then children in such a position — like Sidney — will learn to communicate in an unclear, contradictory way. And yet it is not just a matter of modeling dysfunctional behavior that determines the development of faulty communication and the onset of overt symptoms. There is more to it, Satir claims. Communication difficulties are also closely linked to problems in the development of one's self-esteem during childhood.

Self-esteem, like maturation, is one of Satir's essential concepts. In fact she acknowledges a fundamental difference in her views from those of psychoanalytic thought when she states:

I do not postulate sex as the basic drive of man. From what I have observed, the sex drive is continually subordinated to and used for the purpose of enhancing self-esteem. . .The need to feel esteem about the self is so important that adult mates will do without sexual satisfaction or fail to demand it in a vital relationship if sexual behavior, or demands for it, lead to threatened self-esteem. One sees this over and over again when counselling marital pairs.*

Satir divides self-esteem into two areas: esteem for the self as a masterful person (able to do for himself) and esteem for the self as a sexual person. We will limit our review to her discussion of self-esteem regard-

---

*Satir, V.: Conjoint family therapy: a guide to theory and technique, Palo Alto, Calif., 1964, Science and Behavior Books, Inc., p. 55.

ing mastery, in which she offers an excellent summary of the formative role of a parent in the emergence of a child's self-esteem. Parents, or at least one parent, she says, are essential to validate a child's developmental growth. Validation occurs when a parent notes the existence of growth, communicates verbally or nonverbally that he notices, and gives the child increased opportunity for using the abilities emerging from that growth. A child learns not only to feed himself, tie his own shoes, go to the store alone; in a larger sense he becomes increasingly able to make decisions, to reason, to create, to form and maintain relationships, to plan ahead, to tolerate frustration and disappointment. In short, his sense of self-mastery expands. Parents must time their validation carefully, Satir warns. To ring true and enhance self-esteem, validation must fit the needs, abilities, and readiness of the child.

The development of self-esteem in mastery can go awry when a parent does not validate developmental growth or offers validation inappropriately. In such instances, Satir states, this unvalidated aspect of a child's growth remains an unintegrated fragment, often labeled in his own mind as that part of himself that is unimportant, incomplete, inadequate, or bad. The lack of parental validation can occur in a variety of ways: a parent may fail to see the emerging ability, allow no opportunity for its emergence, or fail to comment on its emergence once manifest. Validation may also fail when a parent perceives growth prematurely, anxiously urging its expression before the youngster is actually capable. Validation can be seriously jeopardized if one parent contradicts the validating messages of another.

Constructive parental validation meets the following criteria: it fits the needs, abilities, and readiness of the child. It is clear, direct, and specific. It is given in a relatively matter-of-fact way. One parent does not contradict or depreciate the validation of another.

With such constructive parental validation, a child's self-esteem flourishes. Satir feels strongly that adequate self-esteem is essential if a child is to grow toward independence, if he is to realize his potential and his individual uniqueness, and if he is to develop a functional style of communication with the people in his world.

Without feelings of competence and mastery, individuals experience considerable anxiety and uncertainty. Unfortunately self-esteem for them is based on what others think, and a sense of autonomy and individuality is thus seriously compromised. Yet a person so crippled often works hard at disguising feelings of low self-esteem from others, especially from those deemed important to impress such as a parent, a spouse, or a future spouse. The individual with low self-esteem is very uncomfortable in any situation that calls for compromise and commitment to a joint outcome (that is, marriage), since any additional sacrifice of self seems an intolerable diminution of something already in short supply — the self. He/she appears poised to receive any evidence of differentness in someone close as a personal insult, a sign of being unloved. Thus differing opinions, feelings, and thoughts have a way of becoming larger than life and so problematic that they may be constantly argued over, or even worse, treated as though they do not exist.

In either case dysfunctional communication as defined earlier is the tragic outcome, for in the name of self-protection, the individual summarized in the preceding paragraph must relinquish any hopes for stating his/her case clearly, clarifying, asking for, or being receptive to feedback from others. Risking the exposure of one's differentness or uniqueness, which is entailed in communicating clearly, is just too great.

Unfortunately, as Satir points out in a chapter titled "Low Self-Esteem and Mate Selection," two individuals with mutually low self-esteem usually seek out one another in relationships, with the predictably unhappy outcome of dysfunctional communication for themselves and for their children as a way of life.

The induction process

As stated, Satir believes that dysfunctional communication between spouses arises from mutual feelings of low self-esteem caused by a failure of parental validation during the childhood of each; however, one still needs an explanation of the connection between the dysfunctional communication of such parents and subsequent symptom development in their child. She postulates for this purpose an induction process, unwittingly utilized by the parents, the keystone of which is "the double-level message." Double-level messages (statements that say one thing and mean another) are ubiquitous:

"I can't stand watching this TV program." (while continuing to watch)
"You little devil!" (with a smile and a hug)
"Oh, I really shouldn't have another piece of pie." (holding out a plate for seconds)

Often quite harmless and entertaining, they are a part of everyone's repertoire in communication, and they do not necessarily lead to difficulty, particularly in situations where clarification and checking out are possible. "Thus, by itself, double-level communication need not lead to symptomatic behavior. But under certain conditions, especially where children are involved, it can produce a vice-like situational effect which has been termed the 'double bind' "(p. 36).[5]

As mentioned in the preceding chapter, this term "double bind" was introduced in a now classic paper by Bateson and others.[1] Stated in its briefest form, a double bind is a paradoxical injunction. One must be careful not to confuse the terms "double-level message" and "double bind." They are not the same. The former is a message, nothing more, while the double bind is much larger; it is a situation, an environment. A double-level message is based on simple contradiction; one may choose either element of the discrepant message. Thus a logical choice is possible. With the double bind's origin in paradox, no choice is logically possible.

Foley[4] elegantly captures the essence of a double bind in his illustration borrowed from Greenburg:

> Give your son, Marvin, two sport shirts as a present. The first time he wears one of them look at him sadly and say in your Basic Tone of Voice: "The other one you didn't like?"*

For Marvin no choice is possible.

For such no-win situations to have symptom-producing effects on a child, several conditions are necessary:

a. First, the child must be exposed to double-level messages repeatedly and over a long period of time.
b. Second, these must come from persons who have survival significance for him.
   — Parents are automatically survival figures because the child literally depends on them for physical life; later, his need for love and approval from them becomes invested with like meaning.
   — In addition, the way the parents structure their messages to the child will determine his techniques for mastering his environment. It is not only his present, but his future survival which is in their hands.
   — As a result, he cannot afford to ignore messages from them, no matter how confused.
c. Third, perhaps most important of all, he must be conditioned from

---

*Greenburg, D.: How to be a Jewish mother, Los Angeles, 1964, Price, Sloan, and Stern, p. 16.

an early age not to ask, "Did you mean *that* or *that?*" but must accept his parents' conflicting messages in all their impossibility. He must be faced with the hopeless task of translating them into a single way of behaving.*

In such a family the parents often fail to recognize the child's feelings, his emerging abilities, his needs for nurturance, and his validation as a worthy individual—largely. Satir feels, because (1) they themselves are not receiving an appreciation of their own feelings, abilities, and need for support from one another in the marital relationship, nor (2) did they receive such validation in their own separate childhoods.

When these conditions are present over an extended period, all need not be present to ensure a double-binding situation. Even the presence of one is apparently sufficient to put the child in a bind.

The options to a child so bound are three in number. None are very appealing:

> First one concludes the "victim" is overlooking something in the situation. He searches and searches but the more he tries to understand, the more confused he becomes. A second possibility is to become absolutely literal and follow each and every injunction to the letter. The basic premise underlying this approach is that things do not make sense anyhow, so why worry. Anyone familiar with institutional living, for example, the army, will recognize this response. A third option is to withdraw from human involvement so that all incoming material is blocked out. The "victim" is caught because he cannot discuss the messages with an outside party. He cannot . . . talk about his communication and thus escape his field. The "victim" therefore remains trapped and unable to escape.†

When an individual in response to feeling double bound adopts, over time, a style of relating that is predominantly confused, literal, or withdrawn, others in his world are bound to remark eventually, "Frank sure is acting funny." Such behavior then comes to be labeled "sick," "crazy," or "bad." The induction process is completed with the appearance, first in the family and eventually in the doctor's office, of an identified patient.

---

*Satir, V.: Conjoint family therapy: a guide to theory and technique, Palo Alto, Calif., 1964, Science and Behavior Books, Inc., p. 36.

†Foley, V.: An introduction to family therapy, New York, 1974, Grune & Stratton, Inc., p. 15. By permission.

Schematically the induction process can be shown as follows:

Mate (husband)	*Mate (wife)*
Individual A	*Individual B*
Lack of parental validation	Lack of parental validation
↓	↓
Low self-esteem and	Low self-esteem and
dysfunctional communication	dysfunctional communication

Pained marital relationship

↓

Dysfunctional parenting
Dysfunctional communication with
child

↓

Especially double-level messages

↓

Double bind situation

↓

Child with symptoms
The identified patient

Implications for the interviewer

Since in this model symptomatology is so directly related to faulty styles of communication within a family, Satir sees family therapy as a study and subsequent alteration of maladaptive family communication methods:

> If illness is seen to derive from inadequate methods of communication
> (by which we mean all interactional behavior) it follows that therapy
> will be seen as an attempt to improve these methods . . . The empha-
> sis will be on correcting discrepancies in communication and teaching
> ways to achieve more fitting joint outcomes. This approach to therapy
> depends on three primary beliefs about human nature:
> — First, that every individual is geared to survival, growth, and get-
>   ting close to others and that all behavior expresses these aims, no
>   matter how distorted it may look. Even an extremely disturbed
>   person will be fundamentally on the side of the therapist.
> — Second, that what society calls sick, crazy, stupid, or bad behavior
>   is really an attempt on the part of the afflicted person to signal the
>   presence of trouble and call for help. In that sense, it may not be
>   so sick, crazy, stupid, or bad after all.
> — Third, that human beings are limited only by the extent of their
>   knowledge, their ways of understanding themselves and their abil-

ity to "check out" with others. Thought and feeling are inextricably bound together; the individual need not be a prisoner of his
feelings but can use the cognitive component of his feeling to free
himself. This is the basis for assuming that a human being can
learn what he doesn't know and can change ways of commenting
and understanding that don't fit.*

This, of course, is an optimistic mouthful, however, one that communicates well Satir's strong belief in the capacity for growth in every individual and her reluctance to view symptoms within a disease or psycho-
pathology framework. People are not sick or bad; rather it is communication and interactional rules that are bad and that produce family pain.
Medical and psychiatric labels have no usefulness in her work. In fact,
avoiding their use is essential for a very practical reason. As summarized
by Foley:

> To take the label off a person and to put it on a way of interacting is to
> defuse a potentially volatile situation. Instead of saying that John is the
> cause of the family's problem, saying that some rules in the family are
> causing a problem has a twofold effect. First, it takes the label of scape-
> goat off John and makes him part of the family system and not the
> cause of its pain. This gives him some breathing room and opens up the
> possibility of his changing. Second, the parents do not have to feel that
> they have been failures in their parental role. They have been guilty,
> perhaps, of overlooking certain procedures in the family, but they no
> longer have to feel guilty of failing as human beings . . . they can re-
> tain their feeling of self-worth as persons and as parents. The distinc-
> tion is important because instead of locking the system into itself by
> reinforcing the labels of identified patient and failing parents, it opens
> up the possibility of change in the system.†

And this perhaps more than anything else is at the heart of Satir's work:
revealing to families their own possibilities for change and facilitating
their awareness of how to change.

A therapist utilizing her approach functions as a resource person, an
impartial observer who can report to the family what he or she sees and
hears. A therapist also provides feedback regarding that which the fami-

---

*Satir, V.: Conjoint family therapy: a guide to theory and technique, Palo Alto,
California, 1964, Science and Behavior Books, Inc., p. 36.
†Foley, V.: An introduction to family therapy, New York, 1974, Grune & Strat-
ton, Inc., p. 101. By permission.

ly seems unable to see and hear. This same therapist operates as a model of clear communication with the family, using functional communication in transactions with family members and explicitly teaching individuals the rules for functional interchanges. How all of this actually happens in an interview situation is in some part a function of an individual's particular interviewing style, but regardless of style, certain things are essential. Unclear communications must be clarified:

"I don't understand what you mean."

"Would you boil all of that down into one sentence and then say it directly to your son."

Feedback is both demonstrated and encouraged:

"I like the strength in your voice as you discuss this issue."

"I see confusion in your face. Am I reading you right?"

Double-level messages are explicitly labeled:

"You just said to Frances that you didn't mind, and then you turned away with your body."

"The tears in your eyes don't match your words that it's not important."

"If you are angry at Debbie, why has your voice to her gotten so small?"

All the (previously listed) false assumptions of communication are challenged:

"What do you mean he should know how you feel? He is not a mind reader."

"Ever, never, always — those words have a way of putting folks on the defensive. Try telling Margaret again, leaving those words out."

Each individual is encouraged to take responsibility for his own actions, thoughts, and feelings:

"Neil, start over again and begin your sentence with the pronoun 'I'."

In these ways and others the process of communication is repeatedly being examined, altered, and redirected. While the therapist is commenting on what he hears, sees, and feels in the family's midst, he is also teaching them new ways to communicate.

Such an approach requires considerable activity on the part of the interviewer. He is essentially directing the interview. Satir agrees; in her own work she considers it extremely important to establish quickly that she will be in charge of the interview. When children are involved she much prefers that parents set limits for the children in the interview. Even so, she has specific rules that she explains early to a family:

I do make it my responsibility, however, to communicate clearly the rules of behavior that apply in my own bailiwick, the therapy room
- No one may hit or play with the microphone or the recording equipment.
- No one may destroy any chairs, window blinds, tablecloths, etc.
- No one (including parents, for that matter) may speak for others.
- Everyone must speak so he can be heard.
- Everyone must make it possible for others to be heard. 'You are hurting my eardrums' I will say, or 'You will have to take turns talking or I can't do my work.'
- The parents will often ask me to set a rule about leaving the therapy room. Mother will ask, 'Is it all right if he leaves?' I will say, 'Yes,' and then instruct the child on how to find the water fountain or the toilet.
- I also set rules on how often a child may leave the therapy room. Usually one trip to the toilet and one trip to the water fountain will give Johnny or Patty all the chance they need to explore.
- I also shorten the length of the therapy session to conform to the ages of the children.*

For Satir, therapy with a family has a reliable developmental pattern. Initial contact is usually with one family member on the telephone. She gathers enough information to understand in brief the stated concerns and to set up the first appointment, usually with the parents alone. In fact, Satir writes in her original book, the first two appointments are most often with parents and without the children in attendance, to underscore her notion that the parents are the "authorized leaders" of the family. In the first session she asks questions to establish what the family expects from treatment. Each spouse is asked separately: "What would you like to accomplish here?" or words to that effect. She then explains the importance of a family view with comments such as the following: "No one person can see the whole picture because he is limited to his own perspective. By having everyone together, we can get the whole picture more clearly. Every person has a unique contribution to make that cannot be duplicated by anyone else." She explores with the spouses their concerns and complaints, usually about their child, "the problem," and concludes by acknowledging the parents' confusion and good intentions regarding the child, his behavior, and their efforts.

*Satir, V.: Conjoint family therapy: a guide to theory and technique, Palo Alto, Calif., 1964, Science and Behavior Books, Inc., pp. 139-140.

Satir then proceeds in what remains of the first and second interviews to what she calls a family chronology, an extensive exploration with the family of their history as individuals and as a family group. It begins with each parent as a child and his/her own relationship with parents. Aside from providing her with a large amount of information, Satir feels it is an invaluable device for helping families to relax and become less frightened. Recollection of the past, particularly of those pleasant times before the family's present trouble started, is often reassuring, and for some it signals the rekindling of hope that things may once again be better.

We have not utilized this aspect of Satir's approach routinely, preferring to begin with families and their problems in the present. We return to historical events only as the situation warrants and not as a matter of course, nor as an introduction/preparation for therapy. This direction on our part is largely due to the influence of Frederick Perls and his stress on "staying in the now." We will discuss Perls and his clinical approaches to human problems through Gestalt therapy in a later chapter. It should also be stated that we no longer routinely conduct initial interviews without the children. In fact, when it is a child's behavior that brings a family to us for help, we generally insist that the whole family attend the first meeting. It seems to us that one may still emphasize that the parents are in charge of their family with the children present, and since we are most interested in helping families with their problems in the present, children—symptomatic or not—are part of the family's present and need to be included. Satir also suggests some rules regarding which children in a family are to attend interviews. For instance, children over 4 years of age attend most sessions. Children under 4 generally attend at least two family sessions. She includes older adult children from the first interview. Our rules are somewhat less complicated: everyone comes for the first interview. Attendance at subsequent interviews will be dictated by the situation and the problem.

Returning to Satir's model, she notes that once the children are included there are specific issues that she hopes to confront right from the first encounter. She would like the family members to recognize that they are individuals and are different from one another. She would like them to recognize that they also have disagreements. She would like them to communicate with one another more clearly. She is careful to integrate the children into the interview process, individuating children by greeting them separately, honoring all questions from them, and asking each youngster specific questions about the reasons for his/her coming to the family interview. She often ends the first family interview on a positive note by introducing the idea that each family member must acknowledge good feelings when he or she is pleased by what another has done or said. For many families this is a decided departure from their entrenched style of blaming and criticism. Such groups have forgotten how to offer positive feedback.

After this beginning phase, family therapy for Satir settles into a middle period; during this time a therapist has his work cut out for him. He must create a setting in which people can, perhaps for the first time, take the risk of looking clearly and objectively at themselves and their actions. He does this is several ways. The therapist demonstrates that whereas the family is fearful, he is not, particularly when it comes to asking questions and taking responsibility for finding out what it is he doesn't know. In this way he demonstrates clear communication and also that he is going somewhere in the interview. The therapist also works to show the patients how they look to others. When he asks for and gives information, the therapist does so in a matter-of-fact, nonjudgmental, light way. He endeavors to build self-esteem in family members through his own validation of their appropriate behavior. He lessens the sense of threat that family members feel toward the interview situation by setting clear rules for interaction in the session. In thus making the interview a relatively safe place, he discourages the need for defenses among family members. At the same time he is very cautious and conservative with material that is obviously charged and loaded, proceeding slowly at such times. During this time of establishing the therapy room as a place of safety and honesty for the family, the therapist is also encouraging family members to assume a sense of personal responsibility and accountability such that each comes to stand on his own two feet in both communication and behavior. He does this by, among other things, reminding individuals of their ability to be in charge of themselves. Statements of blame toward others are discouraged, and each family member's use of the pronoun "I" is encouraged. In this respect Satir and Perls travel the same road: responsibility for the self is essential for the formation and maintenance of functional relationships.

For Satir the concept of using and behaving as an "I" is so important that she considers it in determining when treatment can end.

Treatment is completed:
- When family members can complete transactions, check, ask.
- When they can interpret hostility.

—When they can see how others see them.

—When they can see how they see themselves.

—When one member can tell another how he manifests himself.

—When one member can tell another what he hopes, fears, and expects from him.

—When they can disagree.

—When they can make choices.

—When they can learn through practice.

—When they can free themselves from harmful effects of past models.

—When they can give a clear message, that is, be congruent in their behavior, with a minimum of difference between feelings and communication, and with a minimum of hidden messages.

. . . In short, treatment is completed when everyone in the therapy setting can use the first person "I" followed by an active verb and ending with a direct object.*

REFERENCES

1. Bateson, G., and others: Toward a theory of schizophrenia, Behav. Sci. **1:**251, 1956.
2. Bing, E.: The conjoint family drawing, Family Process, **9:**173, 1970.
3. Chess, S., and others: Behavioral individuality in early childhood, New York, 1963, New York University Press.
4. Foley, V.: An introduction to family therapy, New York, 1974, Grune & Stratton, Inc.
5. Satir, V.: Conjoint family therapy: a guide to theory and technique, Palo Alto, Calif., 1964, Science and Behavior Books, Inc.
6. Satir. V.: Peoplemaking, Palo Alto, Calif., 1972, Science and Behavior Books, Inc.

---

*Satir, V.: Conjoint family therapy: a guide to theory and technique, Palo Alto, Calif., 1964, Science and Behavior Books, Inc., pp. 139–140.

CHAPTER 3

Structural views of the family

THE MALONEY FAMILY

She was 9 years old, and butter wouldn't melt in her mouth. That was the pediatrician's impression of Jennifer Maloney as she sat in his office with her parents for the first time. She was quite pretty, nicely dressed, the sort of child that Jessie Wilcox Smith used long ago in her illustrations for books such as *A Child's Garden of Verses*.

Her parents would not have described her in such beatific terms that day. This was the sixth physician and/or therapist whom they had consulted regarding their only child's difficulties — difficulties that stretched in an unbroken chain over the past 7 years. Mrs. Maloney was near tears as she told their story; Mr. Maloney appeared to the doctor either very indifferent or very frightened.

Jennifer had developed "a sleeping problem" even before she was 1 year old, often drawing up her legs in sleep and seeming fretful. The parents thought and were told by their first pediatrician that she had "colic," and frequent changes of formula were made. The behavior continued. By the age of 2, her parents were convinced that she was having "nightmares," episodes late at night when she would scream out in her sleep. Mrs. Maloney would go immediately to her bedside and try to comfort the child, but Jennifer was "very hostile" during these episodes, and comforting seemed out of the question.

By the time she was 5 years of age, these nocturnal episodes came as often as three times a week. By this time, according to the parents, several physicians, including a family doctor, a pediatrician, and a child psychiatrist, had advised that these spells were most probably night terrors and that Jennifer would eventually "grow out of it." She did not. If anything, the episodes increased in frequency. Frequent enuresis began to

43

accompany them when she was 6 years old. A neurologist (the second) described in his report: "The usual sequence of events is that the girl goes to bed at 7:30. Somewhere around 11:30 to 12:30 the girl begins to 'holler—thrash in her bed—looks frightened—speaks but no one can understand her.' Mother usually goes to her side but is unable to comfort her. This episode may last from a minute to on one occasion 15 minutes. She then resumes sleeping."

Additional problems began when Jennifer reached school age. She became alarmed and anxious about the smallest details of school: what clothes she would wear, how she would perform that day in reading, whether her paper was neat enough, what would happen on the playground, how she would get along with friends, whether the teacher would like her, and so forth. In fact she was an excellent student and did reasonably well with peers and teachers, but she became so anxious regarding all aspects of her school career that she began refusing to go— and school was directly across the street from the Maloneys' driveway. The school counselor was contacted, and some mornings Jennifer would literally be dragged by Mrs. Maloney to the street separating house and school, there to be transferred to the firm hand of the school counselor, who would then continue the coercion into the school building itself. Many mornings Jennifer just didn't go at all—"too upset." Night terrors, enuresis, school phobia—the list was growing.

Mrs. Maloney was desperate, as had been the physicians. The inevitable result was that medication, imipramine for the bedwetting and other tranquilizers for the anxiety, was prescribed. Psychotherapy was also suggested, and for the past 6 months Jennifer had been in twice-weekly individual play therapy with a child psychologist.

In the parents' eyes progress had been minimal, and the mother told each doctor that she felt as though she were on a treadmill in which no one really understood what the family was going through, and the only course became referral from one specialist to another. Until now no one had met with the entire family together.

Several things became clear during this initial family meeting with a pediatrician trained in working with families. He observed that first of all Jennifer enjoyed talking about her "anxieties and worries" and her "therapist." She was quite willing to pursue in detail her experiences and symptoms of the past several years. She clearly saw herself as, and actively sought the role of, "patient." Her parents agreed; Mrs. Maloney added to this image with a lurid, extended, hand-wringing description of Jennifer's difficulties. The sleep situation became the whole focus, reified as though Jennifer's illness had become another family member to be nurtured and reckoned with.

Mr. Maloney, as mentioned, appeared somewhat indifferent. When the doctor would directly ask his opinion, two interesting events occurred each time the father spoke: (1) Jennifer would roll her eyes ceiling-ward as if in eloquent disapproval, and (2) Mrs. Maloney would follow with an interruption and restatement or correction. The pediatrician had previously noted that the father was the last of the three to enter his office, that he seemed to be holding back. What was first assumed by the pediatrician to be a gallant "ladies first" attitude now appeared quite different to him. In addition, the father had seated himself at some distance from the two females. They, on the other hand, were grouped together with frequent touching and much eyeing of one another. Mr. Maloney was not in his wife's field of vision. Jennifer occupied it all. The father's position in the interview and in the family then appeared to be casual, remote, and disregarded.

On the other hand, Mrs. Maloney and Jennifer seemed to be closely allied with one another, even though the connecting ties between them were often those of frustration and conflict. Seating arrangement, body posture, eye contact, and the content of the interview itself underscored their closeness and involvement with one another. Jennifer had a way of visually checking with her mother each time before she spoke. Very often this seemed a triggering mechanism for Mrs. Maloney to enter the conversation and finish Jennifer's sentence. At other times the mother would speak for Jennifer: "Now, Doctor, I know Jennifer won't tell you this, but she's not at all sure about this meeting with the whole family. She would rather see you alone. She really prefers to have her own doctor to talk to." Since this statement was repeated three times by Mrs. Maloney in the course of the first interview, it was clear that someone, and not necessarily Jennifer, was extremely uncomfortable with the notion of a family meeting.

When asked, the family discussed their version of the nighttime scene. In many respects their tale fit the description previously reported by their pediatric neurologist. It was true that at about 11:30 P.M. Jennifer would begin screaming hysterically in her room, and Mrs. Maloney would rush in and then find herself unable to soothe her daughter, eventually becoming worn down by the experience. However, the pediatrician heard additional pieces of information, and he felt they were important for consideration:

Mother: Well, you see, Doctor, my husband and I don't always agree on what should be done. Do you realize, Lester, what could happen to that child? She could injure herself. She gets so physically violent, Doctor, that she actually throws herself out of bed. She did hurt herself that one time . . . I can't let that happen.

Father: I know, that's right. But I still think you go in there too soon. We've never tried just leaving her alone.

Doctor: Tell me a little more about what you have done and what you're doing *now* when it happens.

Mother: When she screams out like that, I do go, I do, I admit; I can't let her scream like that. She's not even awake. When I try to quiet her, then she gets angry with *me*, really violent sometimes, slaps, kicks . . . I bring her a glass of water, and she throws it at me. Then of course the commotion gets really loud. And he hears it and thinks, 'Oh, geez, they're at it again.' And so he comes in like Godzilla and terrifies her. You just can't do that with children, Doctor. Then she ends up being scared of her own father. No patience, he has no patience. Then I have even worse problems getting her settled down after her father comes in. He's shouting at me . . . at her . . . I'm shouting . . . Jennifer's screaming. Sometimes we're up for hours like that.

The pediatrician concluded the hour by telling them that they certainly had a family problem, that he would like very much to help them to help themselves, and that he would continue his help next time by seeing the parents alone in 1 week.

Mrs. Maloney saw her chance: "But Doctor, what will *we* do in 2 days when Jennifer goes back to school? That's our next crisis. How will *we* get ourselves to school?" In a very small voice Jennifer responded, "Maybe I'll just have to go alone."

Father: Right.

Mother: Are you sure you're really ready?

Doctor: Mrs. Maloney, I would like you instead to tell Jennifer, "I am confident that you are ready."

Mother: Oh, I do want to have confidence in her.

Doctor: Will you tell her *now*.

Mother: (to Jennifer) I do have confidence about your going to school?

Doctor: Could you say it once again and remove the question mark from your voice.

She did. The doctor was still leery. The hour ended.

The next day the doctor received a telephone call from Mrs. Maloney. She was frantic; things had deteriorated badly after their visit. Jennifer had had a terrible sleep disturbance that night. The two of them had been up together from 3 to 6 A.M. The child was furious, saying to her mother, "How dare that man say this is a family problem! It's a mother-daughter problem!" Mrs. Maloney then, sotto voce, asked for an appointment alone. "There are just so many things I wanted to say that I couldn't say in front of my husband."

The pediatrician refused to be manipulated and added: "However, Mrs. Maloney, I certainly agree that the family is in a serious crisis at the moment. I don't believe things can wait for a week. I would like to see you and your husband tomorrow."

Mother: Absolutely, Doctor. And if my husband can't come, I could come alone?

Doctor: No, Mrs. Maloney. I will need you both here.

Mother: All right. But now what will we do about our sleeping problem? I don't think we can go through another night like last night.

The pediatrician assured her that he realized that it was a trying time for all and that immediate solutions would indeed be helpful. He had none, except to suggest that if she were spending more than 15 minutes in Jennifer's bedroom at night, she was spending too long. On that note the conversation ended.

The next day Mrs. Maloney arrived on time for the appointment—alone. She relayed her husband's unwillingness to come for this more immediate appointment, making sure that the doctor understood it was a basketball game on television that took priority. The physician held his ground, literally, at the door and politely refused to see her or begin working with the family without him. She accepted his refusal with grace and a glance that said, "At least now you know what I have to put up with at home."

Both parents arrived for their next scheduled appointment. They began and proceeded with a discussion of trust; neither trusted the other in his/her management of Jennifer. Father saw his wife as oversolicitous and ineffectual. Mother stated she was convinced that her husband was an angry, overreacting ogre with children.

After listening, the doctor unfolded his therapeutic strategy consisting of the following:

1. He acknowledged Mrs. Maloney's frustration and obvious exhaustion at dealing with the problem almost single-handedly for years and years. In his medical opinion he did not feel that she could continue much longer. It was not humanly possible.

2. He further felt that Mr. Maloney was crucial to the survival of his wife and family and that only he could help to solve this family problem. His role was essential. It could be done by no one else.

3. However, Mr. Maloney could do it only with the assistance of his wife. In this sense Mrs. Maloney was also crucial to the solution. She was in a uniquely important position, one in which she could enable her husband to teach Jennifer one of the most important lessons that fathers can teach their daughters. Specifically the doctor wanted Mr. Maloney to teach Jennifer respect for men. Only he could impart this to the child. And only mother could provide the opportunity. Did she want her daughter to learn this lesson? Mrs. Maloney, of course, readily agreed that she did.

4. She was then to allow her husband the management of Jennifer's sleep disturbance and to recede into the background. Such a move would accomplish two important goals: it would allow Jennifer to see her father's competence and nurturing abilities, thus enhancing the child's respect for him, and it would provide Mrs. Maloney with a much needed rest for her near-exhaustion.

When asked, both parents agreed, tentatively perhaps, but they agreed. The discussion then turned to specific ways in which Mr. Maloney would proceed with Jennifer at night. He outlined his approach: He would make sure she was not suffering physically and then leave her bedroom, assuring her that all was well and that he trusted her own ability to settle herself down. He acknowledged that he would be willing to do that several times a night if necessary. He also assured his wife that he would not be either physically or verbally abusive, that in the past (he was now realizing for the first time) his lack of control had arisen out of (1) his impatience with his wife's efforts and (2) disappointment with himself that he had tolerated such a peripheral role in parenting. The pediatrician acknowledged Mr. Maloney's feelings and his new realizations.

Mrs. Maloney, while willing to relinquish the manager role to her husband, admitted, in a hopeful show of honesty, "I'm not sure I could handle it if she was crying out for me while you were in there, Lester. I might have to leave the house." The doctor applauded this suggestion heavily, telling her that he wished he had thought of it, and asking if she would indeed be willing to go for a short ride in the car if necessary. "I would have to," she agreed. The second hour ended with a return interview scheduled.

In 2 weeks the parents returned. Mother looked rested and decidedly less frantic. Father looked pleased. They reported that the plan developed in the office had been presented to Jennifer primarily by father with mother in attendance. There had been *no* sleep disturbance since that time. They vaguely remembered 2 or 3 nights of transient whimpering, which Mr. Maloney treated by staying in his own bed.

Mrs. Maloney recalled an interesting episode a few days before this third appointment. The family for years had had accustomed seats when riding in the car. Jennifer was always placed between her parents on the front seat. She now considered that "my place." On this particular day she came to the car to find her mother and father for the first time sitting next to one another; Jennifer was offered a window seat. She was outraged: "I know what that doctor's trying to do; he's trying to get you two together!" Clearly Jennifer was having mixed feelings: anger at losing first place and (as her nighttime behavior indicated) relief.

During this third interview, therapeutic strategies for rehabilitation of Jennifer into regular school attendance were discussed. Flushed with their nocturnal victory, they agreed to follow the same basic plan: decentralize mother, enhance father, and increase Jennifer's feelings of adequacy regarding herself and the management of her own behavior. The concept was never quite so explicitly verbalized with the parents. The next stages of the plan were discussed instead in these terms:

1. Jennifer would be required to attend school daily.
2. Between waking and 9:25 A.M. would be her own time at home. She could use it to dress herself in her own choice of clothes. (Mother had previously been picking out her clothes the night before and dressing Jennifer in the morning.) She could also use the morning time to eat breakfast and do anything else she wished.
3. At 9:25 she would be expected to go out the door for school, period . . . with or without clothes, with or without breakfast. This would be Jennifer's choice. Mrs. Maloney would see that Jennifer left on time.
4. If difficulty developed, Mr. Maloney would be called at work to

come home and assist. Mrs. Maloney would not be required to handle the problem alone any longer.

At the fourth interview Mr. and Mrs. Maloney reported that Jennifer had become hysterical with the presentation of this plan. Nonetheless, they held their ground united and were obviously pleased that school attendance had been regular and without incident ever since. Mr. Maloney had not had to be called. Mother felt successful; father felt relieved.

By the fifth interview everyone was feeling better. Father was freely discussing his desire to continue taking a decisive stand in the work of his own family. Mother was pleased beyond words that she was once again finding a man, husband, and father in the family's midst. Consequently she found less and less need for her previous nagging, critical stance. Their daughter appeared visibly more relaxed; she was sleeping reasonably well and having no difficulty with school attendance. Her parents were able to let her go and turn their energies toward helping her enhance relationships with peers in such things as staying over at a friend's house, heretofore vigorously refused by Jennifer owing to "my problem at night."

Sessions were mutually terminated after ten visits. There was no recurrence of symptoms.

The therapeutic work and a successful outcome with Jennifer and her parents did not rest only on the use of a communication model as presented in the previous chapter. The physician also relied heavily on ideas concerned with the structure of a family. Two individuals, Salvador Minuchin and Jay Haley, have been particularly influential in the growth of so-called structural family therapy. Differences between Minuchin and Haley do exist, even though for several years and until recently both men worked at the same institution (Philadelphia Child Guidance Clinic) and have been generally regarded as belonging to the same "school," that of structural family therapy. A summary of the views of each man will illustrate their similarities with, and divergence from, one another, and the relationship of each to interviewing based on communication theory a la Satir should become apparent also.

SALVADOR MINUCHIN AND STRUCTURAL FAMILY THERAPY

Our group with its pediatric orientation first became interested in the work of Minuchin when we learned that he was engaged in the effective treatment of primary anorexia nervosa through short-term family therapy. This illness, as most pediatric readers can appreciate, has over the years struck panic and despair in the hearts of many clinicians. All therapies, be they medical, endocrinological, psychoanalytic, behavioral, nutritional, or voodoo, have by and large failed when faced with an emaciated, stubborn, starving adolescent and her desperately anxious parents. Therefore it was refreshing to read in some of Minuchin's reports that short-term family therapy (median course of treatment 6 months) was successful in over 80% of cases referred to him for treatment.[7] We began to view his work with interest.

In 1974 a summary of his approaches to families, anorectic or otherwise, appeared in a work titled *Families and Family Therapy.*[5] This volume succeeded his previous major work, *Families of the Slums: An Exploration of their Structure and Treatment.*[6]

The two publications are important for different reasons. The older text describes in detail a research and teaching project evaluating the use and selection of specific family therapy techniques in working with families of the slums. Clinicians involved in the care of such families may find it useful reading. The 1974 text is more generic, articulating Minuchin's views of families in general and tracing the therapeutic strategies he has developed from a structural orientation. His views in this second text will be reviewed here. (Minuchin's most recent publication appeared in 1978.[7] Primarily concerned with his family work in psychosomatic problems, that volume will be discussed more extensively in Chapter 11, "Psychosomatic Conditions.")

Therapy based on a structural framework, Minuchin states, is directed toward changing the organization of a family. He describes structural therapy as a therapy of action, "the tool of this therapy is to modify the present, not to explore and interpret the past."[5] The target of intervention in the present is the family system. The therapist joins that system and then uses himself to transform it. By changing the position of the system's members, he changes their subjective experiences. Minuchin defines family structure as that invisible set of functional demands that organizes the way in which family members interact. For him a family is a system that operates through transactional patterns. Repeated transactions establish patterns of how, when, and with whom one relates, and these patterns support the family's system. In all of these respects he joins other family theorists, including those primarily interested in communication. He too then would seem to be comfortable with the previously elaborated metaphor of a "mobile."

When the structure of the family group is transformed, the positions of members in that group are altered accordingly, and as a result, each individual changes. Agreeing with every other family therapist that man is not an isolate, he further states that therapy with a family rests on three axioms:

1. An individual's psychic life is not entirely an internal process.
2. Changes in a family structure contribute to changes in the behavior and the inner psychic processes of the members of that system.
3. When a therapist works with a patient or a patient's family, his behavior becomes part of the context. Therapist and family join to form a new, therapeutic system, and that system then governs the behavior of its members.

These three assumptions—that context affects inner processes, that changes in context produce changes in the individual, and that the therapist's behavior is significant in change—underlie his approach to therapy. To illustrate the structural therapist's view, Minuchin cites the example of Alice in Wonderland:

> In Wonderland, Alice suddenly grew to a gigantic size. Her experience was that she got bigger while the room got smaller. If Alice had grown in a room that was also growing at the same rate, she might have experienced everything as staying the same. Only if Alice or the room changes separately does her experience change. It is simplistic, but not accurate, to say that intrapsychic therapy concentrates on changing Alice. A structural family therapist concentrates on changing Alice with her room.*

Subsystems and boundaries

Every family system is further characterized, in Minuchin's view, by subsystems or subunits of the family. A subsystem may consist of one individual, two persons (husband-wife, mother-child, and so on), or more (three children, two children with one parent, and so on). The specific subsystems are separated by boundaries. The term "boundary" is fundamental to structural theorists. (The reader will note that the terms employed in this chapter are more concerned with space, place, and mapping than with communication, message, and feeling.) Minuchin defines the boundary of a subsystem as that collection of rules that de-

---

*Minuchin, S.: Families and family therapy, Cambridge, Mass., 1974, Harvard University Press, p. 11.

fines who participates and how. A boundary simultaneously defining a spouse subsystem and a parental subsystem is declared, for instance, when a father tells his son: "Albert, I will be with you in 15 minutes. Until then I would like you to leave us alone. This is a time when your mother and I would like to talk alone."

The above is an example of a boundary that is clear. Boundaries may also be diffuse (unclear) or rigid (too clear and unyielding), in which case they may produce relationships characterized by overinvolvement, conflict, or coalition. Minuchin feels that the boundaries of subsystems must be clear for proper family functioning. He postulates that all families fall somewhere on a continuum, the opposite extremes of which are (1) inappropriately diffuse boundaries or (2) overly rigid subsystem boundaries. Most families fall somewhere between, in what he terms the "normal range of clear boundaries." Other families, operating at either of the two extremes of boundary functioning, he terms "enmeshed" (overly diffuse boundaries) of "disengaged" (overly rigid boundaries).

Almost all families, at some point in normal development and in some aspect of their subsystems, exhibit qualities of enmeshment and/or disengagement. As children grow and begin to separate from the family, for example, disengagement is certainly appropriate, following a prior time when enmeshment had been preeminent and satisfactory. This is normal in Minuchin's view.

It is, however, a persistent and unshifting stand at either extreme that produces family symptomatology and dysfunction. Minuchin summarizes it this way:

A highly enmeshed subsystem of mother and children, for example, can exclude father, who becomes disengaged in the extreme. The resulting undermining of the children's independence might be an important factor in the development of symptoms.

Members of enmeshed subsystems or families may be handicapped in that the heightened sense of belonging requires a major yielding of autonomy. The lack of subsystem differentiation discourages autonomous exploration and mastery of problems. In a child particularly, cognitive-affective skills are thereby inhibited. Members of disengaged subsystems or families may function autonomously but have a skewed sense of independence and lack of feelings of loyalty and belonging and the capacity for interdependence and for requesting support when needed.

In other words, a system toward the extreme disengaged end of the continuum tolerates a wide range of individual variations in its members. But stresses in one family member do not cross over its inappropriately rigid boundaries. Only a high level of individual stress can reverberate strongly enough to activate the family's supportive systems. At the enmeshed end of the continuum, the opposite is true. The behavior of one member immediately affects others, and stress in an individual member reverberates strongly across the boundaries and is swiftly echoed in other subsystems.

Both types of relating cause family problems when adaptive mechanisms are evoked. The enmeshed family responds to any variation from the accustomed with excessive speed and intensity. The disengaged family tends not to respond when a response is necessary. The parents in an enmeshed family may become tremendously upset because a child does not eat his dessert. The parents in a disengaged family may feel unconcerned about a child's hatred of school.*

The clarity of boundaries within a family thus becomes a useful parameter for the evaluation of family functioning. Some families turn in upon themselves, developing their own "safe" world, with a consequent increase of communication and concern among family members. As a result, distance decreases and boundaries are blurred. The differentiation of the family subsystems becomes unclear. Such a system may become overloaded and lack the resources necessary to adapt and change under stressful circumstances. Another family may develop overly rigid boundaries. Communication across this family's subsystems becomes difficult, and the protective functions of the family are handicapped.

Minuchin lists three subsystems for which boundaries should be clearly defined and respected if a family is to function properly:

1. The spouse subsystem: this system must achieve a boundary that protects it from interference by the demands and needs of other systems. This is particularly true when a family has children. The adults must have a psychosocial territory of their own—a haven in which they can give each other emotional support.
2. The parental subsystem: a boundary must be drawn that allows a child access to both parents while excluding the child from spouse functions. Across this boundary some of the most intense family conflicts arise. Parents cannot protect and guide without at the same time controlling and restricting. Children cannot grow and

*Minuchin, S.: Families and family therapy, Cambridge, Mass., 1974, Harvard University Press, p. 55.

become individuated without rejecting and attacking. The process of socializing is inherently conflictual. Conflict or no, a family with clear parental subsystem boundaries never loses correct sight of who is parent and who is child.

3. The sibling subsystem: within this system children experiment with peer relationships. Children learn how to negotiate, cooperate, and compete in this setting, and here they prepare for similar experiences eventually outside the family, hence Minuchin's term that the sibling subsystem represents the child's "first social laboratory."

Mapping the family

Through an assessment of family subsystems and boundary functioning, says Minuchin, the structural family therapist develops a rapid diagnostic picture of the family. This in turn orients his therapeutic interventions.

Observing a family in action, the therapist notices interactions and repetitive behaviors among different family members such that he is developing in his mind's eye (and later on paper) a family map. This family map, changing with time and additional information, allows the therapist to organize the material he is observing and points the way toward specific therapeutic interventions. Certain symbols are used:

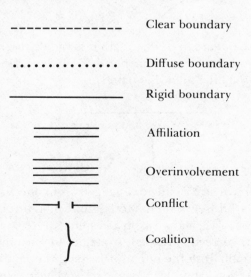

Clear boundary

Diffuse boundary

Rigid boundary

Affiliation

Overinvolvement

Conflict

Coalition

M	Mother
W	Wife
F	Father
H	Husband
$C_1 C_2$	First child, second child
Th	Therapist

Thus appropriate functioning with clear boundaries in a two-parent family with children would be mapped as follows:

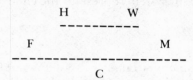

The Maloneys would not fit such a configuration. The reader will remember that Mr. Maloney was peripheral in his fathering and was often in conflict with his wife. Mrs. Maloney, heavily overinvolved with her daughter, shared a relationship with Jennifer that if nothing else fuzzed over any vestige of a clear parental boundary. There are several ways to diagram such a collaboration:

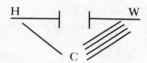

Here wife and husband are in conflict; father is rigidly disengaged from his child; mother and child are overinvolved. A rigid triad develops. The Maloneys would also fit the following pattern:

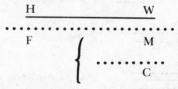

Here husband and wife are rigidly disengaged from one another. Their spouse subsystem is diffusely bound. Mother and child through a diffuse boundary are united in a coalition against father.

Once a family is correctly mapped, strategies to rearrange structure are carried out, usually with the intent of helping the family eventually achieve a configuration with clear boundaries. There may be several transitional configurations along the way to allow for a final structuring that shows clear boundaries for spouses, parents, and siblings.

According to Minuchin the therapist, once he begins work, must include himself in any family mapping that takes place. At this point his third axiom regarding family therapy becomes most demonstrable. That third axiom, the reader may remember, was as follows: "When a therapist works with a patient or a patient's family, his behavior becomes part of the context. Therapist and family join to form a new therapeutic system, and that system then governs the behavior of its members."[5]

The therapist intervenes in such a way as to unbalance the existing system, breaking up repetitive patterns, changing alignments, and allowing for constructive problem solving. To illustrate, with the Maloneys the therapist had specific goals: to engage the father more actively in parenting and to diminish the spousal conflict, enhancing the relationship between husband and wife. He also hoped to demarcate more clearly a boundary between mother and daughter and to diminish their mutual coalition against father. The therapist achieved this in a series of moves utilizing himself to unbalance the system. He first affiliated with the father, then blocked mother-child transactions by conducting sessions without the child and suggesting mother's withdrawal from Jennifer at night; he also encouraged mother and father in a coalition against the child. This may be diagrammed as follows:

$$\text{Th} ===== \text{F M}$$
$$-------------$$
$$\text{C}$$
$$\text{and}$$
$$\text{Th} \quad \text{F M}$$
$$\underbrace{\qquad}$$
$$\text{C}$$

When the Maloney family terminated counseling after ten sessions, their map had developed from these intermediate stages, which included the therapist, into a configuration with clear boundaries. A therapist was no longer necessary.

Joining and accommodation

At this point the reader may have concluded that structural family therapy is little more than a rude chess game with a callow therapist who moves people about willy-nilly. There is an element of "the contest" in the writings of both Minuchin and Haley. Both authors are explicitly concerned with strategies, manipulations, moves, and "operations." Haley addresses this theme, among others, in a chapter of *Problem-Solving Therapy* entitled "Ethical Issues in Therapy."[4] It is recommended reading. However, little is willy-nilly in the approaches of either man. Haley states:

> If successful therapy is defined as solving the problems of a client, the therapist must know how to formulate a problem and how to solve it. And if he or she is to solve a variety of problems, the therapist must not take a rigid and stereotyped approach to therapy. Any standardized method of therapy, no matter how effective with certain problems, cannot deal successfully with the wide range that is typically offered to a therapist. Flexibility and spontaneity are necessary. Yet any therapist must also learn from experience and repeat what was successful before. A combination of familiar procedures and innovative techniques increases the probability of success.*

For both men successful therapy depends on very specific and learnable principles.

For Minuchin the therapist's job is to facilitate the transformation of the family system. The process involves three major steps:

1. The therapist joins the family in a position of leadership.
2. The therapist unearths and evaluates the underlying family structure.
3. The therapist creates circumstances that will allow transformation of the structure.

The timid should take careful note — Minuchin states clearly his view of the responsibility of the therapist: "When the therapist joins the family, he assumes the leadership of the therapeutic system. This leadership involves responsibility for what happens . . . . The family will be the matrix of the healing and growth of its members. The responsibility for reaching this state, or for failing to do so, belongs to the therapist."[5] In our experience therapists have too often dismissed their therapeutic failures with the salvo, "Well, what could I expect; the family wasn't really motivated, wasn't ready for help . . . too resistant." Yet when patients do well in counseling, the therapist is usually credited; why then, when they do not do well, is that failure generally ascribed to the patient, not to the

---

*Haley, J.: Problem-solving therapy: new strategies for effective family therapy, San Francisco, 1976, Jossey-Bass, Inc., p. 9.

therapist? Minuchin (and Haley even more so) appears to deplore such summations as irresponsible therapy. We would agree that this is often the case.

Sensitivity, balance, and time are important in helping a family alter their structure:

> The concept of transformation deals with large movements in therapy, which take place over time. The therapist must know how to map his goals. But he must also know how to facilitate the small movements that carry the family toward those goals. He must help them in such a way that they are not threatened by major dislocations. A person's ability to move from one circumstance to another depends on the support he receives; he will not move toward the unknown in a situation of danger. Therefore, it is vital to provide systems of support within the family to facilitate the movement from one position to another.*

The goal, of course, with the Maloney family was to diminish Jennifer's sleep disorder and fear of school. That represented the "large movement" in therapy. Many small movements were required to set this in motion: mother was supported and given a rest, father was requested to enter the scene more actively, Jennifer was excluded from sessions, mother and father were encouraged in a cooperative effort, and so forth.

Minuchin does define certain processes that, regardless of individual therapeutic styles, he considers essential for successful work with families. The methods used by a therapist to create a therapeutic system and to establish himself in a position of leadership are known as "joining and accommodation operations." Minuchin states these are the foundations of therapy, and without them restructuring cannot take place. "Joining and accommodation are two ways of describing the same process."[5] Joining is the process of engaging with the family, touching them and being touched by them in turn. It requires that the therapist follow their path of communication, discovering what is open, what is partly closed, what is entirely closed. He must attend to individual dilemmas and pain, experiencing as best he can all the pressures of the family system before him. He must be able to disengage himself from the system, maintaining enough freedom to develop effective therapeutic goals with the family. Joining a family thus requires of the therapist a capacity to adapt. Such

---

*Minuchin, S.: Families and family therapy, Cambridge, Mass., 1974, Harvard University Press, p. 119

adaptation Minuchin terms "accommodation." Specific accommodation techniques are varied. Minuchin cites three: maintenance, tracking, and mimesis.

Maintenance refers to the technique of providing planned support of the family structure as the therapist perceives it. The physician's validation of Mrs. Maloney's good intentions, hard work, and exhaustion provides an example of such a technique, that is, validating existing patterns within the family. Likewise when a therapist openly enjoys a family's humor or expresses affection for them, he is using maintenance operations. Maintenance has to do with confirming—individuals, subsystems, or the entire family.

Tracking requires a therapist to follow the content of a family's communications and behavior, encouraging that the members continue. "In its simplest form, tracking means to ask clarifying questions, to make approving comments, or to elicit amplification of a point. The therapist does not challenge what is being said."[5] Tracking confirms the family members by eliciting more information. The therapist does not initiate an action; he leads by following. Keep in mind that this technique is presented as a joining procedure. Alone it is scarcely enough to promote family change. A family session in which only tracking was used by the therapist would likely end in boredom for the interviewer and frustration for the family. We mention this because tracking has often seemed a safe retreat for our beginning therapists, particularly "content-oriented" physicians; they tend to elicit reams of information, tracking as it were until the cows come home. The cows may come home, but the family doesn't move. In such cases joining has occurred to the exclusion of any restructuring within the session.

Mimesis (literally, imitation) is used to accommodate to a family's style and affective range. The interviewer adopts the family's tempo of communication, slowing his pace or quickening it depending on how the family operates. He may utilize personal aspects of himself to blend with the family: "I can't stand carrots either," or "my own mother was like you in that respect." Such statements from the interviewer "increase sense of kinship, indicating that both therapist and family members are . . . more human than otherwise."[5]

Restructuring techniques

Restructuring refers to the process of utilizing therapeutic interventions that confront and challenge a family to make change. It is a different process from joining. Joining diminishes distance between therapist and family; it soothes. Restructuring confronts and is often far from soothing. In joining operations the therapist becomes an actor in the family play. In restructuring, while still an actor, he becomes the director — creating, suggesting, confronting, changing. These procedures are the highlights of therapy, and their success depends on a prior satisfactory joining between therapist and family.

Restructuring techniques come in at least seven varieties, according to Minuchin.

Actualizing family transactional patterns. When a therapist assumes a leadership role — as he must — in the family sessions, he runs the risk of becoming the recipient of all communication. The family tends to view him as the expert through whom all transactions must pass for judgment, correction, approval, and so on. In such instances the therapist becomes the passive recipient of endless descriptions and complaints from family members, and messages intended to pass from one family member to another are channeled through the therapist. He then functions like a telephone switchboard. The results can be stultifying:

Doctor:	Georgie, did you know that your mother has strong objections to your wetting the bed?
Georgie:	#&+?*!
Doctor:	Mrs. Ayres, did you know that Georgie doesn't give a damn?
Mrs. Ayres:	(sob)
Doctor:	Georgie, did you realize that statements like that make your mother mad?

We agree with Minuchin that describing, whether it be from family to interviewer or vice versa, is to be avoided. First of all, it constricts the therapist; if he is perpetually involved in a dialogue first with one member of the family, then with another, he is prevented from pulling back and observing; busy as a yo-yo he will be less able to formulate goals or plan and execute strategies. Second, families tend to become repetitive in their usually well-rehearsed verbal descriptions of "the problem." An effective therapist moves beyond such verbal descriptions and gives directives, enabling actual transactions to take place between family members in the interview. "There is considerable value in making the family enact instead of describe. The therapist can gather only limited data from the family's descriptions. To amplify his data, he must help them transact, in his presence, some of the ways in which they naturally resolve conflicts, support each other, enter into alliances and coalitions, or diffuse stress."[5] Minuchin refers to this as "enacting transactional patterns," and a therapist can use many devices to bring it off. He may create specific family dialogues by directing certain family members to interact with one another around a given issue, explicitly requesting, "That's an issue that involves you and Susan. I would like you two to talk with one another about that now." In some instances families are very obliging when directed to discuss issues directly with one another. Often, however, they are not, perhaps because they fear a confrontation, or that they won't be listened to, or that they need the therapist to hear their side first. For this reason the therapist must be persistent in his request and have several methods available for encouraging their face-to-face communication with one another. The dialogue with a family hesitant to pursue direct communication in a session might go like this:

> *Doctor:* That's an issue that involves you and Susan. I would like you two to talk with one another about that now.
>
> *Mother:* Oh, Doctor, Susan and I have discussed this thing many times at home, haven't we, dear?
>
> *Susan:* (mumble, shuffle)
>
> *Doctor:* I'm sure that you have. In fact it's one of the reasons that you've asked for my help. Will you discuss it once more, this time in front of me, so that I can hear you and help you figure out a solution.
>
> *Mother:* I feel so silly. It's so . . . artificial.
>
> *Doctor:* I agree (silence).
>
> *Mother:* (pause) Oh . . . you still want me to say something?
>
> *Doctor:* (Now simultaneously pushing his chair back 2 feet and choosing not to look at any family member, he stares at his shoe.) Yes, even though it's silly, talk to your daughter now about this most important aspect of her growth, stealing from your purse.
>
> *Father:* Doctor, I was wondering . . .
>
> *Doctor:* Mr. Thompkins, it's probably very hard to sit silently by. At the moment your wife and Susan need to discuss this. Can you allow them to?
>
> *Father:* Of course.
>
> *Mother:* (long silence, then tears as she begins) Oh Susan . . .

This procedure with variations may have to be repeated gently and firmly many times until the family learns that direct communication is required in the sessions.

As already mentioned, a family's seating arrangement in the office offers important information about their relationships and their structure, their alliances and their coalitions. The manipulation of their chosen family space is another technique for helping the family to enact, rather than describe. For instance, in the above example if Susan and her mother are seated on either side of Mr. Thompkins, it would be quite useful to remove him from the middle, requesting that he move his chair over next to the therapist so that "Susan and her mother can more easily talk directly to one another." (It will enable the therapist to place his hand on Mr. Thompkins and gently quiet him when he interrupts their transaction for the second time.) Also, "positioning can be an effective way of working with boundaries. If the therapist wants to create or strengthen a boundary, he can bring members of a subsystem to the center of the room and have other family members move their chairs back so that they can observe but cannot interrupt. If he wants to block contact between two members, he can separate them, or he can position himself between them and act as go-between. Spatial manipulation has the power of simplicity."[5]

Marking boundaries. The therapist may have to protect not only subsystem boundaries but individual boundaries as well. Here Minuchin and Satir clearly speak the same language. Both agree that the following should be established early in the course of an interview: the therapist and family should listen to what a family member says and acknowledge his communication; family members should talk to each other, not about each other; family members should not answer a question directed to another, nor talk about other family members, those present and especially those not present; family members should not require one member to act as the memory bank for all the family.

Marking subsystem boundaries can take place in a variety of ways. In the case of Jennifer Maloney, the therapist marked the spouse boundary by excluding the child from sessions; he simultaneously encouraged a more appropriate boundary between father and daughter by placing Mr. Maloney in charge of the nighttime episodes. He strengthened a parent boundary between Jennifer and her mother when he applauded mother's own suggestion that she withdraw by taking a ride in the car at night.

Escalating stress. The purpose of increasing stress in an already stressed family is to give the therapist "and sometimes the family members themselves, an inkling of the family's capability to restructure when circumstances change. His input and his expert prodding produce new contexts, or changed circumstances, to which the family must adapt under his eye."⁵ Minuchin suggests four methods. The simplest maneuver the therapist can use is to dam the flow of accustomed communication. When Mr. Thompkins is persistently silenced so that his wife and daughter can discuss stealing without interruption, something different may come of that conversation. This is called "blocking transactional patterns." A therapist may also increase stress by "emphasizing differences and disagreements": "Whew, you two obviously don't agree on that issue! Will you discuss it now?"

A family often has ways of minimizing or avoiding open conflict in a subtle, yet regular and predictable fashion. A therapist may want to get around this automatic "derailing" by the family and increase their stress through what Minuchin terms "developing implicit conflict." A child, for instance, who persistently interrupts when his parents approach conflict with one another may need to be silenced. A wife may need to be encouraged to stand her ground, not give up so quickly, and so on.

This suggests Minuchin's fourth method for escalating stress, "joining in alliance or coalition." In the example immediately preceding, the wife and therapist would be temporarily joined in coalition. This, Minuchin states, requires careful planning and an ability to disengage, so the therapist is not sucked into the family war and alliances. It is also chancy, since coalition with one family member risks alienating other family members, and the entire family may not return. Alliances with individual family members should always be viewed as transitional and temporary steps. The use of such maneuvers requires considerable adroitness and careful thought.

Assigning tasks. A therapist may utilize tasks within the session, and he may also assign tasks as homework. When he requests that two individuals "talk about it now," he is assigning a task. He may request that the family participate together on a nonverbal task such as the conjoint family drawing mentioned in the preceding chapter. When the family responds to tasks assigned to be done at home by accomplishing what is asked, "they are in effect taking the therapist home with them. He becomes the maker of rules beyond the structure of the session."⁵ Tasks must be carefully developed to fit the family and further the therapeutic goals. Such was the case with Jennifer's family. The task assigned was a new method for handling nighttime sleep disturbance. It required a careful appraisal of the family's structure and a goal for what sort of restructuring might be useful. The use of tasks in family counseling is discussed in more detail in the succeeding review of Haley's work.

Utilizing symptoms. Symptoms can be handled in a number of ways by the therapist. One may focus on the symptom. This is probably a most familiar role for physicians, and it is also one that the family takes to, since so very often everyone is convinced that "things in our family would be perfect if Jennifer would sleep through the night and go to school." In some situations a focus on the symptom is clearly essential; such things as fire-setting, school phobia, starvation, or refusal to take lifesaving medication cannot be ignored. Focusing on the symptom still requires careful attention to family structure, however. A careful blending of the two—attention to symptom *and* attention to family structure— is illustrated elegantly in a now-famous case from Minuchin's group at the Philadelphia Child Guidance Clinic. Haley was the therapist's supervisor in the case. It is summarized in the writings of both men and is also available as a film. As Minuchin tells it:

> A child comes into therapy with a dog phobia that is so severe he is almost confined to the house. The therapist's diagnosis is that the symptom is supported by an implicit unresolved conflict between spouses, manifested in an affiliation between the mother and son that excludes the father. His strategy is to increase the affiliation between the father and son before tackling the spouse subsystem problems. Therefore he encourages the father, who is a mailman "and therefore an expert in dealing with dogs," to teach his son how to deal with strange dogs. The child, who is adopted, in turn adopts a dog, and the father and son join in transactions around the dog. This activity strengthens their relationship and promotes a separation between mother and son. As the symptom disappears, the therapist praises both parents for their successful handling of the child. He then moves to work with the husband-wife conflicts.*

Clearly it is Minuchin's view, and ours, that a focus on symptoms as an entree into the family system of interactions will produce more than superficial changes.

A therapist may even want to exaggerate a symptom at times. In an interview by one of our staff with the family of a child hospitalized for psychosomatic nausea and vomiting, each time parental conflict was approached, the child retched and disrupted the interview, and chaos ensued. The therapist quickly encouraged the child's vomiting, handed him a wastebasket, and even asked him to vomit more, deliberately re-

---

*Minuchin, S.: Families and family therapy, Cambridge, Mass., 1974, Harvard University Press, p. 153.

questing the family to wait while John threw up—all while urging the boy to increase his efforts. The vomiting stopped and did not return for the remainder of the interview.

De-emphasizing the symptom at times is also useful, according to Minuchin. A most elegant implementation of this strategy is found in his work with anorexia nervosa: "At times it is possible to use the symptom as an avenue away from the identified patient. The technique of having lunch with an anorectic patient and his family, for example, facilitates the creation, within the field of eating, of a strong interpersonal conflict, which then takes precedence over the symptom."[5] With most anorectic patients, Minuchin conducts a family luncheon interview in the early stages of therapy. He and the family eat together, usually before the child's discharge from the hospital. In the course of this interview many noneating issues are addressed. For example, the child's failure to eat may be discussed as a reflection of the parents' mutual coalition in defeat, that is, their inability to make their daughter eat. In the process of what is often a heated interview around such topics, the anorectic patient frequently begins to pick at her food and eventually puts some in her mouth. This action, striking to watch in videotaped examples of Minuchin's work, is not usually directly commented on by the therapist.

One may use symptoms in other ways as well. A therapist may move to a new symptom. For instance, a child's school avoidance brought a family to the doctor. In discussing it mother revealed her own reluctance to be home alone during the day. The interviewer then moved to this issue. A therapist may occasionally want to relabel a symptom. A child who runs away from home may benefit (and so may the parents) from having her action described by the therapist as a desperate maneuver to get close to her parents through the reunion that ocurred when she was found.

Manipulating mood. Delineating a family's predominant mood—joyful, sad, angry, tentative, and so on—is part of the work of elucidating its structure. A therapist can use this knowledge sometimes for restructuring. For instance, he can exaggerate a family mood to illogical extremes. In our own work two overprotective parents were encouraged to such an extent in their efforts by the therapist that even they wanted to back off after a time:

Mother: I want her home 20 minutes after school is out. Children should not be unsupervised. They get into trouble.

Doctor: Maybe 20 minutes is too long unsupervised, Mrs. Jarvis.

Mother: Well, she has to have some time to get from school to the house. It's several blocks.

Doctor: But 20 minutes . . . I don't know. I agree with you; kids can get into a lot of trouble and in less than 20 minutes. Have you considered picking her up in the car at school?

Father: Excuse me for interrupting, Doctor, but I think you're wrong there. First of all, Madelyn works and couldn't possibly pick up Ellen. And second, Ellen has to learn that we trust her by herself. Twenty minutes! . . . That's such a little while. If you can't trust your own child for 20 minutes . . . !

Mother: Exactly.

Doctor: I see. Since you brought that up, what are some of the other ways in which you are letting Ellen know that you trust her own abilities?

Support, education, and guidance. Support, education, and guidance are self-evident. Minuchin includes them last in his list of restructuring techniques and gives them less than a page. Yet these maneuvers are among those most familiar to physicians. They are not to be minimized; however, since they can be frustratingly ineffective with a dysfunctional family, neither should they be used to the exclusion of other techniques. Support is essential in work with families; it isn't enough by itself to do the trick.

JAY HALEY AND PROBLEM-SOLVING THERAPY

Haley is, obviously, another individual who has strongly influenced the development of our clinical approaches with pediatric patients and their families. His previous involvement in the elaboration of communication theory has already been mentioned. As a family therapist he became interested early in power struggles among family members, but more particularly those between a therapist and his patient (family). In a 1963 book, *Strategies of Psychotherapy*,[1] he suggested that any relationship is by definition a power struggle, that people so involved are constantly struggling to define or redefine their relationship. The relationship between a therapist and a patient is equally a power struggle, one in which the therapist must win or be in control if change is to occur. His *tactics* (the word is his) for producing change are rooted in paradox and hypnosis. He acknowledges his debt to Dr. Milton Erickson and that man's innovative development of indirect hypnotic methods in psychiatric treatment.[2,3]

It is not this phase of Haley's work, but rather his more recent views (admittedly an outgrowth and refinement of his earlier emphasis on paradox, hypnosis, and communication), that we wish to review here. His current thinking is summarized in a book titled *Problem-Solving Therapy*.[4] In this work he elaborates a therapy approach that:

> focuses on solving a client's presenting problems within the framework of the family . . . The therapist's task is to formulate a presenting symptom clearly and to design an intervention in the client's social situation to change that presenting symptom . . . . The approach here differs from other symptom-oriented therapies in that it emphasizes the social context of human problems.*

What is important for Haley is "solving problems," and he doesn't beat around the bush: "The first obligation of a therapist is to change the presenting problem offered. If that is not accomplished, the therapy is a failure."[4]

Giving directives

A cornerstone of Haley's therapeutic approach lies in developing the ability to give directives successfully to families. Giving directives or tasks has several purposes. First, since he feels the main goal of therapy is to get people to behave differently, directives are a way of making such changes occur. Second, directives may be used to intensify a relationship between a family and their therapist. "By telling people what to do, a therapist becomes involved in the action. He becomes important because the person must either do or not do what the therapist says."[1] Third, directives are used to gather information. A family reveals itself according to how it responds to directives given.

Just what is a directive? It is essentially anything done in therapy by the therapist to the family—from a simple nod to an elaborate homework assignment:

> Some therapists are uncomfortable about giving directives because they feel perhaps they should not take the responsibility for telling someone what to do. It is important to emphasize that directives can be given directly or they can be given in a conversation implicitly by vocal intonation, body movement, and well-timed silence. Everything done in therapy can be seen as a directive. If an individual or a family in an interview is talking about something and the therapist says, "tell me more about

---

*Haley, J.: Problem-solving therapy: new strategies for effective family therapy, San Francisco, 1976, Jossey-Bass, Inc., p. 50.

that," he is giving a directive. If the therapist only nods his head and smiles, encouraging them to continue, that is also a directive. If someone says something the therapist does not like, he can tell the person not to say that anymore — and that is telling him what to do. If the therapist turns his body away from the person and frowns, he is also telling the person that he should not say that sort of thing.*

There are several types of directives, which are outlined in the following categories:

A. Telling people what to do when the therapist wants them to do it
  1. Telling someone to stop doing something
  2. Telling someone to do something different
     a. Giving good advice
     b. Giving directives to change the sequence in a family
B. Telling people what to do when the therapist does not want them to do it — because the therapist wants them to change by rebelling

Each of these types will be discussed.

Telling someone to stop doing something is one of the most difficult directives to enforce, Haley states — not impossible, but difficult. "If the therapist tells someone to stop usual behavior, he must usually go to an extreme or get other family members to cooperate and change their behavior to support him in this task. Often it is like trying to stop a river from flowing; one can try to block it, but the river will go over and around the block and the therapist will drown."[4] He is even more pessimistic about giving good advice. "Giving good advice means the therapist assumes that people have rational control of what they are doing. To be successful in the therapy business it may be better to drop that idea."[4] In our experience also good advice is often useless in helping families change.

Therefore if one is interested in having a family follow through on a task, one is left with giving a directive that will change the sequence in a family, one that will motivate people because there is some gain in following it. The reader will remember that Jackson refers to "family homeostasis"; Satir uses the term "family system"; Minuchin says "family structure"; and now Haley introduces "family sequence." The terms, while very different, are quite related; they have to do with how each of the above individuals has conceptualized the family unit. Homeostasis

*Haley, J.: Problem-solving therapy: new strategies for effective family therapy, San Francisco, 1976, Jossey-Bass, Inc., p. 50.

suggests a balancing process; system has to do also with balancing through communication patterns; structure suggests an emphasis on configuration and organization. Sequence reflects Haley's particular wrinkle on the same piece of cloth. He feels that family members operate with one another in knowable, repetitive sequences. Such sequences are based on each family's specific organizational pattern. A therapist, hoping to effect change in a family, must determine the family's sequence (or homeostatic pattern, system, structure, depending on the term preferred) and change it. Certain family sequences, as noted by Haley, are so ubiquitous and utilizable in helping families to change that they will be elaborated later in this chapter.

Haley offers some advice for designing tasks. When a therapist first gives tasks to families, designing them may seem difficult. With practice and experience the process becomes easier. Whatever the task, it should be simple enough that the family can do it. The best task is one that uses the presenting problem to make a structural change in the family. With this approach, the focus is on respecting and utilizing what the family considers important (the presenting problem) and what the therapist thinks is important (an organizational change). The steps in designing a task are to think about the presenting problem in terms of the sequence in the family and to find a directive that changes both.

For instance, a common problem is that a child (like Jennifer Maloney) refuses to go to school. Haley suggests that a necessary first step in such a situation is to be sure that the problem is not a school situation in which for good reasons the child should not go.

Secondly it is necessary to motivate the parents to work together by having them agree that the child is falling behind and must go to school. At this point it is made explicit that a decision as to whether the child goes to school is not up to the child but up to the parents. The therapist needs to pull the parents together in relation to the child.

He then gives a directive that takes the family's usual sequence around the problem into account. The Maloney's sequence was as follows:

1. Father insisted that the child go to school; he then left for work.
2. Jennifer manifested anxiety.
3. Mother, alone with Jennifer, felt overwhelmed and gave in.
4. Father subsequently criticized his wife for her helplessness.
5. Mother protested that father was insensitive.
6. Father continued to insist that the child go to school, and again left for work.

Various directives are possible in such a sequence. The responsibility for taking the child to school might be given to father, or it might be given to mother. Or the therapist might say that mother must see that father does it. Or it could be appropriate that both parents escort the child to class. With the Maloneys, responsibility was given to mother for getting Jennifer to school, with father readily available for help (not criticism) as needed. In a straightforward task such as this, Haley states that a crucial issue is anticipating what will happen. The therapist can review with each parent how he or she will take the child to school. The parents are then asked to discuss how the child will probably behave—temper, tears, upset stomach, and so on. The mother is asked what she will do when the child becomes upset; likewise the father is asked to consider his reactions in the face of escalating behavior by the child. The contingencies are all discussed beforehand as the plan is talked through in a "dry run" in the office. The family may even be asked to practice the task in front of the therapist.

Haley offers specific suggestions for motivating a family to follow a directive. He may urge them directly to follow through, acknowledging that they and he want the same thing, a solution to their dilemma. As the reader is aware, even families in profound pain are not always cooperative; in these situations more indirect methods may have to be used. For instance, one may encourage family members to "talk about how desperate their situation is. Rather than reassure them it is not so bad, the therapist can agree with them that it is quite bad. If the situation is made to appear desperate enough, they will listen to the therapist and do the task he offers."[4] The therapist must also fit the task to the particular family. Some families with a flair for the dramatic and crisis will warm to a task if it is described as "huge, of overwhelming importance." A resistant family, on the other hand, may find a "small task" easier to stomach. Attention to a family's general style—informal, organized, cautious, and so on—will also suggest directions for presenting a task successfully. For instance a family that is hopelessly pessimistic and negative may be pushed into success if the therapist agrees with their pessimism: "I do not think that this family will be able to carry this off. I am suggesting it, but I want you to know that I have grave doubts that you can do it at this time."

The therapist should also be precise and specific in his directions. Directions should be clearly given rather than suggested. "I would like you to . . . " brings more success than "You might like to think about . . . " Specificity is important for two reasons: it helps to get the task done, and if it is not done, the therapist needs to be sure that it has not gone unfinished simply because the instructions were confusing.

The best directives involve all family members. For Jennifer's school difficulties, everyone was assigned some job: Jennifer was responsible for her own time before school, Mrs. Maloney was responsible for getting her out the door at 9:25, and Mr. Maloney was assigned the task of being available by telephone to assist as needed.

> A good task has something for everyone. Even if the therapist specifically asks someone to stay out of the task, this request is still giving the person something to do. The task should be structured like any other piece of work. Someone is needed to do the job, someone to help, someone to supervise, someone to plan, someone to check to see that it gets done, and so on.*

Haley also recommends that family members review what they are to do before leaving and in front of the therapist as further assurance that the task is understood. One should actually anticipate noncompliance on the family's part and handle it in advance by beating the family to the punch, that is, reviewing with them the many ways in which each might defeat successful completion of the task. A therapist may do this by asking each person, "How could you contribute to the failure of this project? What are some of the ways?" If none are forthcoming, the therapist may make his own suggestions regarding sabotage efforts. Once these efforts are explicitly and openly discussed before the event, they are seldom subsequently used to defeat the task.

When a therapist has given a task, he should always ask for a report at the next interview. Haley suggests that if the family has done the task, congratulations are in order and the interview should go on from there. If the family has only partially done their job, an exploration of this partial failure is necessary. Haley feels strongly that failure to do what a therapist asks should never be treated lightly. To allow a family to do so suggests that what the therapist has requested is not important. This then makes the therapist less important and also makes it less likely that they will do the next task assigned. He is particularly strong in this view if the family has not done the task and does not have a valid excuse:

> The best attitude for the therapist to take is that they have failed. It is not that they have failed the therapist, but they have failed themselves.

---

*Haley, J.: Problem-solving therapy: new strategies for effective family therapy, San Francisco, 1976, Jossey-Bass, Inc., p. 59.

One way to deal with task failure is to tell the family members that the task was very important and that for their sakes it is too bad they did not do it. The therapist can tell them that now they cannot know how beneficial it would have been to them. If they say they did not think the task would do any good, the therapist can say they can never know that now, because they did not do it. Throughout the interview when they bring up problems, the therapist can point out that naturally they have those problems because they did not do the task. His goal is to get them to say they would like to have the opportunity to try again and do the task. If they do say this, the therapist can tell them that the opportunity is gone and can never come again—they cannot do the task now. In this way, he sets up the situation so that the next time he asks them to do a task they will do it.*

If the reader has momentarily paled at the touch of audacity that seems to be necessary in utilizing Haley's approach for successful directives, that same reader will positively blanch at Haley's suggestions for the use of paradoxical tasks, that is, telling people what to do when the therapist does not want them to do it, because the therapist wants them to change by rebelling (see B. in outline, p. 69). This approach is based on the idea that some families who come for help are resistant to the help that is offered. Indeed with all families, some resistance to change is met along the course of treatment. "The members are very good at getting a therapist to try and fail. The therapist is then pulling at the family members to improve, while they are resisting and provoking him to go on pulling. This situation is frustrating for both the therapist and the family."[4]

A paradoxical task always has two levels: "change" and, simultaneously, "don't change." A brief example from our own work may illustrate the technique. A family arrived asking for help with their two boys, ages 7 and 9. The boys fought constantly, to the parents' chagrin; nowhere was it more troublesome that at the dinner table. Usually inside of 10 minutes the entire family was engaged in a brouhaha, with resulting alienation and indigestion among all four. The therapist suggested that clearly this family needed to fight for some reason, and since their fights were so energy-depleting, they should never fight on an empty stomach. Therefore he was asking them to fight even more, particularly at the dinner table. He designed a task with them in which they were to have a

*Haley, J.: Problem-solving therapy: new strategies for effective family therapy, San Francisco, 1976, Jossey-Bass, Inc., p. 64.

serious fight at the dinner table every night for 14 consecutive nights. Specific roles were assigned to every family member. The family failed magnificently at the task. Two meager altercations were all they could show for their efforts, and they had noticed that they were no longer so involved in arguments with one another at other times either. The therapy subsequently moved to other issues. and fighting did not return as a family issue.

Haley believes that families such as this achieve the goal of therapy to prove to the therapist that they are as good as other people. He regards it as essential that the therapist accept the change when it happens and let the family put him down by proving him wrong.

> If he wants to ensure that the change continue, he might say to the members that probably the change is only temporary and they will relapse again. Then the family will continue the change to prove to him that it is not temporary . . . He can do the same by encouraging a relapse. He can say to the family, "I can see you've changed and are over the problem, but I think this has happened too fast. I would like you to have a relapse and this week go back to the way you were before . . ." To make this directive reasonable to family members, the therapist might say that too fast a change is upsetting.*

Regarding his therapeutic uses of relapses, Haley acknowledges the considerable influence of Milton Erickson.

Haley cautions, and we certainly agree, that considerable skill is necessary in using a paradoxical approach. Even though issues are serious and distressing, the therapist must be able to conceptualize them in playful and fanciful ways. Haley lists eight stages of a successful paradoxical intervention:

1. As in all directive therapy, the therapist works toward establishing a relationship defined as one to bring about change.
2. The therapist helps the family to clearly define the problem to be treated.
3. The therapist clearly sets the goals of treatment.
4. The therapist offers a plan, a rationale that makes the directive reasonable in the family's view.
5. The therapist gracefully disqualifies the current authority on the problem. That authority may be a spouse, a mother, or some other family member. (Usually someone is trying to help the pa-

---

*Haley, J.: Problem-solving therapy: new strategies for effective family therapy, San Francisco, 1976, Jossey-Bass, Inc., pp. 69-70.

tient solve the problem. That person must be defined as not doing the right thing.)

6. The therapist gives the paradoxical directive.
7. The therapist observes the family's response and continues to encourage the usual behavior. If the family improves and is less symptomatic, the therapist labels that as not cooperating.
8. As changes continue, the therapist avoids credit for the change. Otherwise relapses will occur.

In our own work, we are finding the use of directives very effective; the majority of directives we employ are those in which we intend the family to do what we ask. Our use of paradoxical tasks with families is considerably less frequent.

Family organization and hierarchy

Haley notes that the people in a family, with their common history and future, follow organized ways of behaving with one another. To be so organized means that they follow patterned, redundant ways of behaving; they thus come to exist in a hierarchy with one another. A family hierarchy at its most simple level consists of a generation of parents who nurture and discipline a second generation, the children, who in turn become parents and nurture and discipline a third generation. Whatever the specific arrangement in a family, that family must deal with the issue of organizing itself in such a hierarchy, and rules are worked out regarding who is primary in status and power and who is secondary. When an individual shows symptoms, Haley believes, the family organization has a hierarchical arrangement that has become unclear and confused. "If there is a fundamental rule of social organization, it is that an organization is in trouble when coalitions occur across levels of a hierarchy, particularly when these coalitions are secret. When an employer plays favorites among his employees, he is forming coalitions across power lines and joining one employee against another."[4] In this illustration by Haley, the hierarchy has become unclear. So it is with families. When family members cross hierarchical, generational boundaries to form coalitions, the family is in trouble, and symptomatology in one or more family members may be the result. (Mrs. Maloney and her daughter had certainly, with their coalition, toppled the generational organization and hierarchy of the Maloney family.) How do coalitions across generational lines produce symptoms? To answer this question, one must understand what Haley has to say about family sequences. A summary of his views on that subject follows.

Family sequences

We have earlier referred to Haley's use of the term "sequence" in describing a family's behavior. He feels that family members organize themselves around repetitive sequences of behavior with one another and that these sequences ultimately develop into repeating cycles within the life of a family. These sequences can reflect dysfunction when the following conditions are present (in a family of at least three individuals) and interfere with the usual clear hierarchy of a family's organization:

1. The three people responding to one another are not peers but of different generations.
2. The member of one generation forms a coalition across generations with another family member and against a generation peer.
3. The coalition across generations is denied or concealed.

Certain problem sequences are very common in Haley's experience. One involves three generations:

> The classic situation is made up of grandmother, mother, and problem child. That is the typical one-parent family situation among the poor and middle-class when a mother has divorced and returned to her mother. In the classic example, the grandmother tends to be defined as dominating, the mother as irresponsible, and the child as a behavior problem. The typical sequence is as follows:
>
> 1. Grandmother takes care of grandchild while protesting that mother is irresponsible and does not take care of the child properly. In this way grandmother is siding with the child against the mother in a coalition across generation lines.
> 2. Mother withdraws, letting grandmother care for the child.
> 3. The child misbehaves or expresses symptomatic behavior.
> 4. Grandmother protests that she should not have to take care of the child and discipline him. She has raised her children, and mother should take care of her own child.
> 5. Mother begins to take care of her own child.
> 6. Grandmother protests that mother does not know how to take care of the child properly and is being irresponsible. She takes over the care of the grandchild to save the child from mother.
> 7. Mother withdraws, letting grandmother care for the child.
> 8. The child misbehaves or expresses symptomatic behavior.*

And so on. This sequence incidentally had been deftly executed by the

---

*Haley, J.: Problem-solving therapy: new strategies for effective family therapy, San Francisco, 1976, Jossey-Bass, Inc., p. 110.

heroine of Chapter 1, Joan Locksley, along with her mother and grand-mother.

Haley feels that this same sequence can present itself in a family with-out a grandparent—one in which there is a single parent and many children. In such families, often one child, usually the oldest, is designated a "parent-child," that is, a parent figure to the younger children. This child, like the mother in the previous example, often finds himself tem-porarily in charge of others, only to be labeled as irresponsible and in-competent; the above sequence then asserts itself and repeats.

Two-generation conflicts also produce recognizable and symptomatic sequences; the most common involves one parent in coalition with a child against the other parent. This sequence is as follows:

1. One parent, usually the mother, is in an intense relationship with the child. By intense is meant a relationship that is both positive and negative and where the responses of each person are exaggeratedly important. The mother attempts to deal with the child with a mix-ture of affection and exasperation.
2. The child's symptomatic behavior becomes more extreme.
3. The mother, or the child, calls on the father for assistance in resolv-ing their difficulty.
4. The father steps in to take charge and deal with the child.
5. Mother reacts against father, insisting that he is not dealing with the situation properly. Mother can react with an attack or a threat to break off the relationship with father. The threat to leave may be as indirect as "I want a vacation by myself," or as direct as "I want a di-vorce."
6. Father withdraws, giving up the attempt to disengage mother and child.
7. Mother and child deal with each other in a mixture of affection and exasperation until they reach a point where they are at an impasse.*

For Haley, family therapy in any of these situations involves the abil-ity to change the sequences, once identified. Therapy of this sort is best done in stages, he maintains. The therapist combines his observations of the family's hierarchy and repetitive sequences and then devises strate-gies for bringing about change. His goal is to change a sequence by pre-venting coalition across generational lines. When these coalitions are prevented, the family is required to function differently.

---

*Haley, J.: Problem-solving therapy: new strategies for effective family therapy, San Francisco, 1976, Jossey-Bass, Inc., p. 115.

A RETURN TO THE MALONEY FAMILY

We have mentioned that the earlier summarized counseling work with Jennifer Maloney and her family represents a blending of the approaches suggested by both Minuchin and Haley. Minuchin's influence in that case has already been commented on. Regarding Haley's view, the Maloneys are easily recognized as a prototype of the family he describes as having a "two-generation conflict," that is, an overintense parent-child dyad that alternately includes and excludes the other parent. In this instance Haley suggests that a therapist may initiate changes in the family sequence by either using the peripheral person (entering through the father-child relationship), breaking up the dyad with a task (entering through the mother-child relationship), or entering directly through the parents with a focus on their relationship. Jennifer's pediatrician chose the first, using the peripheral person, in this case Mr. Maloney. He used him by suggesting that Mr. Maloney enter the nightime scene, handling Jennifer's "night terrors" and thus providing his wife with a rest. Mr. Maloney had indeed tried to deal with Jennifer previously and had met with opposition from his wife, she proclaiming that he didn't "understand the child." He in turn had often criticized Mrs. Maloney for her overprotection, reinforcing in her eyes the belief that he could not possibly have the sensitivity to understand the situation. Activating the father once again by the therapist therefore required careful thought so that mother would not be antagonized. She could not be made to feel, for instance, that Mr. Maloney was being brought in because she had failed. In order that Mrs. Maloney accept her husband's participation, the doctor did several things:

1. He validated her efforts to date.
2. He sympathized with her exhaustion.
3. He supported her key position in the suggested task—only her husband could teach her daughter respect for men, but only she could provide the opportunity for that to take place between them.
4. He appealed to her sense of good mothering by asking her cooperation in having her daughter learn one of life's essential lessons, respect for men.

The pediatrician, the task, and the family were, as reported, successful in producing a decided change in this family's sequence. Jennifer and her parents ultimately passed through three stages with the therapist before sessions were terminated ten interviews later:

1. Stage one: coalition among therapist, peripheral person, and child
2. Stage two: involvement between therapist and adults, without child
3. Stage three: disengagement of the therapist from the adults and from the family

Haley notes that these stages are required in most instances of problem-solving therapy. The process of change cannot be made in one leap.

With regard to the Maloney family, stage one was extensively discussed in the summary of their treatment; that is, Jennifer, Mr. Maloney, and the doctor became involved in an activity, while Mrs. Maloney was gently shifted to the periphery. The second stage involved mother, father, and pediatrician while Jennifer dropped out of the adult struggle and was free to pursue life with her peers. This was not elaborately discussed in the earlier description. The reader is aware that Jennifer was dropped from sessions after the initial interview; that was one indication of stage two. But stage two also included four or five sessions devoted to husband-wife discussions of their marital relationship and how each could derive more satisfaction in that relationship. Their increasing satisfaction with one another led logically to stage three, when the doctor could disengage from the couple, leaving them involved with each other and with the feeling that they no longer needed the pediatrician's help. Jennifer continued to develop relationships with her friends.

REFERENCES

1. Haley, J.: Strategies of psychotherapy, New York, 1963, Grune & Stratton, Inc.
2. Haley, J.: Advanced techniques of hypnosis and therapy: selected papers of Milton H. Erickson, M.D., New York, 1967, Grune & Stratton, Inc.
3. Haley, J.: Uncommon therapy: the psychiatric techniques of Milton H. Erickson, M.D., New York, 1973, W. W. Norton & Company, Inc.
4. Haley, J.: Problem-solving therapy: new strategies for effective family therapy, San Francisco, 1976, Jossey-Bass, Inc., Publishers.
5. Minuchin, S.: Families and family therapy, Cambridge, Mass., 1974, Harvard University Press.
6. Minuchin, S., and others: Families of the slums: an exploration of their structure and treatment, New York, 1967, Basic Books, Inc., Publishers.
7. Minuchin, S., and others: Psychosomatic families: anorexia nervosa in context, Cambridge, Mass., 1976, Harvard University Press.
8. Rosman, B., and others: A family approach to anorexia nervosa: study, treatment, and outcome. In Vigersky, R., editor: Anorexia nervosa, New York, 1977, Raven Press.

CHAPTER 4

Gestalt therapy and the family

THE WHEELER FAMILY

Kevin Wheeler had been described by everyone, including his parents, as a "hellacious 8-year-old." Complaints that he was destructive, willful, and arrogant, together with the fact that he had recently set two grass fires at home, resulted in several visits to the pediatrician for him and his parents. It had become clear in these interviews that mother felt thwarted in her efforts to set some limits with Kevin by the laissez-faire attitude of her husband. In the third session father was speaking:

Father: You're too hard on the boy, Ethel. I don't think parents have a right to act like prison wardens with their kids. It just isn't right. That's how you are with Kevin, I know you don't agree with me, but . . .

Mother: You're right, Gary. I don't. The boy almost burned down our garage . . . I think . . .

Kevin sat glumly on the sidelines, kicking his toe into the carpet, saying nothing during this interchange. The pediatrician was about to hear for the eighth time in three sessions that the parents could not agree on a course of action for Kevin's recent spate of fire-setting. The boy's behavior did sound worrisome. The doctor wondered silently what was preventing Mr. Wheeler from seeing the danger and responding appropriately.

Doctor: How did that dimension go with your own parents, Mr. Wheeler?
Father: What do you mean?
Doctor: Were you treated fairly as a kid as you look back?
Father: Oh boy, let's not get into that one!
Doctor: What's your objection?

80

Father:	I don't even like to think about my own parents.
Doctor:	Again, what's your objection?
Father:	(angrily) My mother and father should never have had children in the first place! It's just that simple. They didn't understand the first thing about kids. They never did.
Doctor:	And what price did you pay for that?
Father:	Well, I left home at 17 and didn't return for 20 years, for one thing.
Doctor:	What else?
Father:	Isn't that enough? I cut myself off from my own flesh and blood because I couldn't stand what they were doing to me. I don't even think about it anymore. I think we need to get back to Kevin.
Doctor:	I agree. And I want to do it this way . . . which of your parents do you feel was most unfair in his or her treatment of you?
Father:	Huh? . . . Well, both . . . I don't know.
Doctor:	Pick one of the two.
Father:	My mother, I guess.
Doctor:	All right. Now I am going to ask you to do something somewhat unusual (pushing an extra chair into position facing the father). First, I want you to assume that your mother is sitting in this chair. Next, I want you to compose a mental picture of her sitting right there in front of you. Get the image in your brain.
Father:	This is silly.
Doctor:	I still want you to do it. Describe out loud the woman you see facing you.
Father:	(after some additional balking) Now, or when?
Doctor:	Pick a time in your life when the "unfairness" was particularly intolerable for you.
Father:	That's easy . . . When I was 16. That was when I decided I would have to run away.
Doctor:	Describe your mother, now sitting in front of you as she looked at that time.
Father:	Well, she had short hair, I guess it was still brown, not gray yet . . . and . . .
Doctor:	One more thing. I want you to describe her in the present tense, even though it was actually many years ago that she looked this way. Describe her as if she is sitting right *now* opposite you.
Father:	Well, she was . . .
Doctor:	Use the present tense. "She is . . ."
Father:	Right. She is wearing a . . .

Mr. Wheeler was able to formulate aloud a present-tense description of his mother.

Doctor: Good. Now I would like you to have a conversation with your mother who is sitting in that chair.

Father: You mean right here?

Doctor: Yep.

Father: This is stupid.

Doctor: Do it anyway.

Father: I don't have anything to say to *her.*

Doctor: Then tell her just that.

Father: She wouldn't listen. She never did.

Doctor: Then this is your chance.

Father: Well, it's not like the real thing.

Doctor: Do it anyway.

Father: Where do I start?

Doctor: Wherever you choose.

Mr. Wheeler was silent for a long time, during which he looked uncomfortably at his son and wife, then at his shoes. He was obviously searching for a way to initiate the conversation and silently making beginnings in his head.

Doctor: Say your silent thoughts out loud.

Father: I was just thinking . . .

Doctor: Don't tell me. Tell her (pointing to the empty chair).

Father: (turning to the chair) I was just thinking.

Doctor: I *am* just thinking . . .

Father: I am just thinking how I never had . . . never *have* a serious discussion with you because I have no hope of your listening.

Doctor: Go on.

Father: And now that I have your attention . . . I don't even know where to begin. I'm not sure what I want to say to you.

Doctor: (says nothing)

Father: . . . except . . . I am a human being, dammit. Yes, I'm a kid, but I'm a human being. I'm not a thing. I have feelings. Why can't you just once see my side . . . or even admit that there's a kid's side! Why can't you just once in your life be fair and treat me like what I think and what I want is important . . . not necessarily right, but important.

Doctor: Tell your mother specifically how she treats you as unimportant.

Father: (now needing no help from the doctor) I'm coming to that. You won't even let me attend my ninth grade graduation! Why can't you see how important this is to me? I don't care about your damn rule about being out of the house after dark. Just this once I ought to be allowed . . . to go to my own graduation!

Doctor: How would your mother respond?
Father: She'd say something like . . .
Doctor: Say it as she would, using her tone of voice and inflection.
Father: "You always exaggerate everything . . . . Besides parents *make* the
rules; kids follow them. That's the way it is in our house."

In this example the pediatrician was in the process of helping Mr.
Wheeler face an unfinished business from his own past, an unfinished
business that the pediatrician thought now stood in Mr. Wheeler's way of
effective parenting with his own son. The doctor surmised that the lack
of "fair treatment" by Mr. Wheeler's parents may have affected and dis-
torted his current limit-setting approaches with Kevin. The doctor's
hypothesis that this was the case and the strategies he chose for helping
the father and the family in this area were taken from the writings of Dr.
Frederick (Fritz) Perls and from the body of knowledge and thought
now generally called Gestalt therapy. We have found the principles of
Gestalt therapy useful in our pediatric work, especially when family
issues seem to be connected to more than interactional difficulties, that
is, when intrapsychic or individual dilemmas seem to be significant
obstacles to the resolution of family conflict and stress.

FREDERICK PERLS AND THE DEVELOPMENT
OF GESTALT THERAPY

Gestalt therapy seemed to spring from the tumult of the 1960's. At
that time it was generally associated with the simultaneous development
of the "human potential movement" in American psychiatry, a movement in evidence initially on the West Coast and centered at the Esalen
Institute at Big Sur, California. It is true that Perls was in residence at
Big Sur for several years during that time, working not only there but
also extensively throughout the San Francisco Bay Area. It is also true
that he was essentially responsible for the development of the basic principles underlying Gestalt therapy. However, his work in this psychological area antedated the establishment of the Esalen Institute by more than
a few years. He began writing on the subject during World War II; his
first book, *Ego, Hunger, and Aggression,*[2] was written in 1942 while he was
living in South Africa. In later years, after he came to the United States
and had emerged as a well-recognized innovator in the field of psychological thought, two other books appeared: *Gestalt Therapy Verbatim*[3] and
an autobiography, *In and Out of the Garbage Pail.*[4] A fourth volume con-
taining some of his previously unpublished writings appeared shortly

after Perls's death. This last book is entitled *The Gestalt Approach: Eyewitness to Therapy.*[5] *Gestalt Therapy Verbatim,* however, provides the most complete description of Perls's own views. Our summary, which follows, is derived principally from that source.

The persistence of an unfinished gestalt

Perls's education and early professional experiences brought him in contact with the ideas of Gestalt psychology and existentialism in the first quarter of the century. These ideas were then being developed by a group of German psychologists. One of their tenets that interested the young physician-psychoanalyst was that man did not seem to perceive stimuli as unrelated isolates. Rather he would organize them during the perceptual process into meaningful wholes, into something more than the sum of the individual components. For example, they observed that a man coming into a room full of people would perceive the room and the people in it as a unit, that is, as a gestalt. Within that unit, one element selected from the many present would stand out, while the others would recede into the background. The choice of which element would stand out was made as a result of the man's interest. As long as there was interest, the whole scene appeared to be organized in a meaningful way for that individual. Perls decided that man handles his own behavior in this same way. Bits of behavior are also organized by human beings into meaningful wholes, deriving meaning and prominence in a person's experience and awareness on the basis of interest to that individual. Those aspects of behavior without interest become relegated to background and are eventually discarded as unimportant, without meaning.

In the same way that Gestalt psychologists had become interested in the relationship between the perception of stimuli as figure versus the perception of stimuli as background, Perls too became fascinated by figure-ground relationships, but in terms of human behavior, not just perception. He noticed that certain experiences tend to remain as foreground for individuals while others recede, at least temporarily, into the background. Generally the experiences that remain as foreground are those with interest and meaning, especially those that are considered incomplete or unfinished experiences. It is the incompleteness, he felt, that invests an issue with dominance and foreground status, since these experiences are those that an individual continues to confront, attempting to close, complete, and resolve. Perls maintained that although all human beings experience innumerable, simultaneous physiological and social needs, they can respond to only one such need at a time. Hence man develops a hierarchy of values, attending to the one dominant need at a particular time that is perceived as essential for survival. Man then strives through his behavior to satisfy that specific dominant need, to "close the gestalt," before moving on to other behavior.

Thus an incomplete gestalt, an unfinished business, will push repeatedly to the forefront of an individual's behavior, pressing for completion and closure and sometimes producing symptomatic behavior. For instance, Mr. Wheeler, in the introductory clinical example of this chapter, had never satisfactorily completed an important unfinished business with his own parents regarding their treatment of him as a child. That unfinished business was continuing to emerge in his behavior years later and now threatened his effectiveness as a parent with his own son.

Environmental support versus self-support

All life and all behavior are governed by a process of homeostasis. This term, by now familiar to the reader, is shared by all the major theorists whom we describe in this book, including Perls. Homeostasis is a fundamental concept for deriving an understanding of human behavior, whether one is talking about communication, family structure, sequence, or an unfinished gestalt, although in each instance the term may have a slightly different connotation. In Gestalt therapy, homeostasis is the process by which man satisfies his needs and maintains his equilibrium with his environment. Both psychological and physiological needs are constantly and simultaneously present. Since only one need can be satisfied at a time, an individual establishes a hierarchy of values, attending to what he perceives as the dominant need facing him. Thus the dominant need of the individual becomes the foreground figure, while other needs recede, at least temporarily, into the background. As the dominant need (unfinished business) is satisfied, it too recedes and is replaced by one that is considered next important. All life is characterized by this balancing process within a hierarchy of needs between man and his environment. For satisfaction of needs or resolution of an unfinished business to occur, an individual must be able to (1) sense just what he needs for completion of the unfinished business and (2) know how to manipulate himself and his environment so that completion takes place. Needs can only be satisfied, according to Perls, through this homeostatic interaction between an individual and his environment.

A premise of Gestalt therapy is that no individual is self-sufficient; he exists always in an environmental field. Therefore the nature of a man's relationship between himself and his environment becomes an important phenomenon. Essentially, what takes place at this interface — the contact boundary — between an individual and his environment will determine his behavior. In many ways Gestalt therapy is a study of man's activity at that contact boundary. An individual reaches out toward the world through two systems, the sensory system and the motor system. The sensory system provides an orientation; the motor system furnishes a means of action. These concepts are important for understanding symptomatic behavior. If, for instance, an individual is unable to sense his dominant needs or to act on his environment in such a way that his needs are satisfied, that individual may behave in a disorganized and ineffective way. Perls referred to this disorganized, ineffective behavior as "immature."

The converse, "mature," or maturation, Perls defined as the process of transformation from environmental support to self-support. This concept is a familiar one to the authors, reaffirming the writing of Dr. Frederick Allen, one of the early influences on our clinical approaches.[1] Allen maintained that a child's behavior most often reflected that child's striving for "growth toward independence." Hence this aspect of Perls's work has seemed a logical extension of Allen's previously articulated "growth" model for understanding a child's behavior. Perls, like Allen, postulated that during childhood and the process of maturation, there are basically two choices. A child either learns to use his own abilities to overcome frustration (self-support) or he learns to be "spoiled" (environmental support). He may learn to be spoiled as the result of a number of circumstances. His parents may persistently and too readily answer all his questions, whether correctly or incorrectly. His parents may anticipate all his needs, providing satisfaction for every voiced desire, perhaps because "this was never done for me as a child; my own children will not suffer as I did." Or perhaps his parents may simply not know how to use frustration positively or may not understand that frustration (that is, allowing a child to delay gratification) does serve a useful function in the promotion of growth and maturity. Without frustration there is no experience with facing an unmet need, no reason to mobilize one's resources and to discover that one can do something on one's own. Of course frustration, always an uncomfortable experience, is understandably avoided if possible by every young child. In the Wheeler family, the child's environment conspired with the boy to make it too possible, too easy, to avoid frustration (setting limits on his impulsiveness) most of the time. He was supported in his acting-out, fire-setting behavior because of Mr. Wheeler's unresolved conflicts with his own parents. The result of this consistent avoidance of frustration was that Kevin had learned to use his growth potential for manipulation and controlling his environment (adults) rather than for learning to develop the means of satisfying his own needs and controlling his own behaviors. Instead of mobilizing resources for managing himself, Kevin was creating a dependency on others, looking to others to control his impulses, rather than to himself. It is a childhood lesson that eventually could become an accustomed style of relating for him, even as an adult. Such an individual learns to manipulate his environment for the support and control that he is unable to muster from within himself for himself.

How does such a child, and later the same person as an adult, manipulate his environment? Perls said there are many ways. An individual can demand directional support and manipulate by questions (for example, "What do you think I should do?"). He may play the role of "crybaby" if he doesn't get his way. He may pretend to comply and bribe the adult. Or he may above all play stupid or helpless (for example, "I can't help myself. Poor me. I am so impulsive. You have to help me, you are so wise; I'm sure you can help me.") Each time this individual "plays" helpless, he creates a dependency. He then may crave praise and validation from everyone, making everyone his judge. In the long run he manipulates not only his environment but himself, conning both into believing that he is helpless and unable. He behaves with his world as though he lacks one of the essential qualities that promotes survival: self-support. Problems may arise for an individual lacking this quality. Such an individual cannot see his own survival needs clearly and therefore cannot meet them. This person may be unable to establish any sort of equilibrium between his personal needs and the demands of his society.

As the process continues, the individual's means of manipulation become elaborate. He can talk, sulk, promise, break promises, be subservient, sabotage, play deaf, forget, lie, move others to tears, irritate, flatter, or wound. He can particularly manipulate with questions; Perls states that questions are one of the immature individual's main tools for not coming to grips with his own problems. He seeks answers in someone else rather than in himself.

Since the environment can never provide such an individual with enough unfailing support all of the time, the immature person comes to feel that the environment is hostile and not to be trusted. He develops a hypersensitivity to his world and is always ready to outguess, outfeel, and outwit others. He dreads rejection and disapproval from his environment, so he may put on the appearance of one who is "good, submissive, and compliant" in the hope that others will be even more supportive and nurturing. Since his self-concept provides him with essentially none of his support, he expects little from himself or his own resources. Rather he engages in self-nagging, self-disapproval, and a squashing of genuine self-expression. In the process he exhausts not only himself but also the resources of the environment for provision of support. He has projected onto others what should be his own means of self-support to such a degree that a pat on the back is absolutely necessary and very welcome, but it is never enough. He is unable to assimilate praise, remaining dissatisfied with whatever external validation he does receive. When the environment withdraws, concluding that the individual is insatiable and unpleasable, it is a confirmation of the immature person's view that the environment is not to be trusted. He then steps up his efforts to find need satisfaction from some other element of the environment, perhaps as yet untapped. And the cycle begins again.

The individual who has adopted environmental support as a way of life without developing significant elements of self-support in his behavior is, as the preceding suggests, constantly struggling and warring with some aspect of his environment. In the course of this struggle he will develop one or more specific defenses to protect himself, according to Perls. These defenses are introjection, projection, confluence, and retroflection.

Introjection

During the growth and maturation of an individual, he comes to accept or reject what his environment offers. Growth will occur if, in the process of taking, the individual digests and assimilates. This is literally true (physical growth depends on the digestion and assimilation of foodstuffs from the environment) and figuratively accurate as well (emotional and intellectual growth depends on the selective assimilation of thoughts, attitudes, and feelings present in a person's environment). Thus the psychological process of assimilating is very much the same as its physiological counterpart. Concepts, facts, standards of behavior, morality, and ethical, esthetic, or political values — all these come to the individual originally from his environment. They must be digested, altered, and absorbed if they are to become truly the individual's own, a part of his personality. If a person instead accepts them entirely and uncritically — swallowing them whole — they become undigested attitudes, ways of acting and feeling; such undigested bits of behavior and thought Perls referred to as "introjects." Introjection is the mechanism whereby an individual incorporates into himself standards, attitudes, ways of acting and thinking that are not truly his. When the introjector says, "I think," he often means instead, "they think."

Projection

Projection is the tendency for an individual to hold the environment responsible for something that actually originates within himself. Such an individual seems unable to bear the responsibility for his own wishes, feelings, and desires, attaching them instead to objects or people in his environment. This individual makes assumptions based on his own fantasies and hunches; he fails to recognize that they are only assumptions.

Utilization of this defense causes a person not only to disown his own impulses but also to disown parts of himself. In a sense he gives these disowned parts an objective existence outside himself so that he can make them responsible for his troubles without facing the fact they are actually a part of himself. As a result, the projector becomes a passive object, the victim of circumstances or other people rather than an active participant and shaper in the business of his own life.

Confluence

We have already mentioned the contact boundary, that interface between an individual and his environment. When a person comes to feel that no boundary exists between himself and his world, when he feels that both are one, he has succumbed to confluence. This defense can have serious consequences, not only for the individual but also for those around him. For with confluence, the individual demands likeness and refuses to tolerate differences. Parents in this predicament often insist that their children are merely extensions of themselves. Such parents do not tolerate the fact that their children may be unlike them in significant ways. When the children dare to confront such parents with obvious differences, they are often met with parental rejection and alienation. An individual utilizing confluence is very fond of the pronoun "we." Unfortunately one is never certain just who is included in that collective pronoun, since the individual has lost his sense of boundary vis-à-vis others.

Retroflection

Retroflection, the fourth defense mechanism mentioned by Perls, refers to "turning back sharply against." Essentially an individual using retroflection does to himself what he would like to do to others. This is contrasted with the previous three defenses already described: (1) the introjector does as others would like him to do, (2) the projector does unto others what he accuses them of doing to him, and (3) the confluent individual doesn't know who is doing what to whom.

•   •   •

How do these four mechanisms manifest themselves clinically? Introjection shows itself in the use of the pronoun "I" when the actual meaning is "they." Projection displays itself in the pronoun "it" or "they" when the real meaning is "I." Confluence, as already mentioned, is characterized by the use of the pronoun "we" when the correct pronoun is in question. Retroflection is shown by the use of the reflective "myself," as in "I have to force myself to do this job," as though the individual and himself are two different people.

These four defenses are generally adopted by an individual who is experiencing difficulty balancing his needs and his interactions with his environment. This difficulty may arise in the first place because of the continuing presence of unfinished business from his past. Such unfinished business has a way of freezing an individual to an outmoded way of behaving in certain situations, rendering him incapable of facing problems and meeting needs in the present. He will then be unable to find a homeostatic balance between satisfaction of his own needs and his environment. He may begin to feel overwhelmed by either one or the other, or both. The above defenses are then developed and utilized by the individual as a protection against this threat of feeling overwhelmed.

Implications in clinical situations

The reader may well ask what these principles have to do with either clinical pediatrics or pediatric family interviewing. One of the stated aims of Gestalt therapy, developed out of the foregoing principles by Perls, is to promote growth (maturation) and develop human potential. Pediatrics is also very concerned with growth and the development of maturation. Maturation in Gestalt therapy terms, as already stated, is the process whereby an individual learns to shift from environmental support to self-support. Gestalt therapy seeks to facilitate the discovery by an individual that he can do many things, much more than he had previously believed.

In the course of family interviewing with pediatric patients and their families, regardless of the presenting problem, we have often been struck by the observation that one or more individuals in a family is relying on the environment for his support rather than behaving in a self-responsible fashion and using his own resources for satisfying his needs. This dependence on environmental support by an individual frequently has a direct bearing on the whole family's behavior and style, and it may even be contributing to the persistence of the child's particular presenting symptom. For instance, one family member may persist in dwelling on past history, refusing to let go of old resentments, irritations, fears, and so on that represent unfinished business from the past, to the continuing frustration of everyone else in the family. Or a family member may repeatedly avoid taking responsibility for his own behavior, blaming either others or himself for his "inability to change." As a result, growth of the family in general is prevented. Or a family member may, using a lesson learned in childhood, persistently manipulate others to such an extent that they feel used and exploited and therefore angry and resentful. Or a family member may resist change either in himself or in the family unit because of a reluctance to face imagined, dreaded catastrophic expectations, originally developed long ago and perhaps currently untrue.

In any of these situations, helping a family toward resolution of problems not only may depend on an alteration of family interaction in communication, structure, and sequence but will also require internal shifts within the individual so that he learns to develop his own support, rather than relying on, manipulating, and blaming the environment (family). We have therefore come to utilize some of the principles and techniques of Gestalt therapy for human dilemmas that appear to require intrapsychic attention. Gestalt approaches are called upon for problems located "inside one's skin." The family approaches developed by Satir (communication), Minuchin (structure), and Haley (sequence) are chosen for interactional issues, those localized "outside one's skin," that is, between two or more individuals. Frequently in families both areas are in disarray and in need of the pediatrician's attention.

Application of Gestalt therapy principles

The essence of Gestalt therapy has been said to lie in two adverbs: "now" and "how." *Now* covers all that exists at the moment, in the present tense. The past is no more; the future is not yet. A patient in Gestalt therapy work is encouraged to stay in the present, to become aware of his thoughts, actions, feelings *now*, as they are presently affecting his behavior. Since each of us carries around considerable unfinished business from earlier years and childhood, staying in the present can be extremely difficult. This was demonstrated by Mr. Wheeler's behavior at the start of this chapter. As noted, an incomplete gestalt from the past was interfering with his present behavior and influencing his son's behavior as well. Even here, the doctor simulated a shifting of the problem into the present, encouraging Mr. Wheeler to confront his mother *now*, in the present, with that old unfinished business of years ago. A Gestalt therapist listens carefully to the tenses of verbs used by patients and encourages them to express past events, feelings, and ideas in the present tense. Patients are urged to deal with their problems in the "here and now." For instance:

> *Father:* (describing his desertion as a child by his own father) He just left. That's all. And he promised me, I remember that, he promised me that he would come back. I didn't forgive him for that.
>
> *Doctor:* You *don't* forgive him for that?
>
> *Father:* What's that? . . . Yes, you're right. I still don't forgive him for that.
>
> *Doctor:* Tell him that directly. Put him in front of you and talk to him about that.
>
> *Father:* You mean right here?
>
> *Doctor:* Sure.
>
> *Father:* I can't. That was 25 years ago.
>
> *Doctor:* I know. That's OK. Do it anyway. Right now.
>
> *Father:* I can't.

Here the doctor noticed that the father was avoiding self-responsibility in another sphere. He was playing helpless by saying and assuming that "I can't." The doctor challenged this assumption.

> *Doctor:* Change that to, "I won't."
>
> *Father:* Huh?
>
> *Doctor:* "I won't confront my father."
>
> *Father:* (silence) I won't confront my father?
>
> *Doctor:* Well, it's your choice whether you do or not. But don't tell me that you can't.
>
> *Father:* I know I *can* . . .
>
> *Doctor:* Whether you do or not is up to you.
>
> *Father:* Well, what would he say if I did?

Again the doctor notices the patient's tendency to "play helpless," this time through questions.

Doctor: Don't ask me. Do it here and see how it goes.

Father: (to himself) Well, why not? . . . I never have forgiven you for lying to me. I don't think I ever will.

Several Gestalt therapy strategies were being implemented by the physician here. First of all the patient was being encouraged to view a past problem in the present, to bring it out of the past and into the present so that the situation was available for resolution now. He was also being encouraged to be self-responsible as he approached the issue; his tendency to be helpless and ask questions was discouraged and frustrated so that a view of himself as independent and capable of his own problem-solving was repeatedly introduced. He was not allowed to manipulate the listener through "helplessness" as he had been accustomed to doing very successfully over the years. He was experiencing one very slight shift in his usual total reliance on environmental support as opposed to self-support.

While these strategies are basic to Gestalt therapy approaches, they are not unique to this view. Both Minuchin and Satir also emphasize the importance of helping patients stay in the present, and they, too, promote direct confrontations and communication, discouraging a patient in his efforts to "talk about" or describe. Active, experiential work is to be preferred.

Another important area of agreement exists among Perls and the other theorists summarized in this book. All agree that use of the pronoun "I" is an extremely important concept. It is the hallmark of one's ability to take responsibility for one's thoughts, feelings, and actions. A persistent avoidance of the pronoun "I" calls for an intervention by the physician. To illustrate:

Mother: Men just never understand women!

Doctor: What men, what women? I need you to personalize that.

Mother: I mean, men just never seem to figure what women need, that's all.

Doctor: Do you include yourself in there somewhere?

Mother: Well, of course . . . I'm a woman.

Doctor: Then make it a statement about yourself, not women.

Mother: But I think it's true of all women.

Doctor: At the moment I am not concerned about all women. I am concerned about you. Say it about yourself.

Mother: Oh, all right. Men never seem to know what I need.

Doctor: Good. Now which men?

Mother: (looking down at her feet) Most men.

> *Doctor:*   Are you including me in most men? If so, I would like you to tell me directly.
>
> *Mother:*   No . . . actually it's not you so much . . . I mean Harry (indicating her husband).
>
> *Doctor:*   Harry is right here. Tell him directly.
>
> *Mother:*   (after hesitation) Harry, you never understand . . . me.
>
> *Father:*   (angrily) What are you talking about?
>
> *Doctor:*   I would like you, Helen, to tell Harry what you want from him in this regard. One rule: start your sentence with "I."

After continuous spadework by the doctor and many false starts, Mother finally said:

> *Mother:*   I would like you to say that you care about me.

This interchange revolved almost entirely around the mother's avoidance of the pronoun "I." Such avoidance not only signaled her reluctance to take responsibility for her own wants, it also played havoc with the communication process taking place between Harry and Helen.

Gestalt therapy with its emphasis on "now" tends to be an experiential therapy, that is, the individual is encouraged to experience as much of himself as possible in the here and now. Since past unfinished business continually gets in the way, it may be difficult for him to participate fully in the present. Nonetheless the patient is asked to turn all his attention to what he is doing at the present, during the course of the session — right here and now. He is asked to become aware of gestures, breathing, facial expressions, tone of voice, and so on as he struggles with mastery of situations in the present. Returning to the preceding example, the doctor noted that the patient was tensely wringing her hands and trembling as she said to her husband, "I would like you to say that you care about me."

> *Doctor:*   I want you to pay attention to what you are experiencing at this very moment, Helen.
>
> *Mother:*   Very tense. I'm very tense . . . it's silly; I almost feel afraid.
>
> *Doctor:*   Look at your husband. (She does.) Do you see anything that frightens you?
>
> *Mother:*   No. In fact he's listening to me . . . for once. That's nice. Then why . . . why am I frightened?
>
> *Doctor:*   (suggesting that Helen take responsibility for her own feeling) Not why, but how . . . how are you frightening yourself?
>
> *Mother:*   I don't know.

The doctor assumed at this point that since, according to the patient, there seemed to be little in the present situation to frighten her, perhaps

Helen was introducing a past fear (an unfinished business from another time, another encounter) into the current interchange. He decided to test this and said:

> *Doctor:*   Pick someone else in your life to whom saying that sentence would be very risky.
> *Mother:*   What sentence?
> *Doctor:*   "I would like you to say that you care about me."
> *Mother:*   (beginning to have tears) My grandfather.

Thus the doctor was suggesting that old unfinished business be brought into the light of the present for examination and resolution. He had also furnished an example of an additional Gestalt therapy strategy. Rather than bombarding the patient with "why" questions and allowing the patient herself to act helpless through "why" questions to others, he chose instead to question her, "how?" "How are you frightening yourself?" The question so worded could offer a different route of inquiry than the more traditional, "Why are you frightened?" The latter would suggest first of all that it was being done to the patient by some force outside her, permitting a continuing avoidance of self-responsibility, and second, the doctor's answering the "why" question would only furnish a cause, a reason. The patient would not necessarily be any further along in either altering her behavior or taking charge of herself. On the other hand, the question, "How are you frightening yourself?" could communicate two important ideas to the patient: first of all that she was producing the feeling herself, that she was responsible for it and had some control over the behavior; she was not the victim or passive recipient of the feeling from elsewhere. Second, "how" in the question implied that a process was underway. Such a process, under the patient's control, was potentially amenable to alteration and change if she chose. One can't really change a reason, which is the usual response to "why" (for example, something happened because . . .). However, processes (for example, how is the patient contributing to the behavior) are dynamic and fluid; they can be shifted and modified by the patient.

The impasse

In the two immediately preceding clinical examples the patients were approaching what Perls called "the impasse," that place in the patient's life and experience where he feels stuck and immobilized and beyond which he feels emotional and perhaps literal survival is not possible. This impasse takes form originally when as a child the individual cannot get the support that he requires from the environment, nor is he yet able to provide his own support. At this point, this moment of impasse, the child begins to mobilize and manipulate the environment in an effort to get what is deemed necessary. From that situation, always experienced as unpleasant, unfinished, and frightening, certain attitudes and behavioral patterns arise, so that in later years when a similar situation presents itself, the patient tends to behave in the same manner as when first confronted with an inability to have his needs met either by the environment or by himself. He reacts in these subsequent times with helplessness, manipulation, fear, confusion, panic, and so on. It is as though he is facing the initial experience all over again, as if he were a young, helpless child. Since the situation, the impasse, was never successfully negotiated in the first place, the patient has no reason to believe that he can succeed subsequently. As a matter of fact, the patient facing an impasse has generally constructed elaborate and terrifying catastrophic expectations regarding what might happen if he were to push beyond. These terrible expectations are generally connected to the patient's notion that he is helpless and without the resources necessary to successfully master whatever lies beyond the impasse. Since Gestalt therapy is directed toward maximizing one's own growth and self-support, it is not surprising that clinical work is directed toward helping and directly supporting individuals to face their impasses without running away or avoiding, so that they may experience their own strengths and supports, learning once and for all that they are capable of guarding their own survival. The catastrophic expectations so feared are usually fantasies, fears that the individual has often projected onto the world (for instance, "If I speak up to my father, he will hate me.") and with which he has excused himself from taking current reasonable risks that are part and parcel of growing and living. The impasse then is seen as mostly a matter of fantasy, no matter how it arose originally in childhood. It doesn't exist in reality in the present. A person only *believes* that he does not have his own resources to handle the situation successfully. He uses catastrophic expectations to prevent an experiential confrontation with this imagined "stuck place."

How does one proceed to assist an individual to face and then move beyond his impasse? First, it requires from the physician a combination of sympathy and frustration. With sympathy alone the physician becomes as trapped as the patient, manipulated by that individual's helplessness. With frustration alone, the physician will soon be viewed as just another part of the "hostile environment," about which the patient already knows too much. Hence both sympathy and frustration (for example, not giving answers or solutions, thus helping the patient to use his own resources) must be employed. Especially one must frustrate the patient's attempts to control the interviewer through manipulations. Frustration of this sort will enable the patient to develop self-support. Second, the physician provides the patient with an opportunity to discover just what it is he needs for the development of his own self-support, that is, those missing parts of himself from which he feels alienated, having given them over (through projection) to the world and to the therapist; it is the loss of these disowned parts, incidentally, that has rendered the patient "helpless" in his own view. At such times the doctor provides the direction toward and the situation in which the individual may grow, an opportunity to experience his impasse. During this experience the doctor frustrates (does not give answers) and directs the patient in such a way that he is forced to discover his own possibilities, reown his previously discarded parts of himself, and learn that what he has been expecting from the doctor in terms of help, answers, and solutions, he is just as able to provide for himself. The patient thus learns about his own competence in handling his own growth and survival needs.

For an example, let us return to a previous clinical illustration, the mother, Helen, who was trembling at the thought of saying to her grandfather: "I would like you to say that you care about me."

Doctor: Say some more.

Mother: Oh, this is so dumb. I shouldn't be crying like this. (using self-blame to interrupt herself)

Doctor: Give yourself permission for your tears, and continue.

Mother: Oh . . . Oh, I don't even know what I meant to say to my grandfather. I don't know why I picked on him. . . where was I? (now beginning to interrupt herself with confusion and helplessness, often a reliable sign that an individual is approaching an area of impasse)

Doctor: (remains silent)

Mother: Isn't there some way . . . I'm not sure that he . . . Oh, I just get all confused when I cry.

Doctor: Then say out loud, "I use my tears to confuse myself."

Mother: No . . . no. (Her crying ceases.)

Doctor: I certainly can't force you to. (long silence) What would you need, do you suppose, to feel more comfortable in speaking directly to your grandfather?

> *Mother:* Oh, you would have to know him, Doctor. He was something!
> *Doctor:* Describe him to me.
> *Mother:* Well, he was . . .
> *Doctor:* Close your eyes and describe him in the present tense.

She does so.

> *Doctor:* What are you experiencing at this moment as you picture him?
> *Mother:* (silently shakes her head and begins to sob)
> *Doctor:* (gently) I assure you, Helen . . . it is safe in this room to tell him what you are feeling at this moment.
> *Mother:* I . . . I am so sorry, Gramp. Why can't we talk, ever? Just once even. Just once if you could say that you even care whether I live or die. I can't help it that Momma died . . . and I feel that you blame me for that.

Now sobbing heavily the patient continued to "speak to" her grandfather, stating that she had always sensed that he blamed her for the death of his daughter, her mother, from measles encephalitis, contracted following a light case of the same disease in Helen herself at age 6. Helen spent her growing-up years in the grandfather's household, walking on eggs, plagued by her own assumption that he blamed her for the death, and yearning for some refutation of that worry through a caring message from her grandfather. A closed individual regarding feelings, he never committed himself one way or another on the issue; it was never discussed, and Helen was terrified of asking directly about his caring for her, certain that her awesome worst fear would be confirmed in his answer, that she would be openly blamed and then rejected.

> *Doctor:* Now, I want you to say your opening sentence to him here, now.
> *Mother:* What was it? . . . Oh, I need you to say that you care about me. I do. I really do. (She is no longer avoiding. She is actively confronting the image of her grandfather.)
> *Doctor:* All right. Now, Helen, I want you to get up out of your chair and move over into the chair where you have placed your grandfather. I want you for a moment to be your grandfather and to respond to the child, Helen, who has just spoken to you.

As this sounded somewhat outlandish, there was some temporary balking, handled by gentle persistence on the doctor's part. Eventually Helen seated herself in the opposite chair.

> *Doctor:* (speaking as if to grandfather) Helen has just told you that she needs you to say that you care about her. Respond to that.

Mother: I don't know what he would say.
Doctor: Don't tell me. Be your grandfather and speak to Helen.
Mother: I don't know what to say, Helen.

The pediatrician then encouraged mother to move back and forth between the two chairs, literally playing both parts of the dialogue, first herself, then her grandfather, as the theme of verbalizing caring messages was discussed. At length, mother in the grandfather's chair said:

Mother: Helen, it's not that I don't love you. Those things are hard for me to say, always have been. (A smile crosses mother's face as she says this.)
Doctor: Now return to your chair. What are you experiencing? Right now?
Mother: It just struck me . . . . I think maybe he did care. He never could tell anyone — not even Grandma — anything about feelings. (She continues to smile.)

The work continued beyond this point, but we will end the excerpt here. With a combination of sympathy and frustration offered by the doctor, Helen was able to persist in facing an impasse from her childhood, reexperience the event in the present, survive it, and move beyond. Later she began slowly in other areas of her life to state her own needs more successfully in relationships with others, particularly her husband, and she became gradually much more efficient in learning to stand on her own two feet, without constant demands for validation from her environment.

Certainly this sort of clinical work with impasse resolution is more than many pediatricians will be undertaking in the course of a clinical practice. However, it should be mentioned that even when a pediatrician is simply employing "practice sessions" in his pediatric counseling (for instance, having a mother practice in the office how she will set limits with her child), he is actually employing some of the techniques of Gestalt therapy mentioned in the preceding illustration on impasse resolution. Indeed we have found many of the strategies and techniques used in this chapter to be easily transferable into many pediatric family interviewing situations. Particularly useful concepts have been:

Now and how
The pronoun "I"
Responsibility for the self
Transformation from environmental support to self-support
Blending of sympathy and frustration

Unfinished business
Closing a gestalt
We recommend their clinical application in pediatrics.

REFERENCES

1. Allen, F., Psychotherapy with children, New York, 1942, W. W. Norton & Company, Inc.
2. Perls, F.: Ego, hunger, and aggression, New York, 1969, Random House, Inc.
3. Perls, F.: Gestalt therapy verbatim, Lafayette, Calif., 1969, Real People Press.
4. Perls, F.: In and out of the garbage pail, Lafayette, Calif., 1969, Real People Press.
5. Perls, F.: The Gestalt approach: eyewitness to therapy, Palo Alto, Calif., 1973, Science and Behavior Books, Inc.

PART II

CLINICAL APPLICATION

CHAPTER 5

Designing the clinical setting for family interviewing

ATTENDANCE ISSUES

In developing a clinical setting for the interview of a family, one faces almost immediately the dilemma of who, inside and even outside the family, should attend the interviews. For years it was assumed that, when it came to behavioral problems in children, fathers were unavailable, uninterested, unwilling, uninvolved, unaware, and uncooperative. At best a father was portrayed as a hard worker, singlehandedly upholding the economy of his family while his unbroken attendance record at work was declared essential to the family's financial well-being. At worst he was pictured as a wild man, an insensitive brute who might slap people around at the mention of behavioral difficulties with his son. There was no point in even suggesting his participation in the interviews at the doctor's office. Justification for his absence was often supplied by the mother. If not by her, no matter; the physician interviewer was so conditioned to view Dad as remote that he anticipated difficulty and poor cooperation from a child's father whether this was in fact actual or imagined. Hence either mother or doctor was equally willing to finish Sentence A with one from Column B:

Sentence A	*Column B*
No, my husband couldn't possibly come in; you see, Doctor	1. He's working — 12 hours a day, 7 days a week.
	2. He hates doctors.
	3. He doesn't feel Percy's self-mutilation is anything to worry about, especially for anyone *outside* the family.

No, my husband couldn't possibly come in; you see, Doctor . . . .

4. He doesn't know I've come in.
5. He and I don't agree on this issue at all.
6. He doesn't speak English.
7. He's really the problem.
8. He and I are getting divorced.
9. He's terminally ill.
10. He refuses to discuss anything with me.
11. He thinks you're a jerk.

Whether these pronouncements were rooted in fact, in mother's desire to tell the story her way without contradiction, or in the physician's unstated discomfort at working with father, is open to debate. In our experience fathers are not nearly as hopeless as we had been led to believe; they appear to have been more victims of bad press than anything else. It seems reasonably clear that attendance at family interviews is a direct function of interviewer expectations. Of course there are instances when a father refuses to participate, when no amount of interviewer persuasion is successful in bringing him in, or when work circumstances make his presence in the interview room impossible, but these times are decidedly infrequent. We expect, our trainees expect, and even our secretaries expect that fathers will attend family interviews. And they do.

Clearly stated expectations by the doctor are not used as a threat with families and fathers. Rather our intention is to communicate the importance of a father's role in his family and the essential contribution of his view and his perspective. We find, as Satir states (p. 5): "Once the therapist convinces the husband that he is essential to the therapy process, and that no one else can speak for him or take his place in therapy *or* in family life, he readily enters in."[2]

We have become considerably more cautious in accepting at face value a mother's vigorous stand — usually on the telephone before the first interview — that her husband won't attend. It has too many times, in retrospect, indicated her own need to control the structuring of the interview, her family, and the interviewer. In these circumstances we usually indicate that we would like to speak to the father directly and that we are quite willing to call him at work or in the evening, at which time our kindly insistence on the need for his input and help with a solution often succeeds in gaining his attendance for at least the initial interview. That, like the first olive out of the jar, is the most difficult. His subsequent participation will depend on the problem and on the therapist's ingenuity at accommodating and utilizing father in a solution of the family's difficulty. Concessions such as late afternoon and evening appointments usually manage the commonly invoked conflicts with work responsibilities. We have utilized these freely; a majority of our family interviews take place after 4 P.M.

Even with a divorced couple, we encourage that both parents attend the initial session, especially if both individuals are geographically available and actively involved in the parenting of their children. The therapist must use his discretion as to the advisability of continuing participation by both ex-spouses in subsequent interviews.

Family therapists argue mightily over what particular children, if any, are to be included in family interviews. Satir begins by seeing parents alone for one or two sessions, to establish what they want from therapy and to shift the focus from the identified patient to the family as a whole. She subsequently includes the children, often determining by age who will become regular participants in ongoing family interviews. Other therapists, believing that children's observed behavioral difficulties basically reflect a marital neurosis, prefer to exclude children from the beginning and to continue work without even seeing them. Still others prefer to work with only the identified patient and parents, bringing in other children as the situation warrants. Our preference, briefly stated earlier, is that both parents and all children attend at least the first interview. Subsequent attendance is influenced by the problem and the circumstances. We agree with Aponte that "those who are asked to attend are those necessary to get the job done."[1]

We ask the entire household to come initially for several reasons. Since a therapist is quite often working to diminish the scapegoating of one family member, the identified patient, he may defeat his own purpose in requesting that only that particular child and the parents come to his office. What other messages can George, age 6, and his parents receive than that he is being singled out for scrutiny and that the physician, just like his parents, sees him as "the problem"? The elimination of scapegoating is made more likely when the interviewer demonstrates through his actions, from the very first contact, his interest in the family as a whole.

Second, if helping a family involves getting a fix on its system, its "mobile," its structure, nothing serves this function better than getting a glimpse of that system in operation with no missing pieces. It should come as no surprise to the reader who has progressed this far that in our view even an "asymptomatic" child serves some purpose in maintaining the family's precarious balance of relationships. It is quite helpful, for instance, to see firsthand that 7-year-old Robbie, unmanageable at home, never has access to his mother because her lap and her energies are taken up by the 3-year-old darling of the family, rosy-cheeked Charlie.

Third, asking all children to attend the first interview occasionally brings some surprises. The Bensons originally asked for help with their 8-year-old daughter, Brenda. Brenda was refusing to attend school. No mention was made of James aside from the fact that he was Brenda's twin brother. Once in the interviewing room, however, James's withdrawal and depression were most apparent and of considerable concern to the interviewer.

If grandparents or other relatives are living at home and appear to be a part of the family's structural apparatus, they too are encouraged to attend the first interview. Some family therapists, particularly the noted Carl Whitaker, place special emphasis on the three-generational aspects of most families. He includes grandparents as often as possible in his work.[5]

It is a logical extension of the family systems notion that therapy with an individual should at times encompass all those important to that person's basic structure of relationships; an individual's "family" is not necessarily limited by bloodlines. This approach, called network therapy, most expertly developed by Speck and Attneave,[3] involves work with that unit designated as the family network and may include upwards of 10 to 20 individuals—those within the family and outside it who are strongly involved in the patient's life situation. Network therapy is not a concept that we have attempted to use ourselves or to teach pediatricians. Our own temerity and need for order has interfered with any suggestions by us to our trainees that they interview such crowds.

TIME AND MONEY ISSUES

Before the reader throws this book aside in an angry display of pique at the ravings of impractical idealists far removed from the workaday world of clinical medicine, let us say that we agree that the ideas and approaches suggested in this text cannot be compressed into a 10-minute visit, which already includes an interval history, reexamination of a 3-year-old's recently treated bilateral otitis media, her refusal to provide a urine specimen, three telephone interruptions, and a message from the office nurse that that 18-month-old admitted to the hospital last night with *Haemophilus influenzae* meningitis is going sour. They cannot be, and do not need to be, squeezed into such a setting.

One of our first rules for trainees entering a family interview is that they must provide for their own comfort during work with the family. We call it "making room for oneself." Unless the interviewer attends to his own needs — and fast — the session disintegrates into at least boredom and at most chaos. This rule applies equally to the physician in a clinical practice setting. His attention to time will be essential for both his comfort and his success in the interview. It may mean that he must redesign his office procedures in certain ways.

Family interviews do take time. Ours are generally 1 hour long, although there is nothing sacrosanct about the 60-minute hour; in some situations 30 minutes works reasonably well, especially with very small children. There have even been situations when 2-hour appointments have clearly facilitated the work a family was doing. It seems to take a certain period of time in each interview for a family to get down to business, even if it's the fifth or the tenth interview and even when the interviewer is diligent in his work. An hour usually allows for this settling-in process. Whatever time period is arbitrarily chosen, however, it must subsequently be protected by the physician and other office staff. We do not accept calls or interruptions, except for emergencies, during the course of a family interview.

We also recognize that time is a precious commodity for the pediatrician. One may be able to make considerable "room for oneself" regarding office time but continue to be decidedly uncomfortable if the office rent is not being paid. Hence we are not suggesting that a doctor see families for 60 minutes and, as many do, charge only for the customary 15-minute follow-up visit. The physician is entitled, and indeed has a responsibility to himself and his staff, to charge for his time, which may mean the equivalent of a bill for four 15-minute appointments. To the often-raised question of whether families will use services so charged, the answer is an overwhelming yes, both from our experience and from that of our pediatric trainee graduates who have subsequently entered clinical practices. Specific settings in which pediatricians have successfully utilized family interviews with a fee-for-service billing system have included university medical center outpatient clinics, private solo pediatric practices, small group pediatric practices, large prepaid health care facilities, state-supported health care clinics, and consultative pediatric practices limited to family counseling for behavioral and developmental disorders.

Families generally expect that a physician has something of value to offer when they request his counsel; the physician must also respect the service that he is able to provide through family interviews. If he is serious in his work, it is substantial. Physicians who persist in refusing to charge (appropriately, not excessively) for their time: (1) are afraid they are incompetent, (2) know they are incompetent, (3) are plagued by pervasive feelings of low self-esteem, or (4) are independently wealthy. The first should get some training, the second should get out of the business, the third would do well to find himself a family therapist, and the fourth should spread it around.

If a doctor is charging appropriately for his services, the worry that he is "taking time away from the practice" diminishes. The decision as to when in the day interviews are best scheduled rests on several variables. Working parents, as mentioned earlier, are generally more available in late afternoons or evenings. Physicians may also want to take into consideration at what time of day their energies are up to wrestling with a family. The realities of other aspects of the practice must be considered. Group pediatric practices, in which individuals often enjoy some degree of flexibility in determining specific time commitments, particularly lend themselves to the institution of one-night-a-week evening clinics. Nursing and other office staff are not really required, and the physician by himself can see two or three families in an evening, in an office setting uncluttered by ringing telephones, coughing kids, and perplexed parents.

OFFICE EQUIPMENT

Happily, family interviewing does not involve heavy expenditures for the interested clinician. Space, a few toys, comfortable chairs — and Kleenex — are really all that is required. Space can be a problem, particularly in an office sleekly designed for efficiency with a multitude of pediatric examining rooms and little else. Such examining rooms have a way of being long, narrow, and inhospitable in appearance. They can handle a family of two parents and three children only if the interviewer is willing to work single file with the group. It is far preferable to have a spot in which the family can spread out comfortably, and also large enough for the therapist to manipulate space with them as needed. In some offices the waiting area can be used for this purpose, especially if interviews are held after regular office hours and if it offers the largest open space and the most comfortable furnishings.

A simple assortment of toys on hand is useful in several ways. It works well as an innocent enticement for reluctant children to enter the room. Also, very anxious and/or hyperactive children are often able to handle an interview with more ease if they can fiddle with interesting things through the hour. In addition, the use of toys and play by the children and their parents can provide very useful diagnostic information: Are the children allowed to play? Do they know how? Is their play age-appropriate? How do siblings handle the competitive and conflictual aspects of play? Do the parents have a capacity for playfulness? How are limits set on the children's play and by whom? What are children communicating to the interviewer about the family through their play? All of these questions can be answered through careful observation of a family's manipulation of toy materials. The materials can be inexpensive: hand puppets, puzzles, blocks, toy soldiers, cars, and drawing materials.

Interviews conducted around a large table are preferred by two of the authors (H.G. and W.B.). Drawing materials—a box of crayons and paper—are available at each session for the children. Even at times when the children appear to be uninvolved and uninterested in the discussion, their drawings are often dramatic illustrations of their nonverbal participation in the topic being discussed. For instance, during an interview with a family of two parents and their two boys, ages 6 and 8, the younger child worked most diligently and silently on his own project at the table. His parents were discussing their recent marital separation and the inability of each partner to control anger with one another or with the boys. Within a few minutes, the young artist, encouraged by the therapist, was describing his picture to the group assembled. He said it was a picture of the hospital clinic building with a huge fire on the second floor (the interview location) "burning everybody up." Four individuals were shown to have perished in the flames. One small figure, a little boy, had leaped out of the window to save himself, but he too was dead on the sidewalk. For reasons such as this, which have occurred repeatedly, we do not consider a child's play irrelevant or just busywork in the session. We urge trainees to set aside time during an interview in which children who have seemingly been occupied in their own play may discuss their particular drawings or play products, incorporating their efforts to communicate through play into the substance of the interview itself.

We have omitted one piece of equipment that may indeed be expensive. We refer to the use of recording equipment. This apparatus may range from the simplest cassette audiotape recorder to an elaborate videotaping system. We utilize both in our training work with pediatricians. For the clinician in practice we also recommend that interviews be recorded (with the family's permission, of course) at least on an audiotape; the use of videotape, although desirable, may be financially and logistically unreasonable. Taping is useful with the family; selected segments of an interview can be played back for them to illustrate specific therapeutic points. Feedback for individual family members regarding communication processes can be effectively provided through tape playback. It is also a way of returning a family to an important topic, earlier strayed from. More than this, we strongly urge the taping of interviews for the interviewer's continuing growth and supervision. Family interviewing is intellectually and emotionally difficult work. Doing it in isolation is an invitation to stagnation and the unwitting development of poor technique and bad habits. We urge against it. Carl Whitaker[6] strongly advises that a family therapist find himself a "cuddle group," a group with whom he can review experiences and from whom he can continue to receive feedback. We agree.

If the interviewer finds himself totally alone, at least he can play back tapes for his own review. This sort of self-criticism and review is better than none. Far better is to find someone, a spouse or co-worker, to share in the process or, better still, to find a group of family interviewers interested in providing mutual feedback and enhancing the individual growth of its members. This last is not a new idea. It was successfully developed by a group of pediatricians in Rochester, New York, as an antidote to the "dissatisfied pediatrician" syndrome. In an effort to enrich their clinical experiences and escape the tedium that many of their cohorts were encountering in clinical pediatrics, these physicians incorporate abbreviated counseling for behavioral problems into their individual practices and met one evening a month to review tapes and techniques. The group grew steadily over a 5-year period and eventually included as many as 25 participating pediatricians. A written description of this project appeared in 1968.[4] One of the authors of this book (B.A.) was a member of that group. It appeared to be highly successful and easily replicable elsewhere by interested groups.

REFERENCES

1. Aponte, H.: Personal communication, 1977.
2. Satir, V.: Conjoint family therapy: a guide to theory and technique, Palo Alto, Calif., 1964, Science and Behavior Books, Inc.
3. Speck, R., and Attneave, C.: Family network: retribalization and healing, New York, 1973, Pantheon Books, Inc.

4. Sumpter, E., and Friedman, S.: Workshop dealing with emotional problems: one method of preventing the "dissatisfied pediatrician syndrome," Clin. Pediatr. **7:**149, 1968.
5. Whitaker, C.: A family is a four-dimensional relationship. In Guerin, P., editor: Family therapy: theory and practice, New York, 1976, Gardner Press, Inc.
6. Whitaker, C.: The hindrance of theory on clinical work. In Guerin, P., editor: Family therapy: theory and practice, New York, 1976, Gardner, Press, Inc.

CHAPTER 6

The initial interview with a family

PRE-INTERVIEW ISSUES
The telephone

Mrs. Ruggles is on the telephone with her pediatrician: "It's Harry this time, Doctor King. . . this is really embarrassing, but I find he's been stealing from my purse and not just nickels and dimes. Last Friday, for the second time, I found $20 gone. . . Can I bring him in so you can talk to him, please? You're so good with all the kids—Harry adores you. Remember when you had to sew up his thumb last summer? Well, he swears to everybody that you're the only doctor who can do that without hurting. What's that?. . . Eight, he's eight now, just starting the second grade. Now I don't dare tell my husband about this. You know Milt. Milt. *Milt* . . . . my husband, Milton. He gets so tense with the kids, and he's just had that surgery in the last year for his ulcer. We don't like to get him upset. . . . This would just kill him. He doesn't know about the other times. What? . . . Oh to be honest, this has been going on 6 months or more I think. I didn't call you—you're so busy, and it wasn't a big thing— I thought I could take care of it . . . yes, the first time was right after Christmas. Harry took $15 that his brother, Greg, had gotten for a Christmas present. He promised that if I didn't tell his father, it wouldn't happen again. . . . We had to swear Greg to secrecy, too. Then there was a second time, but that was only $1.50. . . Now recently this business with the 20 dollar bills from my purse. I just can't get through to him. But now if you could just have a little talk with Harry—the two of you alone—I'm sure he would listen to you. . ."

If Dr. King agrees to a "little talk with Harry—the two of you alone," he is in trouble. So many family issues are on the table: Harry's stealing, of course, but that's not all. What about Mrs. Ruggles's collaboration with her sons and "protection" of her husband? What about her attempts to manipulate the doctor into an approach she prefers, one that will continue the collaboration and include the doctor in her coalition? What about her communications that suggest that she is openly, or unwittingly, encouraging her son's behavior (for example, "then there was a second time, but that was *only* $1.50.")? What about her direct communications to her son regarding his behavior? How is it that she "can't get through to him"? How could the doctor help her — or Harry — by succeeding where Mrs. Ruggles has already failed? What messages has brother Greg been receiving throughout this situation? What about father and his apparent position of weakness and vulnerability in the family? If Dr. King agrees to leave him out of the picture, can it do anything but support the notion of father's fragility? None of these issues could be handled in a "little talk with Harry alone." The family's participation is essential for a resolution of their dilemmas.

The Ruggles family illustrates our view that the initial interview actually begins *before* the family enters the office. For many physicians the first contact is a telephone conversation with one parent, often the child's mother. As illustrated, considerable mischief can occur in that call if the doctor is not prepared.

The caller is often intent on filling the doctor in, giving him the "real story," sharing secret agendas or confidences, enlisting the doctor to take sides and form judgments, presenting views in a light that will favor the caller, and so forth. These maneuvers, if successful, will not only alter the interviewer's perspective of the family but may seriously compromise his effectiveness in the family interview. As an illustration, it would be difficult if not impossible to work with a family in which a child's dishonesty — "lying" — is both parents' concern, and yet the interviewer has agreed in a private conversation with one spouse not to reveal to the other that the child has been stealing.

To minimize the possibility of pre-interview alliances with one family member, we discourage lengthy discussions of a parent's concerns on the telephone, stating that we prefer that such concerns, which are of considerable importance to all, be brought up at the first family meeting. Thus after eliciting a brief description of the reason for requesting assistance and after supportively acknowledging the feelings of the caller, be they concern, confusion, anger, or helplessness, one may firmly and tactfully discourage further discussion of "the problem." The remainder of the call may be used to (1) explain that the first interview must include the entire family, (2) discuss length of appointments, fees, and so on, and (3) arrange a time that is suitable for all. We prefer to make these arrangements for scheduling ourselves rather than through a nurse-receptionist, since this dialogue with the calling family member often yields valuable information regarding that individual's willingness to consider a family approach and his ability to correctly communicate to other family members our interest in working with the family as a group.

Failure to appear for the first interview

Since the family is generally communicating by its pre-interview behavior certain aspects of its system and structure, a failure to arrive for the first family interview should be carefully included in the interviewer's growing data base surrounding that particular family. Their absence usually has a direct bearing on case understanding. How well does the family know the physician? Do they trust him? Does a missed initial family interview indicate that the family collectively is frightened of a *joint* encounter? Or is perhaps just one member afraid and refusing to attend? What combination of influences has led to the family's nonappearance? A missed appointment is not ignored; neither should it be left to the family to reestablish contact. The above questions can be pursued in a follow-up telephone call by the interviewer to the family. We do not find it desirable for such telephone interactions with families to be handled by a receptionist for the reason stated above; that is, the family's behavior, even outside the interview proper, becomes important diagnostic information for the interviewer to gather firsthand as he develops his formulation of the family system and its relationship to the voiced concerns.

Occasionally, even after careful preparation by the interviewer and seeming agreement from the caller that the entire family will attend, only a portion of the family appears at the scheduled time with apologies for the absent member or members. Those present indicate their intention to proceed without the participation of the entire family. When this occurs, the family is often demonstrating in very concrete terms their particular collection of alliances and alienations and their desire to maintain such a system. Interviewers will need to use discretion in deciding whether or not to proceed under such circumstances. In our experience, if the missing person is either a spouse or the identified patient, proceeding with the interview is particularly difficult, and subsequent inclusion of the missing members is often impossible. The interviewer should not hesitate to cancel such an interview before starting, rescheduling it at a time when the absent family member will attend. However, if the missing member is a child, not the identified patient but a sibling with, for instance, another commitment for the same time, we are not averse to beginning family work without that individual. Even here, however, the interviewer may express his displeasure at meeting with the incomplete family and request that subsequent sessions include the absent member.

Depending on the circumstances a physician may wish to charge a family for a missed initial (or subsequent) appointment or an appointment canceled because only a portion of the family arrives in the office. It is acceptable practice that he do so, having first informed the family of this policy. It may even be a necessary practice for sound office economics.

Anxiety: family and interviewer

The previously described pre-interview issues are important; however, we would not like to give the reader the impression that those issues appear in every encounter with a family. On the contrary, most often an opening telephone contact with a concerned parent goes quite smoothly. The parent (it is usually mother) is forthright in her request for help from the doctor, and the suggestion of an initial family meeting is accepted without question. In these instances, which for us are the majority, the family members also manage to get themselves to the office on time for the visit. Therefore let us proceed now from the point at which an entire family has arrived.

Actually for many of our beginning trainees, their major concern is that the family *will* arrive, that nothing short of a natural disaster will stop them. For the beginner, even after observation and preparation, leading a family interview can be a harrowing experience. Perhaps a brief aside is in order to address what's happening on both sides of the interview room. Many authors have discussed the initial interview, initial referring to the fact that it is the family's first time; we intend to do likewise. There is correspondingly little mentioned in the literature about the very first interview in the interviewer's experience. For one of the authors (B.A.), his first family interview is remembered as a ghastly disconnected jumble during which his simple physiological survival and the ability to feign coherence assumed tremendous significance. After review with his supervisor, the event was subsequently and quickly relegated to a remote, seldom-visited area of his awareness. We suspect it has been so for others as well. Hence it is not surprising that this supreme moment has seldom been discussed in the literature.

In the novice's mind there are so many "what if's." As already stated, what if the family fails to arrive? There are others: What if there are ten of them? What if they won't be quiet? Worse yet, what if they won't talk? What if I can't control the situation? What if the family starts to fight? What if I won't be able to figure out what's going on? What if I won't know what to say? What if the family falls apart during the interview? What if the session becomes chitchat that seems to lead nowhere?

Such doubts about competence and performance are common in any new learning situation. The physician has experienced such doubts during his first physical examination, his first lumbar puncture, and so on. It is easier to learn correct venipuncture techniques with the aid of a cooperative, vigorous, 52-year-old male patient with prominent veins in the antecubital fossa, than it is, syringe in hand, to chase a terrified 2½-year-old buzz-bomb around the examining table, with his mother pacing out in the hall or in the examining room. Usually the learning experiences in medical school are provided in this sequence. Likewise the physician interested in developing his family interviewing skills is urged to make it as easy on himself as possible in the beginning. A family with whom the doctor already feels somewhat comfortable and one that presents an apparently "simple" child-rearing issue ("he won't mind, Doctor") would seem a good beginning experience. Venturing into more serious, heavily conflict-laden family problems (for instance, delinquency or anorexia nervosa) should await his growing experience. He may even choose, and appropriately so, not to work with the latter sort of cases at all, even after extensive experience in family interviewing. However, the same principles in interviewing will apply in either the simple or the complex situation. A firm grasp of the principles underlying effective family interviewing and the practice of using them will gradually lessen the physician's anxiety surrounding his performance. A doctor in his training has learned the importance of developing his interview fact-finding (content) skill. Through training and years of experience he has developed this ability to an exquisite degree; it is a skill of which he is very proud and with which he is comfortable. Now in learning to deal with process as well as content in interviews, he essentially has to start over again and thus reexperience anxiety of the same sort that he originally felt during those unfamiliar "firsts" of venipuncture, suturing, and so on.

Until experiential knowledge accumulates — knowledge based on utilization of specific principles such as those summarized in this text — the interviewer will most likely be anxious in anticipation of an interview with a family. We do not say this to scare off potential interviewers. That would be defeating our purpose. Rather we are saying to the beginning interviewer-physician: discomfort, though painful, is appropriate and to be expected. Be assured that you, the doctor, and the family will survive the experience. If you are one who envisions the potential usefulness of a family-oriented approach to many pediatric problems, we suggest that you stay with it long enough not only to feel the anxiety of a first interview but also to enjoy the flush of accomplishment that comes with successful functioning in a family interview. After a particularly good session one of our trainees likened the feeling he was experiencing to his feeling the first time he successfully intubated a premature infant. He called it "pure exhilaration."

The beginning interviewer may find it helpful to know that usually his own anxiety is surpassed by that of the family. Helpful or not, this fact is important to consider; it is safe to assume that this is the case for every family. The family's "what if's" cover an even broader range than the doctor's. Most prominent and generally shared by child and parent alike are: What if the doctor says it's all my fault? What if he thinks I'm overanxious or stupid? What if he doesn't like me and the way I'm treating my child? What if he won't agree with me? Sometimes there are also: What if our family secret is revealed? What if I don't maintain control of myself? What if I don't maintain control of my family? Families are usually frightened and defensive at the beginning of an interview. They are risking exposure to and scrutiny from "the outside." And yet they want help with some sort of difficulty that has prompted their visit. Consequently they often feel two ways about embarking on the venture: eager for help and fearful of the process. When an interviewer acknowledges the family's sometimes sizable apprehension and understands their ambivalence, he can be moderately successful in reducing their anxiety so they can feel safe enough to show themselves and their system and allow work to begin toward a solution.

OPENING STAGE OF AN INITIAL INTERVIEW

The process of making a family comfortable is called the social stage of an interview, and it begins when the family is ushered into the interview room. *Each* family member is greeted separately by name with both eye contact and physical contact (a handshake, a friendly hand on the shoulder, and so on) initiated by the interviewer. The family is allowed to choose their own seating arrangement. A brief period of small talk may ensue. Minuchin refers to this (p. 207) as "living room behavior, conforming to cultural rules of politeness."[3] The interviewer may introduce himself to any family members he has not met and discuss the recording equipment he may be using.

Since we routinely use audiotape or videotape in our interviews, we generally have the equipment running by the time the family enters the office. This obviates the awkward need to flip switches and adjust microphones once the family is seated. Recording is usually presented to the family in this way: "You will note that I am using a tape recorder today. I tape for two reasons: During the interview I may want to play back a certain section for us to review together. I will also use it for my own review at some point after the session is over. I do not keep the tapes on record; they are erased after I review them." Families' objections to the use of tape devices have been extremely rare. However if, following the above, even one family member expresses a reluctance to be taped, the machine is turned off.

During this greeting stage, the interviewer is also making observations. What is the general mood of the family? How do the parents seem to be doing with the children? Are they severe and demanding, or are they ignoring, permissive to the point that the children are out of control? How does the family appear to be organizing itself as the preliminaries of the interview unfold? Who speaks? Who speaks for others? How do they seat themselves? Such observations as these and others mentioned earlier in the section on content and process are important. However, we agree with Haley (p. 18): "It is important to gather information, but it is also important to keep conclusions tentative. The therapist may be misled and therefore ideas should not be too firm. Observation gives information that can be tested as the session continues. A therapist who gets too set in one idea is not free to consider other ideas."[2] Diagnosis is an ongoing process.

DISCUSSION OF CONCERNS, THE SECOND STAGE OF AN INITIAL INTERVIEW

As quickly as the therapist senses that the family can tolerate it, the social stage of the interview should move into the more purposeful second stage of discussion of the presenting concern(s). This must generally be initiated by the doctor. Such an act gives the family the feeling that the doctor is in charge. It is his first entrance into the family system, so to speak. He may choose one of a variety of routes. He may explicitly ask the general question, "What brings the family here today?" or "What help would this family like from me?", these directed toward no one in particular. The response offers not only an answer to the question but also additional information regarding, for instance, who in the family takes responsibility for getting the family going, or who is most concerned, or who is spokesman for the group. Parenthetically we do not often word such an initial question in terms of "the problem." That is, we tend not to ask a family, "What's the problem?" It may seem no different in substance than asking, "What brings the family here today?", yet the former question seems to invite a process in which one family member looks directly at another and with a pointing finger declares essentially, "he is." When this happens, the therapist may well lose the goodwill of the scapegoated family member, and the doctor will be at a disadvantage for the rest of the session with that individual. To be sure, scapegoating of the identified patient may still occur, even when the opening question has been most carefully worded. Blaming is one of the most common dangers and defense mechanisms that a therapist encounters as he helps an interview get underway. After all, the family has generally asked for counsel because of the behavior of one particular individual; their inclination to blame that person is understandable. Unfortunately such an inclination can be extremely damaging for the therapist's work. Children have already and repeatedly been made to feel bad and deserving of punishment at home for the symptomatic behavior that has prompted the visit. If the interview continues this process and parents and even siblings are allowed to continue blaming the child in front of the doctor, the child will quickly withdraw from the interview process and become sullen, silent, and uncooperative.

The simplest way to change a family's blaming stance in regard to their "problem" child is to comment on its first appearance in the session with a statement such as, "You know, Mrs. Gilroy, I am uncomfortable that Alice must be feeling pretty bad about this whole situation. I am beginning to understand your own exasperation as well. Could you rephrase your worry in a way that does not blame her?" This intervention may require repeating often and with others in the family as well.

One may wish to be less ambiguous in the opening inquiry with a family. For instance, an interviewer may wish to begin teaching the family immediately that he intends to broaden his focus from an individual to the family unit. He could do so with the following opening:

"I am glad the entire family was able to come in today. I talked briefly on the phone with you, Mrs. Watson, but not very much. I wanted to wait until we had this opportunity to meet. I consider that each of you has feelings and opinions that are important if things are to get better in this family. I would like to ask each of you, and I will start on this side and go around the room, what brings you here today, what changes would you like to see take place in this family?"

One may thus pose the initial question to no one in particular or to everyone in general. One may also choose a specific family member to receive the opening question. Haley, for instance, often directs his beginning question to that adult who seems less involved with the problem. He further states:

> Generally it is not a good idea to start with the problem child and ask him why the family is there. He will feel that he is too much on the spot, and it may look as if the therapist is blaming him for everyone being there. It is better to deal with him later.*

This has not been our experience, and we have quite often begun this second stage of an interview with a question to the identified patient such as: "Frankie, tell me what you understand about today's visit. How come the family is here today?" This child is usually especially worried, having already learned or sensed at home that "he" is the reason for their appearance. The therapist may thus momentarily increase the child's anxiety by such a forthright spotlighting approach; however, as he continues, he demonstrates through careful listening to the child's words and acknowledgement of the child's uncomfortable feelings that he, the interviewer, is truly interested in the child, in his feelings, and in helping him to relax. Quite often when asked the opening question a child will steal a look at one or both parents and shrug his shoulders, indicating that he doesn't know why the family is sitting in the doctor's office. Hence an entree is provided into a discussion of how the child and other family members were prepared for the initial visit. Were they simply dragged along, or was an attempt made to explain the nature of the visit? One may explore these questions directly — when the child indicates that he

---

*Haley, J.: Problem-solving therapy: new strategies for effective family therapy, San Francisco, 1976, Jossey-Bass, Inc., p. 25.

hasn't the foggiest idea of the reason for the family's presence in the doctor's office, the interviewer may say: "All right, Frankie, I would like you to pick either your mother or father and ask one of them to explain to you what brings the family here today." This request serves several purposes. First of all, the child is not chastised by the doctor for "pretending not to know when in fact he does." He may indeed be confused as to why the appointment has been made, having been told nothing more than, "you will go." Secondly, the child indicates which parent he is willing to approach with the question. Third, a dialogue between these two family members is initiated, a conversation that the therapist can observe from the sidelines, in which he need not participate. Fourth, the interviewer is able to see some of the communication process between the chosen parent and the child. Do they communicate functionally or is it a dysfunctional interchange, laced with, for instance, double-level messages, assumptions, or generalizations? Does the parent talk in a manner appropriate for the child's understanding? Is the explanation congruent with what the interviewer has learned on the phone, or do there seem to alternate versions? In this way the family's actual communication style is demonstrated in front of the therapist.

INTERACTIONAL STAGE OF AN INITIAL INTERVIEW

At this point the family has entered the third phase of an initial interview, the interactional stage—a stage the interviewer has directed and set in motion. As the family talks together, its system and structure are most clearly revealed. Rather than "talking about" their problem with the therapist they enact it among themselves before him, and the doctor is able to observe firsthand how the family members behave with one another.

Some families will begin this process on their own. Without any specific help from the interviewer they are soon discussing among themselves feelings, thoughts, and opinions. However, most do not initiate such discussion, and the interviewer must direct considerable effort toward helping family members interact with one another, preventing their addressing questions to him and discouraging their attempts to have the doctor take sides (for example, "Don't you think I'm right, Doctor?"). This unfortunate tendency of the family to use the interviewer as a central, expert receptor of messages was mentioned in an earlier chapter. It is a role that the interviewer must decline. It is sometimes a hard position for pediatricians to avoid, and once adopted, even harder to give up. A pediatrician is used to being in the "director's chair" in a clinical setting with a child and/or a family. This has most often meant that he is the expert, the information gatherer, the questioner, the answerer, and the dispenser of both medication and advice. He and his patients are accustomed to this style and role. We would like him to stay in the "director's chair," but he must direct somewhat differently. Facilitating the family's own interaction requires that he, after an initial directive, neither question, nor answer, nor dispense. Rather he must be more passive and silent and allow the family to unfold its story and its system. He may feel awkward, and the family may also be less than delighted with such a stance. Nonetheless we feel it is essential for obtaining an understanding of the family structure, relationships, and communication style.

How does a physician accomplish such a shift in what has been his traditional format with patients and families? The simplest maneuver has already been mentioned. The interviewer redirects comments from family members to himself with the firm directive: "That sounds like a message for George. Tell him that now, Gloria." Gloria may do it without hesitation. More commonly she will:

1. Continue talking as though she did not hear
2. State that she does not understand what the doctor means
3. Protest by saying that she and George have discussed it a thousand times previously
4. Protest with an assumption either about herself or about George:
   "He knows what I mean."
   "He wouldn't understand."
   "I can't talk to him about this."
5. Politely put the doctor and his suggestion in its place:
   "That seems so artificial."
6. Not so politely put the doctor and his suggestion in its place:
   "No, I won't. I don't like your telling me what to do."

The interviewer should be ready beforehand for such protest and be prepared to insist on direct communication. It should be apparent that even by this time the family is beginning to reveal its communication difficulties, providing both diagnostic information and material that the interviewer may use in his therapeutic work with the family. For instance, if Gloria protests against speaking directly to George for reason 4, the interviewer has his work cut out for him in helping Gloria drop assumption-making from her communication style.

This maneuver of asking family members to talk to one another rather than to the therapist must usually be repeated and encouraged several times in the first and ensuing interviews, and generally it must be repeated with each family member. With time, family members will become so accustomed to it as an important rule of the interview that the doctor's simply pointing without words to that individual for whom the message is intended will be enough to have the sender turn and deliver it appropriately. A mistake we see beginning trainees make with this strategy is that they give up too quickly. They will successfully redirect an individual at the start and then in a few moments allow that same individual or someone else to resume a style that channels comments once again to the interviewer. Perhaps 20 minutes later the trainee realizes what he has let slip and again attempts a maneuver that encourages the family's communication. It seems more effective for the interviewer to teach the family *persistently* from the beginning that direct communication is required in the session and that he expects that family members will so behave in the interview.

As mentioned earlier, one advantage of direct communication is that the interviewer is freed from his active role in any conversation. He is thus enabled to observe the family's interaction while outside their system, and he has moments to himself in which he may develop his beginning strategies and plans. There is another advantage. Very often a major problem for the family being seen is its marked difficulty in the communication of feelings to each other. Therefore an interviewer is defeating one of his own goals for the family in encouraging or allowing family members to express their feelings to him rather than to one another. For if feelings are expressed to the interviewer and hence dissipated in his direction, they are then never received by the individual for whom they were intended. Thus the family members do not learn skills for direct expression and reception of feelings among themselves; instead they continue to blame and explain while not responding to one another constructively.

Along with the verbal directive that family members talk with one another, an interviewer may need to use other means to underscore his emphasis on direct communication. He may ask two family members to move their chairs so that they are facing one another as they speak. He should request that any family members seated between the two participants move back or away so nothing interferes with direct communication between the two involved members. He may request that the two people hold hands or touch as they talk so that contact between them is maximized, and each clearly has the other's attention. The interviewer and the family will discover that communication in such a position becomes less threatening. If a family is particularly resistant to direct communication, the interviewer may want to move his own chair out of the family circle, demonstrating that he will not participate in the interchange that he has requested.

Once family members have begun to talk directly to one another, the interviewer may begin to reshape their communication style itself. For instance, he may request that each individual concentrate on using the pronoun "I" in talking with others (beginning sentences with "I need," "I see," and so on), thus underscoring that each individual is to assume responsibility in communication for his own thoughts, acts, and feelings. The interviewer may also ask that family members concentrate on present thoughts, present actions, present feelings, rather than resorting to repeated reports and complaints about the past.

All of the above, of course, are done with an eye toward how fast the family seems able to tolerate interventions. With a particularly frightened family one would proceed slowly. However, even with the most tentative family group we generally plug away at encouraging their direct talk to one another. Often it is the first lesson for the family, and it may take several sessions.

There are other techniques for encouraging the family to interact and demonstrate its system to the interviewer. We mention three of them here. They have been used sometimes in an initial encounter with a family and also often in ongoing counseling work after the family has participated in several sessions. The techniques are: (1) conjoint family drawing, (2) family sculpture, and (3) written listing of "appreciations and resentments."

Conjoint family drawing

The reader will remember our mention of this technique in the section on content and process. Aside from its use in resident training we also use it in direct work with families for a number of reasons. First of all, it encourages participation in a task by all family members; the less talkative are not edged out. Second, it is a nonverbal task, and particularly with families who tend to talk excessively or intellectualize, it is a way of cutting through their often obscuring verbiage to see something of their usually more revealing nonverbal behavior with one another. It is an appealing format for children most of the time, and they participate with enthusiasm during the task. It also reveals something of the family's ability to be playful with one another, demonstrating their relative comfort or discomfort with such a "childish" enterprise. Finally, since the interviewer is not participating directly in the task, it is another device for providing him with time to diagnose, organize, and plan strategies within the framework of the sessions, as he observes the action.

This procedure has been used in a variety of clinical situations, including marital therapy,[3] the treatment of schizophrenia,[4] and various other family problems.[6] Specific instructions to the family may vary. One source suggests the following:

> Each family member is to select a felt pen of a different color and is not to exchange for any other color pen. I would like for you as a family to draw a picture as you see yourselves now as a family. You can draw the picture any way you want to, but I'd like to encourage you to be as creative and original as you can in representing yourselves as a unique family. You can draw the persons any size and place them in any position on the paper. They may be drawn touching each other, or separate. You can draw yourselves or each other, whichever you think best describes your family.*

Here the interviewer is rather specific in telling the family what to do. Our own directions to families are considerably more general. A large sheet of drawing paper (approximately 2 feet by 3 feet) is taped on top of a flat table around which a family is seated. A box of crayons is also provided. Each family member is asked to choose a separate color and not to change colors. These instructions are given:

"I would like the family to work together on this sheet of paper for the next 20 (or 25 or 30) minutes. What you draw is up to you. However, there is to be no talking, either with me or with one another throughout this time. We will talk when the time is up. OK, you may begin."

Sometimes at this point individuals express embarrassment at having to expose their allegedly poor artistic skills. The interviewer (after making a mental note of the self-deprecator) may wish to state that the task is not a test of anyone's artistic ability. Other comments, explanations, and suggestions need not be offered, however. The interviewer should instead fall silent, and in a short time the family will do likewise.

With families, just as with trainees, it is less the content of the drawing and more the process during the task that should dominate the inter-

---

*Bing, E.: The conjoint family drawing, Family Process **9:**173, 1970.

viewer's observations and his subsequent discussion with the family. One should note who initiates the drawing, who seems responsible for organizing the task and the group. How are responsibilities shared for developing a theme and carrying it through? Does each individual have sufficient drawing space? How are issues of spatial territory handled on the paper? Do subsystems of the family appear, two or three individuals working jointly on a project that does not include others? Do the children seem to have a say in the development of the drawing? Do they have such a say that the process seems largely under their control, the parents remaining inactive and passive? Or is it the other way around? Does one family member shift from one subsystem to another, seemingly unable to find a place to light and enter in? How are reluctant participants handled and by whom? The answers to these and other questions can be added to the interviewer's growing collection of observations regarding the family and their particular structure.

Once the drawing is completed, the family is usually eager to discuss their experience. For this purpose one should allow perhaps 30 minutes, particularly if the family consists of several children and two parents. In structuring the family's discussion, the interviewer may assist by requesting that each family member offer in turn a summary of his own feelings during and as a result of the task. To get them started, the doctor can ask that each person list three adjectives that describe the experience for him (that is, silly, frightening, revealing, or whatever). The doctor may also ask each person to walk around the drawing, comment on the contribution of each family member, and listen in turn to that member's response. The commenter thus initiates a dialogue with each family member regarding the drawing and the process. Since everyone is given a turn to comment, the interviewer is able to observe the specific communication style for every possible dyad in the family.

Specific content issues of the drawing can be discouraged by emphasizing the use of the word "how" in each family member's description of the experience. In this way the "hows" of the process are discussed rather than the "whats" of the picture itself. Even during this period of discussion family members should be directed to speak to one another, not to the interviewer. If one directs the discussion to a sharing of *how* the drawing took place, one can avoid falling into a trap that many families encourage (and yet probably fear): that of "explaining" the symbolic significance of specific items in the drawing. Such a discussion between a family and the doctor comes dangerously close to sounding like an afternoon in a gypsy tearoom. We recommend that it be saved for that environment and that the family interviewer limit his scope in this task to an understanding and discussion of the family's process during the drawing.

A family may also be encouraged to view the family drawing task as a learning experience for themselves. The interviewer may ask each person to describe something he has learned about himself during the process and something he has learned about how the family works together during such a task.

The conjoint family drawing can be repeated at intervals throughout one's continuing work with a family. It will usually reflect alterations in a family's basic set of relationships, if these have occurred.

The clinical usefulness of this drawing task is illustrated by the following summary:

The Harris family entered family therapy because one child, Kelly, 8, "has no initiative, just won't do anything on her own, is dependent and whiny," especially with her mother. The whole family agreed to participate in sessions, including both parents and two other children, Steve, 11, and Rona, 9. These two children were described as cooperative, resourceful, and independent, in contrast to their "balky, immature" sister, the identified patient. Mrs. Harris openly complained that Kelly's clinging, whining, and demanding were driving her "crazy." Mother felt guilty and ashamed that, because of Kelly's behavior, she found herself often behaving in very rejecting ways toward her daughter, which only made matters worse. The whole family agreed that a veritable battleground had developed between mother and this one child. It was unclear what role the rest of the quintet played in the sequence of events.

During the first family interview, the family completed the family drawing shown on p. 128. They were asked to "work together on this piece of paper without talking for the next 20 minutes." Each had chosen one color: mother, red; father, green; Kelly, light green; Rona, blue; and Steve, black. The position of each family member around the table during the drawing process is indicated in the drawing. Briefly, the drawing had been produced in this fashion: the identified patient was the first to put a mark on the paper, and she enthusiastically began work with a line across her side of the paper, this line destined to become the lawn of her portion of the drawing. Immediately mother leaned across the paper and began drawing the lines of a house on top of Kelly's line. (Mother's complaint had been that Kelly would not leave her alone, yet here was a clear demonstration that it was Mother who was unwilling to leave Kelly alone.) In broad strokes she constructed a house on top of Kelly's lawn and then began to color in the roof, her product beginning to dwarf Kelly's efforts, which were now relegated to the thin strip of paper left on the bottom of the page. Nonplussed, Kelly began to draw family figures in the space left to her. Mother and daughter certainly seemed to be in some sort of struggle with one another for space, but it was Mother, not Kelly, who appeared to initiate and maintain the struggle.

What of the others? For the first few minutes, father and the other two children hung back, watching this nonverbal interchange develop between Mrs. Harris and her daughter. When mother finished her lines on the house in Kelly's area, she resumed her seat to begin drawing flowers on her portion of the paper. At this point Rona began to draw. Although described as resourceful and independent, she was clearly watching her sister very carefully and taking cues from her as to subject mat-

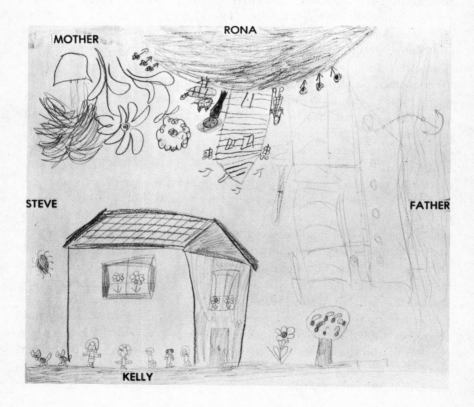

ter. Rona began her own version of a house, family, and lawn scene. It was an obvious copy of Kelly's work with a few original touches. Steve continued to stare uncomfortably at the paper and intermittently drummed his crayon on the paper; beyond the few dots he produced, he drew nothing. Mother was visibly upset at his inactivity, drew some of her flowers in his direction, and motioned with her hand for him to join in. She succeeded only in obliterating his space and leaving him very little room. Father was also continuing to watch rather than participate. However, unlike his son, he eventually began to draw, unrelated to the drawings of the others, the form of a sailing ship. His lines were lighter and less distinct. He became dreamily absorbed in his work, seemingly oblivious to the work of the rest of the family. The most diligent worker of all was clearly Kelly, the child with "no initiative." By the time the drawing had been completed, she had embellished her mother's house with walls, doors, windows, flowers, trees, sun, and people.

The pediatrician initiated the post-drawing discussion:

Doctor: OK, now I would like each of you to come up with one word that describes how you found this task you have just finished. What feelings did you have as you were participating in the drawing? We'll go around the table, and I'll start with you, Mrs. Harris.

Mother: Frustrating, very frustrating.

Doctor: Next, Steve.

Steve: . . . Silly.

Kelly: Fun. I thought it was fun.

Father: Interesting.

Rona: I thought it was fun, too.

Mother: (starting to laugh) That's so funny, Al, that you thought it was interesting . . . you over there on your sailboat or whatever it is, just doing your own thing, never mind what's happening with the rest of us . . . just like at home.

Doctor: Would you tell him directly what you found frustrating about the experience.

Mother: Well, that . . . for one thing. You seemed so removed over there, drawing that boat. That's like where you are most of the time . . . and I was hoping that somehow we would all get together and draw something . . . one picture, not separate ones. That was one part of my feeling. And then Steve—not drawing anything at all! I was very impatient there, wanting him to get going, and I could see that he wasn't going to.

Doctor: Ask Steve what he was experiencing.

Mother: I think I know.

Doctor: Ask him anyhow.

Mother: Well, what was happening with you?

Steve: Well . . . at first I couldn't think of anything to draw, and then all the space started getting filled up . . .

Mother: (speaking for her son) And you decided that if you couldn't have all the space, then you weren't going to use any of it, right?

Steve: Well . . . yeah.

Mother: I knew it. And then I started getting frustrated about that. I knew that's what he was doing, and I couldn't say anything about it, since we had to be silent.

Doctor: It's hard not to speak out?

Mother: Well, yes, I guess it is. They all tell me I have a big mouth. Right, gang?

The children all quickly agreed with mother's last comment.

Doctor: And I was wondering if you all noticed Kelly's independence and enthusiasm, her ability to work creatively and alone.

Father: That's what I found so interesting—not my own drawing, Sally, but that Kelly was so clearly taking off on her own. I wouldn't have expected it.

Mother: Well, she likes to draw, that's all.

The "how" of the drawing—that is, how it came to be—uncovered all sorts of family data, much of it at odds with the stated version of the "family problem" (Kelly's dependency and clinging). For instance:

1. Kelly was, on the contrary, capable of considerable independent activity. However, this activity was hardly validated in the family. It was summarily negated by mother ("she likes to draw, that's all.") and a surprise to father.
2. Mother had loudly complained of perpetual infringement on her own space at home by Kelly. However, in this experience it was clearly mother who intruded on her daughter's area.
3. Mother and father were at odds, specifically about the issue of father's involvement in family matters.
4. Steve was hardly the resourceful, independent, cooperative youngster that both parents had described.
5. Rona, for all the parental praise about her creativity and independence, was little more than Kelly's mimic and follower.

All of this information, which proved accurate, could then be used in subsequent sessions. The drawing had provided an effective entree into the family system, enabling the doctor to glimpse what lay beyond the family's official portrayal of themselves and their difficulties.

Family sculpture

The family sculpture is another means for helping families to interact while avoiding what they are most comfortable doing — endlessly explaining their "problem." The technique borrows much from the field of psychodrama, and like the conjoint family drawing, it is largely a nonverbal task. Peggy Papp of the Ackerman Institute for Family Therapy and the Philadelphia Child Guidance Clinic has been cited as the originator of the technique, and articles concerning its use have appeared in the literature.[5,7] A family sculpture is basically a physical arrangement of family members that expresses their relationship to one another in the family at a particular moment in time. The technique of directing a family to produce such a sculpture in the doctor's office is perhaps best understood through a clinical illustration.

Laura, age 15, had anorexia nervosa. She recently entered the hospital, where the diagnosis was confirmed and where she was now in the process of gaining weight before family treatment would continue through outpatient visits. During her hospitalization on the pediatric ward, her family agreed to begin family counseling by meeting Laura and her doctor in a room just off the pediatric ward. This was the first such session, and thus the pediatrician-interviewer and family were new to one another. Besides Laura, there were two other children, Anna, 19, and Joe, 6. Mr. and Mrs. French, the parents, were also present for the meeting. As the interview began, the doctor was struck by a general feeling of timidity and caution coming from the family. Concerns were discussed in such a bland and general manner that the interviewer felt bogged down in the family's polite and almost too careful regard for one another. Nothing much was happening. At this point he decided to risk injecting some liveliness into the session, hoping thereby to relax the family, move beyond their protective veneer of good manners, and help them to reveal something more of their family system and structure. He began:

> *Doctor:* OK. I would like to do something different with this family. First of all, I would like everyone to stand up and push the chairs back. (He quickly rises and pushes his chair out of the way and assists others in doing the same.) Good. Now I am going to ask you to do what's called a family sculpture. Does anyone know what I'm talking

about? No — OK, I will explain. I would like you to assume that everyone standing in the middle of the room is clay to be molded. One
of you is going to be the sculptor — Laura, I will begin with you. You
are the first sculptor. Everyone will have a turn eventually. I would
like you to consider that everyone in the family is made of clay and
that you are going to mold them into a sculpture, a family grouping
that will show something about how you see relationships in your
family. Do you follow me so far?

Laura: Well, I'm not sure.

Doctor: Let me see how else to put it . . . well, you know that in your family,
just as in other families, certain people are, for one thing, closer
than others. I would like you to show me your version of that — by
physically taking for instance, your mother, moving her body, her
arms, her facial expression, her hands, whatever, into a position
that says something about her place in the family and her closeness
and distance relative to others in the family. You may move her
wherever you feel she is in relation to you and others in the family.
You may want some people to be touching others; you may want
faces to look or not look in certain directions. You may want to
arrange faces in certain expressions. And don't forget to include
yourself in the sculpture.

Laura: (indicates, though tentatively, that she gets the idea)

Doctor: All right, I would like you to start now. Oh, one more thing. There
is to be no talking with one another or with me while you're doing
this. If you want someone to be smiling, don't tell them; move their
facial muscles with your hands. Remember, no talking.

Laura: Well, I don't know if. . .

Doctor: Do the best you can. Give it a try.

Laura's sculpture did indeed help the family and the interviewer
move into a productive area for subsequent discussion and work. She
placed her mother and father side by side, close together and holding
hands. Next to her father, on his left, she placed her younger brother,
Joe. The two males were in friendly contact each with one arm around
the other. Anna, her older sister, was placed kneeling on the floor, facing
front and in front of her parents, with her left hand extended to and
touching Joe, and her right hand stretched backwards into Mrs. French's
hand. Anna's face was positioned looking over her right shoulder into
her mother's face. Laura did not put herself into the picture. When the
interviewer urged her to do so, she inserted herself standing in the middle of this very small family circle. The final configuration then was a

tiny enclosed circle: mother, father, brother, and sister—all touching. Inside, touching no one, was the identified patient. She indicated with a helpless gesture that she did not know what to do with her hands.

The interviewer extended one implication of the sculpture by asking the family to transform the picture into a kinetic sculpture:

> *Doctor:* All right. Now, maintaining the positions in which Laura has placed you, I would like each of you to take just one step—in any direction . . . it doesn't matter where.

They promptly and literally fell over one another. The interviewer was then able to begin working with the family around a specific concept: sometimes when families are tremendously close, as the Frenchs were, there is little room for individual movement and growth. Any attempts at individual steps lead to inadvertent stepping on one another, while no effective individual movement occurs. This metaphor developed into a major theme in the continuing work with Laura and her family.

Perhaps a further word should be said about the French family before leaving them in a heap on the interview floor. There were, of course, numerous other important issues demonstrated by Laura's sculpture: mother and father were not looking at one another; most of mother's posture was directed toward her older daughter; the identified patient, Laura, had no eye contact with anyone in the family. Anna was in a particularly awkward position in the family, on her knees in front of them. Any one of these could have been utilized by the doctor in his beginning stages of work with the family. He arbitrarily chose one issue. However, he did return to the others mentioned as time went on. In any case the technique of having the family interact through Laura's version of a family sculpture provided his entrance into important family issues and helped to nudge the family gently beyond their initial fear and self-defeating need to appear polite.

One may extend the family sculpture in other ways besides asking the family to introduce movement into their static configuration. For instance, one may also introduce speech by asking the sculptor to give each family member a different sentence to say while in the designated position, something that would befit the person and the position. When sentences have been assigned to each individual—and again the sculptor must include himself in this aspect of the task—the interviewer may request that the family in turn repeat their sentences while standing in position. In this way very often a cohesive picture of family functioning becomes apparent to the family and the doctor from these seemingly unconnected bits of verbal and nonverbal behavior. Often what emerges in this section is the possibility of a dialogue between two family members based on the sentences provided them by the sculptor. For instance, let us assume that a mother has been placed in a position with hands on the sides of her head and the words, "I can't stand it anymore," and father has been positioned with legs apart and arms akimbo with the phrase, "Well, what are you going to do about it?" One may ask other family members to drop away for the moment and encourage mother and father to have a conversation with one another, beginning with their assigned phrases and carrying it beyond those statements into a more extended dialogue.

An interviewer may find additional productive results in requesting that each family member, while in the assigned position, assume that this is to be his or her permanent position in the family and in life. Once this is assumed, each member is asked to describe in some detail how such an existence would feel, how life would be in such a position. Frequently and often with some surprise, family members report that their descriptions of life in the assumed position closely match a description of their actual existence. For instance, a mother who was placed by the sculptor, her 14-year-old daughter, with her face to the wall, facing away from the family and into a corner of the room, declared: "I don't have to imagine that this is my permanent position. It is! I feel turned away, isolated, and out of it. I'm in that kitchen, and all I look at is a row of cupboards. I feel very lonely and isolated."

Family sculpture has proved very useful in families such as the Frenchs, who are understandably anxious and are helped by some sort of informal maneuver to break the ice and get started. It has seemed to be a popular device with children generally. Very often the children in a family who have not been selected as sculptor will ask directly for a turn, after they have seen how it goes. We have decided that one reason it is so appealing to children, their basic playfulness and sense of adventure aside, is that it is a sanctioned opportunity for a child to literally push his parents around, and those times don't come very often in life. For every family member, parents included, it is a time when touching is not just allowed but required. For families who have grown out of touch with one another, it may be the first such experience in months or years. We generally give everyone in the family, including parents, an opportunity to sculpt the family. The first family member selected as sculptor may be chosen because he appears to be the most interested, the most open, the brightest, or the most likely to "spill the beans." In any case one should probably start with that individual most likely to aid and not sabotage the interviewer's efforts.

Written listing of "appreciations and resentments"

The technique of a written listing of "appreciations and resentments" for encouraging family interaction in front of the therapist is quite easy to introduce. Satir has often used it. Each family member is given paper and pencil. Everyone is asked to list in writing five things he appreciates about each other family member; following that, each person is to list five things he resents about every other family member. An interviewer may also suggest that each individual include himself on his own list, writing five things he appreciates about himself and five things he resents in himself. The family is given as much time as it requires; often this task takes 20 or 30 minutes. When they have finished, the family members are assisted in sharing their lists with the group, one at a time between appropriate individuals.

Several things are accomplished with this maneuver. First of all, it is clearly a "let's get down to business" message from the interviewer. Second, it allows each family member to organize his thoughts privately and to participate, though silently for a time as he writes, in the interview. Third, it relieves the identified patient of his apprehension that the interview will focus only on him as "the problem," since without a doubt, everyone is going to be involved in the project, that is, every family member is going to be discussed in terms of behavior that is appreciated and behavior that is resented. Fourth, the technique gives explicit permission for family members to appreciate and resent, to feel two ways about others in the family. All too often families in trouble have a way of polarizing members, assigning them restricted roles—the good child, the bad child, the sympathetic parent, the insensitive parent, and so forth. In addition some families have unwritten taboos: one is not allowed to say anything critical of another family member, or conversely, one is not permitted to verbalize positive feelings toward someone else. The task suggests that everyone in the family has attributes and feelings on both sides of the coin. Frequently parents require a decided turn in their thinking processes to first conceptualize, then write down, and finally discuss qualities in the identified patient that they appreciate and like. In short the task is a beginning lesson for all the family that they do have and are expected to have both positive and negative feelings for other family members and for themselves as well and that both feelings are OK.

A discussion of appreciated qualities offers an opportunity for the doctor to teach family members the importance of and ways for effective validation of others, while a discussion of resented qualities allows for expression of anger and frustration in a relatively safe environment, watched over by the interviewer. Here especially, the doctor must guard against the family's communication pattern deteriorating into a tirade of blame and accusations leveled at one another. Family members should understand that they have a right to their feelings of anger and resentment and that in the interview these feelings can be expressed in some form other than blame and personal attack. Perls has accurately indicated that behind resentment is usually an unspoken demand. It may be helpful at this point, when family members are sharing resentful feelings with one another, to direct each to rephrase a specific resentment in the form of a particular request and encourage each to take responsibility for the self by using "I":

Father: (speaking to his wife) Number 3, Marion, on my resentment list, is that you're too unselfish — that goes for both of us.

Doctor: Be more specific.

Father: Well, she . . .

Doctor: Be more specific, but tell Marion directly.

Father: Well, you give 90% of your time and energy to the children. You and I only get 10%, if even that much.

Doctor: Rephrase your resentment in the form of a request to Marion, Elliott. Begin your sentence with the pronoun "I."

Father: I don't like our never having time together.

Doctor: Tell you what, I'd like you to do it once again — this time tell Marion what you *would* like from her, not what you don't like.

Father: I'd like us to have more time together, Marion.

In this situation the doctor has had to intervene four times in an effort to have Elliott transform his resentful statement into a specific request for which Elliott takes responsibility. The statement of resentment, if unchanged, would either stifle any further interchange or initiate a battle when Marion rises to her own defense. Elliott's specific request will at least provide room for a nondefensive response from Marion. The work would continue from this point, the interviewer helping Marion to respond in a nonthreatening, undefensive way and continuing to work with Elliott in making his request more specific, so that some agreement between the two of them could be made. For instance, how much time does Elliott want, and when, and doing what? Elliott will be directed to work out all of these toward a satisfactory conclusion of his diffuse opening line that began, "You're too unselfish."

The resentments that an individual lists about himself are often useful clues to the self-growth for which that person may be hoping. For instance, when someone writes about himself, "I don't show my feelings," often that person desires to bring that issue out in the open in hopes that he can, with help from others, become less fearful and more open in the expression of feelings. Listed self-resentments generally seem to be aspects of an individual's style that he would like to change by bringing them to light in the family discussion.

It should be apparent that this technique of listing "appreciations and resentments" among family members is particularly effective in supplying the interviewer with a wealth of diagnostic and potentially therapeutic material, especially in the realms of communication patterns, expression of feelings, and revelations about self-worth.

INTERVIEWER GOALS IN AN INITIAL INTERVIEW

Every family interview is different; no two ever unfold in exactly the same fashion. This does not mean, however, that a family interview is a haphazard event or that one should be conducted by simply gathering the family together in a room and then blindly hoping for the best. A successful interviewer will have a tentative plan even before the interview begins, and he will continue to elaborate specific goals for the interview as it gets underway and even as it ends. These specific goals to which we refer are those that arise from a study of and interaction with the family, its problem, and its system. They are the goals developed to help a family resolve the situation that has brought them into the doctor's office. Examples of such goals and plans are mentioned throughout the clinical examples presented elsewhere in this book.

There is still another level of goal planning that must take place in the interviewer's mind, particularly during his first encounter with a family. These plans, or goals, transcend the specific problem a family presents and hence have little *directly* to do with, for example, a child's refusal to take her insulin or persistent tension headaches in a 10-year-old about whom everyone in the family is concerned. They are goals that can be applied to any clinical interviewing situation, even those more traditional medical interviews that do not necessarily include a family unit. However, they are especially apt in preparing one's first interview with a family. They should be pursued regardless of the presenting complaint.

These goals, which we review with our trainees before their first interview experience, are as follows. An interviewer needs to: (1) establish that he will be in charge of the interview, (2) develop a beginning formulation of the problem (often unshared with the family initially) and a tentative treatment plan, (3) make the interview a "touching" experience for every family member, and (4) ensure the family's return, if this is indicated. A brief discussion of each of these goals follows.

Establishing who will be in charge

At first blush, it seems obvious that the interviewer will be in charge of the family interview; that is one of his jobs. Unfortunately the family does not always see it that way. Many of the struggles as family interviewing begins actually reflect a basic power struggle for control between the family and the doctor. Consider some of the clinical illustrations we have mentioned so far:

"Oh no, my husband couldn't possibly come."

"I wonder if you and Harry could have a little talk together—just the two of you."

"Even if my husband can't come, perhaps I could come in alone, Doctor."

"You're not going to give her a shot, are you? She hates needles."

These are all efforts by at least part of the family to control the interview situation. And there are many others. A family may reveal its control manipulations through its general behavior in the session:

A child who won't talk

A parent who won't be quiet

A child who won't sit still

Siblings who won't stop fighting

A family member who leaves the room

A family may also demonstrate its intent to control through specific communication methods in the interview:

A family member who speaks for someone else:

"Franklin won't talk, he hates doctors." (Of course, after this prophecy and expectation, Franklin doesn't talk.)

A family member who uses generalizations:

"Gregory, why do you *always* become sullen and difficult the minute we bring this up?" (Gregory, like Franklin, takes the cue and obliges with sullen and difficult behavior.)

A family member who attempts to "mind read":
"I think what you really want to know, Doctor, is whether Frances and I are having problems. Isn't that it?"

A family member who projects his own feelings onto others:
"The doctor is ashamed of you, Stacey."

A family member who cross-examines:
"When was the last time I reminded you about that? Huh? When? Was it on January 8, only 2 nights ago, just as we were ready to leave?"

A family member who attacks and depreciates something that another person stands for:
"Well, Doc, I suppose you feel this family interview is going to tell us something. Well, OK, I guess you should know. After all, you're the doctor. By the way, are you an intern or a real doctor?"

A family member who brings up the past:
"Doctor, I think it would probably help you to have a little background before we get started. Now 12 years ago, the child was only 3 months old, and my husband . . ."

A family member who use intimate knowledge against someone:
"Now, Gene, I know you didn't want me to tell the doctor this, but . . ."

The list could continue for pages. Families are ingenious in their often extraordinary efforts to wrest control of the session from the interviewer. Generally the family's motives do not have an evil origin. They are quite simply frightened—frightened about their "problem," frightened about exposure, frightened about the unknowns of the interviewer and the interview process itself. Exerting control is one way of holding on to the "known."

No matter what the family's motivations are, however, the doctor must win this power struggle if his work with them is to be successful. A family interview in which the family exerts its control over the interviewer is an invitation to disorder and chaos. This is most clearly experienced in an encounter with the sort of family that we have come to call an "uproar" family. Successful interviewing with an "uproar" family is helped if one has nerves of steel and a definite air of sangfroid. Such families do appear in the doctor's office, and once seen they are seldom forgotten. Take the Martins, for instance.

The Martins had asked for some counseling help with their 10-year-old son, David, a boy with a learning disability and an explosive temper. Apparently he was always in hot water, at home and at school. His mother was worried and depressed; his father traveled a lot and was seldom home. There were three siblings: Michael, 12, Rebecca, 14, and Susan, 16. The entire family arrived a little early for their scheduled appointment. Their presence in the waiting room was immediately felt. The four children quickly launched a joint assault on the furniture of the waiting area. Fortunately both the room and the furniture were momentarily empty. Chairs, tables, and lamps were rearranged; magazines were rolled up and transformed into jousting rods, and the kids began to have at one another. The receptionist's effort to settle them was only momentarily successful. Within a few minutes they were fighting again. In one corner of the waiting room Mrs. Martin sat disconsolately, never looking up, trying very hard to find meaning in our office copy of *Curious George Goes to the Circus*. Mr. Martin occasionally roared at the children from his vantage point beside the fish tank. However, he was no more successful in restoring order than the receptionist had been. The doctor then collected the group to begin the family interview, ushering them into the room. His not preceding them was a mistake, for between the first and last family member's entrance, before the doctor was in the room, one of the kids had turned off the tape recorder, another was holding his head under the office faucet getting a drink, and a third was pinching the fourth. Mrs. Martin slid into the nearest chair and actually shifted very little from her previous posture in the waiting room; indeed she was still carrying that book. She continued to say nothing while Mr. Martin roared at the children to behave. They did not heed him.

Families such as the Martins, while perhaps entertaining to describe, are horrendous to work with in an interview itself. As long as they are out of control themselves and thereby controlling the interview process, nothing very productive can happen in the encounter. Their unusual degree of frenzy and confusion may call for equally strong measures on the therapist's part. He may refuse to proceed with them until order is restored, or he can direct the parents to bring their children into line, halting the interview until this has been accomplished and acknowledging to himself that such a step may take the entire session. All will not be lost, however, for he will see played out before him all of the family's difficulties with clear communication around the issue of limit setting, and these observations will be useful in subsequent work, if there is any, with the family. Then he may decide that the entire family cannot continue to be interviewed together and choose to interview subsystems in the family, either parents alone, or children alone, or parents with certain children. Other family members of the interviewer's choosing are then excluded and ushered, bodily by the parents if necessary, from the interview room.

The Martins, while relatively typical of an uproar family, represent an extreme in the issue of control between interviewer and family. Most families are not as flamboyant in their desire to control the situation. What these families lack in drama they more than compensate for in subtlety and effectiveness. A family's control manipulations consist of behaviors that its members are using with one another daily, and each family member has developed his own repertoire into a finely practiced and almost automatic skill. These same control manipulations are turned toward the therapist in the first interview, as he begins to work toward helping the family change its system.

Control manipulations may be either active or passive in nature. The active ones are easier to identify and deal with in an interview situation. Those of a more passive nature require considerable vigilance by the interviewer, if he is to spot them and avoid being manipulated by them.

Those who control through active means are often one of the following:

The Judge:	This individual blames
	accuses
	distrusts
	says "I told you so"
The Bully:	This individual threatens
	humiliates
	argues
	insults
	is sarcastic
	name calls
The Calculator:	This individual deceives
	lies
	tries to outwit
	uses pressure tactics
	blackmails
	bribes
	makes false promises

The Dictator: This individual gives unilateral solutions
gives orders
suppresses
bosses

Those who control through passive manipulations are more likely to be in one of these categories:

The Protector: This individual exaggerates his support
is nonjudgmental to a fault
is oversympathetic
"spoils" others
cares only for others and not for himself
says, "I'm only doing it for your own good"

The Nice Guy: This individual exaggerates caring and loving
is overkind
is always aiming to please
never asks for what he wants himself
apologizes prematurely and unnecessarily
appeases and smoothes over

The Clinging Vine: This individual wants to be taken care of
lets others do his work
cries
plays helpless and confused
demands attention
complains
is easily fooled

The Weakling: This individual exaggerates his sensitivity and is
easily hurt
forgets
doesn't hear
is passively silent
gives up
worries
withdraws

The Intellectualizer: This individual explains and rationalizes
stays with facts, not feelings
uses words to impress and create distance
quotes opinions and authorities

If an interviewer is to remain in charge of the interview process, he must be ready when any of the preceding control manipulations are directed his way. He must stand his ground so that, in the words of Carl Whitaker, "the family members are in charge of themselves, while the interviewer is in charge of the session."[9] That they may accomplish this, we urge trainees to do whatever is required to provide for their own working comfort in the session. We have earlier referred to it as "taking care of oneself" in the interview. If an interviewer feels secure in paying attention to his own needs and establishing the circumstances under which he can best work, he will very likely be in control of the interview. This can mean different things for different interviewers and different families, yet in each instance it will boil down to one essential: it is the interviewer's responsibility and not the family's to determine the rules of the session. The rules may concern the room, the family's communication within that room, or other aspects of family behavior while in the room. The interviewer may want to share such rules explicitly with the family as he begins. Rules may also be introduced as the need arises. Examples of rules often used in family interviews are:

No blaming is allowed.

One person at a time may talk.

The past is not to be discussed; discussion stays in the present, in the "here and now."

The children may play with the available toys; they may not use them as weapons.

Individuals may not run around the room.

The room equipment is off limits.

Each person speaks for himself. No one speaks for someone else.

An interviewer should direct the parents to establish and maintain order with their own children. However, order in the session is ultimately the physician's responsibility. Should the parents be "unable" to bring their children under control, once again the physician must look to his own needs as a guide for his next action. If an 11-month-old infant brought to the session simply won't be quiet long enough to allow a sustained conversation with the rest of the family, and it is clear to the doctor that he cannot conduct the interview, either he should arrange for the child to be cared for outside the interview room by available office staff, or he should terminate the session. Taking care of oneself means knowing under what conditions one is comfortable working and also under what conditions one is unwilling to continue.

Developing a beginning formulation and treatment plan

The goal of developing a beginning formulation and treatment plan goes almost without saying. Trainees are usually clear that figuring out what's going on in a family and helping the family learn what to do about it is the interviewer's business. Perhaps it is important to stress that in an initial visit with a family, a *beginning* formulation is called for. Conclusions must be kept tentative and available for alteration, since both diagnostic formulations and treatment plans are in a state of flux as the family continues with time to provide the therapist with additional information about their systems and their problem. Usually one will not have all the pieces of the puzzle by the end of an initial interview. No more than a beginning formulation is even possible. After all, a family is a very complex and intricate set of relationships. Not only that, specific family members may be withholding important information from disclosure in the session. Therefore not only may these pieces of the puzzle be missing, but the puzzle itself may change; hence the interviewer should keep in mind that his beginning formulations will need testing, perhaps changing, or even discarding when circumstances warrant.

Nonetheless beginning formulations are important, since they will determine early therapeutic interventions with the family, and interventions of some kind must begin quickly. Families seek the doctor's assistance because they are in distress and pain. If one does not set about alleviating some distress within the first session, chances are quite good that the family will lose hope in the process and in the interviewer. They may not return. We believe it is important that the family members leave the session with the distinct feeling that they have received something from the doctor. It is also important for the doctor to feel he has been able to give something of value to the family. The implementation of a beginning therapeutic plan is one means for helping a family feel they are receiving something from the visit: The doctor may propose a task for the family. Or he may begin in the first interview to challenge existing communication styles and teach the family more functional ways of communication, to the relief of some family members. Or the doctor may intervene in the family's structure and begin to disrupt accustomed coalitions and alliance. Any of these are evidence that interventions have started with the family, and the group will feel that they are receiving something more than good advice.

Therefore developing a tentative treatment plan and beginning to use it quickly with the family is important. However, we have some hesitation in suggesting this to physicians, particularly pediatricians. Since we are in the field of pediatrics, we understand the pediatrician's well-developed tendency to offer *something* to patients quickly. It is partly in the nature of the clinician to do so, and it is partly a characteristic of pediatrics itself that children's medical problems often call for rapid and decisive action. We would therefore not like the pediatrician to use our suggestions (that families need to leave the first session feeling that they "received something") as support for a style that promotes "getting them in, getting it solved, getting them out." We mention it because we often encounter such an approach in the beginning family work of our pediatric resident trainees. In their zeal to help a child and his family, they often forge ahead with advice and directive solutions long before the family is able to act on or even understand such advice:

> *Doctor:* You folks are just going to have to be more firm.
>
> *Mother:* Well, I . . .
>
> *Father:* That's what I keep telling her, Doc.
>
> *Mother:* But Frank, you don't understand.
>
> *Doctor:* Fire-setting is a serious problem, Mrs. Anderson. Do you realize, Dwayne, you could have set the garage on fire!
>
> *Dwayne:* It was only a Coke bottle full of kerosene.
>
> *Doctor:* No matter. I want you to promise your parents right now you will not do that again—ever.
>
> *Dwayne:* (silence)
>
> *Doctor:* Now come on, Dwayne. Your parents and I can't leave today until this gets settled. Be reasonable. Think about what could have happened.
>
> *Father:* Sit up and listen to the doctor, Dwayne.
>
> *Mother:* He's so upset.

The advice itself may be accurate and the directive necessary, but it all happens so fast and with such persistence on the resident's part that the family feels they have been programmed and categorized rather than heard. They usually don't return, and the resident feels frustrated that his advice was not followed. In all likelihood the resident's therapeutic urge to make things better and solve the problem in one fell swoop overwhelmed his attention to our suggestion that, solutions aside, he must also take care to make the interview a "touching" experience for each family member. Unfortunately without having attended to this very important matter first, he has found that no well-intentioned and even correct solution will work. Hence our third general goal for an initial interview presents itself.

Making the interview a "touching" experience

One of the most important "somethings" that a family member can take from the first interview is a feeling of relief based on a certain awareness that the physician has heard, understood, and acknowledged his distress. The patient feels heard and "touched." If possible every family member should leave the initial interview with this impression. Such feelings of relief will have a direct impact on a person's level of hopefulness regarding change, on his willingness to work diligently on issues, and, as already mentioned, on his desire to return for future sessions.

To facilitate these feelings in every family member is hard work for the interviewer, especially if the family is large. Nonetheless, one should spend sufficient time with each family member, particularly in the first session, so that each of them has the opportunity to say, at least to himself: "This doctor is listening to me, seems interested in me, and even understands some of what I am feeling inside." That awareness alone may be enough to bring individuals back for a second session when this is indicated.

The techniques for "touching" family members in this way are varied, hugely dependent on an interviewer's personal style and his own means for expressing empathy toward others. Regardless of style, however, one may be guided by this internal thought as he works to touch each family member: "As this family member is talking about _____, what is he/she experiencing inside?" Once that question is answered, the next becomes: "Now, how do I let him/her know that I see and can appreciate those feelings?" A similar mental process must be repeated with each person in the room. The actual touching process, once these questions have been answered, is straightforward and uncomplicated. For example, some acknowledgement of understanding regarding an individual's underlying feelings is expressed:

"Gee, that's tough."
"You look very worried."
"What an awful spot to be in."
"Your eyes look pleased as you tell me that."
"How frustrating."
"Are you feeling pretty helpless about that?"

These communications "touch" the feelings of another. They are the ways in which an interviewer communicates that he has picked up what the family member is experiencing. They are essential in order that the family develop trust in the interviewer as a person who hears. Ironically, until the family sees the doctor as someone who hears, they themselves will be unable to listen. Conversely, as the doctor shows that he hears, family members begin to listen — to him and to one another.

Ensuring the family's return

Generally if the second and third goals have been attended to, the fourth, having the family come back, follows automatically. If an interviewer has been successful in beginning a therapeutic program with the family, and if he has been able to touch most of the family members (especially the parents and the identified patient), the family will return. We are assuming, of course, that a return visit is indicated; most often more than one session is required. There are times when, although a follow-up session appears necessary, the interviewer for various reasons has not been able to offer a beginning treatment plan nor has he yet effectively touched the necessary family members. Under these circumstances it is probably best to make a clean breast of the situation in a statement such as the following:

> *Doctor:* Our time is just about up, and I am feeling very frustrated. You must be feeling it even more. This family came in for some help, and you've not gotten to any solutions yet. I know from what you have said that you were hoping for some specific answers to come out of this session today. Frankly, I feel you and I need more time to understand your difficulties. There are no immediate answers to your dilemma. And frustrating as that may sound, I am asking that you come in again in 5 days so that you and I may continue working on the problem.

This sort of bridge at least demonstrates that the interviewer has heard the family's desire for instant answers. His acknowledgement of their wish and his honesty as to what he can provide may be sufficient to have the family suspend a decision that returning would be useless. In this situation the interviewer will be helped if during the interview he has been able to "touch" even one family member.

ENDING THE INTERVIEW

Good endings, like good beginnings, require planning. We do not feel that an interview should simply ooze to a termination. Neither should it end abruptly because, to use a phrase, "Our time is up." Rather a family interview should be led to a conclusion by the interviewer. Each interviewer must decide—probably differently in each interview—how much time will be required for the winding-up process. The following may be included in that winding-up process:

1. Reviewing the presenting problem with the family
2. Offering a specific directive or task, short or long
3. Planning the next appointment time
4. Selecting the family cast for the next appointment
5. Discussing the expected duration of the therapy process
6. Settling fee issues
7. Providing the family time to recoup after a very unsettling session
8. Discussing what the family and/or the doctor is to do between sessions (for example, contact school authorities)

There may be others, but the point is already clear. One must allow sufficient time with the family to settle important items such as those listed above. It is a useful idea to take stock silently of the interview at the halfway point, 30 minutes after beginning if the session is an hour, and plan how one would like to finish in another 30 minutes. Frequently bringing the interview to a satisfactory conclusion will take half of the remaining half hour. One should remember that a good ending to the interview is also an influence in determining a family's return. As Minuchin states (p. 212): "All therapeutic interventions must be made with the clear knowledge that the first rule of therapeutic strategy is to leave the family willing to come again for the next session."[3]

REFERENCES

1. Bing, E.: The conjoint family drawing, Family Process **9:**173, 1970.
2. Haley, J.: Problem-solving therapy: new strategies for effective family therapy, San Francisco, 1976, Jossey-Bass, Inc.
3. Minuchin, S.: Families and family therapy, Cambridge, Mass., 1974, Harvard University Press.
4. Mosher, L., and Kwiatkowska, H.: Family art evaluation: use in families with schizophrenic twins, J. Nerv. Ment. Dis. **153:**165, 1971.
5. Papp, P.: Family sculpture in preventive work with "well families," Family Process **12:**197, 1973.
6. Rubin, J., and Magnussen, M.: Family art evaluation, Family Process **13:**185, 1974.
7. Simon, R.: Sculpting the family, Family Process **11:**49, 1972.
8. Wadeson, H.: Conjoint marital art therapy techniques, Psychiatry **35:**89, 1972.
9. Whitaker, C.: Personal communication, 1975.

CHAPTER 7

Common behavioral problems

In this chapter we will be discussing common behavioral problems and their treatment by a physician. One may easily slip into conceptualizing behavioral problems in children as discrete "disease" entities that either exist or do not exist, in much the same fashion as pharyngitis; it is either present or it is absent. A sore throat is a sore throat; there is nothing relative about it. However, a behavioral problem is not always a behavioral problem. Let us explain. The physician can surely remember instances when, observing the behavior of someone else's child in the office, this thought has come to mind: "Whew, if that kid were mine, I would be going absolutely crazy!" One's discomfort may be that the child takes "forever" to feel comfortable in new situations, that is, the office; or one may be troubled by the youngster's seemingly excessive persistence. Yet the parents are not particularly worried; indeed they are not even cognizant of the child's behavior that the clinician finds maddeningly difficult. In the doctor's household the child would be a "problem." In the child's own he is not; in some way his behavior fits, meshes with that of his family, and is not problematical. Conversely a physician may recall other times when a youngster has been particularly appealing in some manner. Perhaps the child, like the doctor, is regular as clockwork in all aspects of his functioning, or maybe the doctor enjoys the child's intense, aggressive approach to almost every situation presented. But the parents, far from appreciating such characteristics, are exasperated and dissatisfied with their child's behavior. Complaining, scolding, they are worried about their "problem" child, while the pediatrician would like to take him home for keeps. For him there is no "problem" in the child's behavior.

149

BEHAVIORAL INDIVIDUALITY IN CHILDREN

We have made earlier references to the work of Chess and co-workers.[3] They have shed welcome light on this phenomenon. Their work, beginning in the 1950's with an extensive longitudinal study of children's individual behavior, provided documentation for two essential and basic concepts.

1. Each child has his own specific, individual behavioral and temperamental style, detectable in the first week of life and perhaps persistent throughout the child's subsequent development. Such characteristics, present so early in the child's life, appear to be one of that child's innate contributions to his environment and may often determine his reactions to imposed parental and environmental influences. Parenting approaches can thus take neither total credit nor total blame for many of a child's behavioral characteristics.

2. An understanding of children's behavior cannot be obtained through scrutiny of these specific temperamental characteristics if they are taken alone, nor can such understanding occur by an exclusive focus on the parents and their influences on their children. Behavior becomes understandable through clarification of the *interaction* between a *particular* child and a *particular* set of parents:

Not only does the child screen his environment, he also influences it. Thus it is not alone the parents who influence the child, but the child who influences the parents. The child, by his own nature, "conditions" his environment at the same time that the social and cultural environment affects him. In short, there is a continual effect produced by the child on his world, as well as by his world upon him.*

Numerous excellent clinical examples demonstrating the interaction of nature *and* nurture as an important determinant of children's behavior are to be found in the written work of these investigators. We paraphrase one here for illustration:

Ralph and Jerry, from different families, were very much alike as babies. In any new situation their initial reaction was to back off quietly. With each new experience, the first bath, the first new food, a new per-

---

*Chess, S., and others: Your child is a person: a psychological approach to parenthood without guilt, New York, 1972, Viking Press, p. 21.

son handling them, they either turned solemn or quietly refused to participate. Both children would turn away from a new food or let it dribble out of their mouth. When older, each might run behind mother's back if a strange person greeted him. However, after tasting the new food over and over again, or seeing the new person many times, both children would gradually come to accept the innovation. In short, both boys took a long time to warm up.

By the time they were 5 years old, however, the two children behaved very differently. Ralph was a well-adjusted member of his kindergarten group. He looked forward to going to school, greeted his playmates pleasantly, and visited back and forth with friends after school. Ralph's parents had come to understand very early that his hesitancy about accepting the unfamiliar needed to be honored. They found that rushing him didn't work. They provided him with the necessary time and warming-up period in new situations.

Jerry's early functioning was much like Ralph's. His parents, too, didn't rush him. They didn't care how long it took him to begin to eat solid food or change from four to three feedings a day. But his mother's attitude changed when she started to take Jerry to the neighborhood playground, and he reacted to the new situation and strange faces by holding back and clinging. She was sure that other mothers in the playground were blaming her for having such an "anxiously" timid baby. They probably were. Instead of holding him or giving him a familiar toy to play with until he warmed up to the new setting, she began to push him insistently to play "like the other little boys." The more she pressured, the more he clung. Finally, she gave up taking him to the playground at all and avoided placing him in new situations if possible. When Jerry entered kindergarten, he cried and clung again. In class he rarely spoke above a whisper. Before school each morning he clung to his mother. He had, in fact, become the anxious fearful child his mother dreaded.

From birth on, both Ralph and Jerry were examples of what Chess and co-workers refer to as the child who is "slow to warm up." That particular behavioral attribute was clearly handled quite differently by the parents of each boy. It becomes apparent then that the particular mix of a child's own temperament and that of his parents determines many aspects of behavioral development and often whether or not a "behavioral problem" will arise.

Chess and Thomas say it this way:

Normal and deviant development is at all times the result of a continuously evolving interaction between a child with his individual characteristics and significant features of his intrafamilial and extrafamilial environment. The temperament is only one attribute of the growing child — albeit a highly significant attribute — and must at all times be considered in its internal relations with abilities and motives and in its external relations with environmental opportunities and stresses.*

This view has considerable common-sense appeal. It is also tremendously reassuring to mothers and fathers, providing them with some relief from the traditional finger of blame arising from the view that a child's behavior, good or bad, is his parents' fault. Psychoanalytic theory has been particularly hard on mothers. Dr. Hilde Bruch, herself trained in psychoanalysis, empathizes with the plight of parents:

Modern parent education . . . implies that parents are all-responsible and must assume the role of playing preventive Fate for their children . . . An unrelieved picture of model parental behavior, a contrived image of artificial perfection and happiness, is held up before parents who try valiantly to reach the ever receding ideal of 'good parenthood,' like dogs after a mechanical rabbit.†

In this orientation, when problems in a child arise, a parent inevitably must feel responsible.

The work of Chess and colleagues clearly has as one of its purposes the alleviation of parental guilt engendered by such an approach. Indeed their publication for parents, *Your Child is a Person,* is subtitled, *A Psychological Approach to Parenthood Without Guilt.* We feel they have succeeded in this regard, and they have made a major contribution to the understanding of children's behavior and its determinants.

They found that infants' behavior could be accurately classified under nine headings:

Activity level. Some babies were from early infancy onward much more active than others.

Biological regularity. Babies were found to differ significantly in the

---

*Chess, S., and Thomas, A.: Temperamental individuality from childhood to adolescence, J. Am. Acad. Child Psychiatry **16:**218, 1977.
†Chess, S., and others: Your child is a person: a psychological approach to parenthood without guilt, New York, 1972, Viking Press, pp. 5-6.

regularity of their biological functioning (feeding, sleeping, bowel and bladder function, crying).

Approach or withdrawal as a characteristic response to a new situation. Regarding the child's initial reaction to any new stimulus pattern, be it food, people, places, toys, or procedures, they found that some babies easily accepted these new experiences, while others pulled away.

Adaptability to change in routine. Some babies shifted easily and quickly with changing schedules. In general they changed their behavior to fit in with the new routine the mother wanted to set. Others accommodated more slowly to change.

Level of sensory threshold. Babies with a high "sensory threshold" did not startle at loud noises or bright lights. They did not react to being wet or soiled, for instance. At the other extreme were babies who cried the moment they soiled. A slight sound would attract their attention; they would wake the moment the light was switched on.

Positive or negative mood. Some children cried when they woke up or were put down, and they just generally fussed. Others predominantly cooed, gurgled happily, and smiled.

Intensity of response (in terms of the amount of physical energy displayed). Some babies greeted hunger with loud, piercing cries. Others cried softly. These differences were often apparent in other aspects of their behavior as well. Some babies demonstrated tremendous energy in responses to both painful and pleasurable activities while others showed less energy and were more gentle and less vigorous.

Distractibility. Some babies seemed able to concentrate better than others on feeding or staring at a mobile, for instance, no matter what else was going on around them.

Persistence and attention span. Babies demonstrated great variation in the ability to continue an activity in the face of difficulties or to resume it after interruption.

• • •

The authors referred to the child's preponderant pattern of functioning in these nine categories as the child's temperament.

There is nothing mysterious about temperament. It merely represents a statement of the basic style which characterizes a person's behavior. Some students of behavior have divided psychological functioning into three parts which they call the what, the why, and the how. The what refers to the content of behavior, including intelligence, skills, aptitudes, and talents. The why relates to motivation, or the reasons for behaving in a given way. The how refers to temperament—the manner in which the what and the why are expressed.*

It should be stated also that the usual variability shown by infants and children in these nine categories all reflect normal, healthy functioning. A child who is characteristically negative in his mood and very intense in his response to situations is not necessarily abnormal. Granted he may not have a lot of friends in the sandbox, but his behavior may simply be a reflection of his own specific behavioral repertoire, his temperament. One temperamental style is not better or more normal than another; styles are simply different from one another. Some are easier for parents to manage than others.

Sometimes (in 7% to 10% of babies according to these investigators[4]) a child does demonstrate a specific selection of behaviors from the nine categories, which wins him the dubious title of a "difficult child." Such a child, partly because of his temperamental style, may be more at risk for the onset of behavioral problems than his temperamentally different peers, according to Chess and co-workers. This child demonstrates irregularity in biological functions, especially in the newborn period. He does not establish definite hunger and sleeping patterns that are predictable from day to day. He does not have regular bowel movements. He tends to have withdrawal reactions to new stimuli and situations. In addition he is not easily adaptable, and almost every change in his routine involves a struggle and his own very high intensity of response. Even though this temperamental pattern may smooth out as the youngster grows older, such behavior as an infant can be particularly troublesome, especially for a new mother who could easily, yet erroneously, assume from the above collection of behaviors that something is drastically wrong with her mothering. The combination of irregularity, slow adaptability, withdrawal reactions, high intensity of response, and predominantly negative mood can be perplexing to handle. However, even in youngsters with this temperamental style, the authors stress that they could find no evidence that mothers or fathers of these "difficult" babies were responsible for the child's mode of behavior.

The authors also describe another category, that of the "easy child." Temperamentally this child is regular in his biological functions, is mod-

*Chess, S., and others: Your child is a person: a psychological approach to parenthood without guilt, New York, 1972, Viking Press, p. 32.

erately active, adapts to change quite well, seems always happy, is not particularly intense, yet is not distractible and can persist long enough to complete a task. He is almost always charming, seen as easily adaptable and wanting to please. The combination conjures up notions of a parent's and babysitter's dream, and that is often the case but not always. Chess and colleagues cited one example of such a "model" child who stimulated her parents to accept indiscriminately the child's every move. The result was a child who by age 3 knew how to be charming but very little about how to work and play with others. Those outside the immediate family found her "babyish and immature." Her social style had not progressed much beyond that of infancy.

We have mentioned this concept of behavioral individuality in some detail because we see it as an important variable for consideration by the doctor who chooses to work with families concerning common behavioral problems. Recognition by the doctor of a child's temperamental pattern as it differs from that of the parents and assistance in helping the parents to understand and work more effectively with their child's pattern can be tremendously helpful.

For instance, Chess and co-workers[4] report the case of a mother who had failed to wean or toilet train her 3-year-old daughter or even leave her alone with anyone else for an evening because she "didn't believe in making issues over the crucial steps in development." When it came time for nursery school, the mother found that her daughter would have to be toilet trained to be accepted. The mother became panicky and asked for help from Dr. Chess. The child's temperamental pattern was characterized by biological irrgularity, mild intensity of response, and easy adaptability. It seemed to the authors that, given these characteristics, if her mother had set a schedule for her, she would have been a model child by 3 rather than a whiny child around whose demands the whole family revolved. It also appeared that she could still be readily trained by firm scheduling and consistent handling. Mother was desperate and agreed. By the time nursery school began, the child was trained. In this case an understanding of the child's behavioral pattern suggested appropriate measures for both the doctor and the parents to take.

Hence, along with dysfunctional communication, family alliances, coalitions, homeostasis, predictable family sequences, and so on, the family interviewer can also take into account a child's individual temperament and its impact on the family constellation. It is one additional view of the child, of the family, of the situation that together with other observations will ultimately suggest appropriate therapeutic directions for the interviewer to follow.

PROBLEMS FREQUENTLY ENCOUNTERED

As the pediatric clinician is often painfully aware, in his waiting room there may be as many children with "discipline problems" as those with fever and earaches. Members of both groups are frequent visitors in the office. At a subsequent visit within 2 weeks, the child with an earache, thanks to antibiotics, some aspirin, and a few days home from school, is usually well on the road to recovery. The child looks well, the mother looks relieved, and the doctor looks like a miracle worker. Everyone smiles. The episode is closed. However, the child with difficult behavior, seen originally on the same day as the child with the now-resolving ear infection, has had seven separate temper tantrums at home in the past 2 weeks and is about to experience his eighth in the office waiting area. In this situation no one smiles, and the episode is far from closed.

From this one may then conclude two things: (1) in pediatrics, common behavior problems such as temper tantrums are just that — extremely common — and (2) they often do not disappear as rapidly as everyone would wish; they have a way of being devilishly persistent. The doctor is very often the *first* professional to be consulted in such situations. A "discipline problem" is not the only entity to which we are referring. Parents regularly come to the doctor for advice and counsel concerning any of the following behavioral symptoms in their children:

1. "Minding" and discipline
    The child just won't mind
    steals
    lies
    has been setting fires
2. Sleep
    The child won't sleep in her own bed or alone
    is having nightmares
    won't go to bed
3. Eating
    The child is eating too much
    won't eat enough
    won't eat the right foods

4. School
The child has failing grades
won't go to school
won't behave in school
5. Getting along with others
The child fights with other children
won't play with other children — is a loner
doesn't get along with adults or authority figures
is frightened of boys, or girls, or adults, or dogs

It would be appealing, having broken down these everyday concerns into categories, to proceed now in cookbook fashion with separate recommendations for working in each category — appealing, but impossible. Human beings, and especially children, have never put up with anyone's attempts to categorize them. Thus there is no single correct approach or method to use for "the child who refuses to go to sleep at night," or for "the child who eats too much," or for "the youngster who is always in fights with peers." Defining a child's symptoms alone will not define the necessary therapeutic approach. The doctor will do better to help family members become aware of their particular system of communication and interaction with one another, since it is often this interaction (along with differences in neurodevelopmental maturation and behavioral individuality) that most directly contributes to the development of symptoms for which the child is being seen. Figure out the family system, its meaning and purpose, and one will usually figure out the problem and very often its resolution.

Our previous clinical examples have illustrated the use of this maxim in work with common behavioral problems. In the case of Joan Locksley (Chapter 1), she was not sleeping; that was her symptom. But it would have made little difference had her grandmother instead complained that Joan wouldn't eat or wouldn't mind — little difference, that is, in terms of the pediatrician's eventual direction with Joan and the family. In any case he would still have proceeded by helping the family to understand and then wish to alter its existing system, structure, and pattern of communication with one another, no matter what symptom Joan was presenting. The same holds true for Jennifer Maloney (Chapter 3) and her colorful collection of symptoms: "night terrors," school avoidance, enuresis. A different array would not have altered the therapeutic direction followed by her pediatrician. It was the family system of communication regarding unspoken feelings and fears that required scrutiny and alteration by the family, not the symptom per se. Do not misunderstand: recognition and understanding of the dynamics and purpose of the symptom by the interviewer has its important place in family work. It will often suggest specific therapeutic interventions such as the choice of a particular task assignment given to a family. We are not of the opinion that symptoms should not be discussed in the interview with the parents; nothing seems to offend and alienate troubled families more quickly than such a rule. Families come to the doctor for specific help with a specific problem. Total disregard for their concern by the interviewer or refusal to discuss their stated problem generally sends the family packing and understandably so. The symptom does need to be discussed, but it is a rare circumstance in which a focus on the specific symptom alone will dictate the course of treatment. Gaining an awareness of the family interactions will, however, furnish the necessary diagnostic information and therapeutic direction.

Hence, we will not illustrate the previous list now with a separate clinical example of treatment for each symptom listed. Such an endeavor would be tiresome and misleading: tiresome because the same principles would be reiterated from case to case and misleading because it would suggest we recommend that one proceed in such and such a fashion with a noneater, while the therapeutic direction should be thus and so for a withdrawn loner. Not so. More often than not the symptom presented by a child is merely the "ticket of entry" used by that child and his family to come to the doctor's office and seek assistance.

Instead, we would like to illustrate the use of family treatment in common pediatric behavior problems by arbitrarily selecting one symptom from the above list and discussing in some detail our clinical work with a family who sought help because of that particular symptom. Our arbitrary selection is that of a child who "just won't mind." While the specifics of this family's situation are certainly unique to them, the principles used by the pediatrician in helping them would apply in many other clinical encounters, with the same or with a different common behavioral complaint.

THE THOMAS FAMILY

A friend and fellow pediatrician, Dr. Tom Jones, called asking to refer to the Child Study Unit a child and family for help. He had known of the unit's interest in using family approaches with pediatric problems and often asked for such assistance; indeed, having trained in the unit, he occasionally did family interviews in his office. This family, however, for reasons that are not even remembered now, he chose to refer. Dr. Jones indicated on the phone that the family was concerned about their 4-year-old who "won't mind." He followed up his phone call with this letter:

> I am sending Andrew Thomas and his parents to you for consultation regarding his behavior. This nearly 4-year-old child is a happy, alert, quite verbal youngster who has seemed quite advanced for his years. He is the Thomas's only child. There have been relatively few medical problems except for an episode some months ago of what seems to have been ketotic hypogylcemia, which was appropriately treated with IV glucose and responded well to dietary changes; he has had no further episodes since then. The parents are both professional dancers who lead a somewhat busy life. At the current time they are *very* frustrated about his behavior, that is, his unwillingness to accept any limits or to "behave." They are wondering if he is abnormal in any way—developmentally and emotionally. I would appreciate your comments regarding Andy and the family situation.
>
> With best personal regards,
>
> Thomas Jones, M.D.

Mrs. Thomas subsequently called for an appointment and readily accepted the stipulation that the entire family come for the first interview. A suitable time was arranged. The pediatrician kept the call brief and did not encourage her to discuss in any detail the family's concerns. For the most part she complied. She sounded both frustrated and amused by her son's obstinancy:

Mother: (laughing) He's such a little devil, Dr. Anderson. I just don't know what to do with him (exasperated sigh).

The doctor heard both sides of her message but chose not to comment on the discrepancy. He acknowledged her frustration and filed away his observation of the double-level message for future use, should the family and he get together eventually.

Session no. 1. The family and pediatrician met as scheduled 1 week after the initial call. The family arrived 15 minutes late for their first appointment. Their entrance into the office reminded the doctor of nothing so much as a processional. Andy led the group. He was only 4 years old, but he seemed to swagger into the room. The doctor greeted him; Andy gave him a long, careful look, and then glided straightaway over to the toys in the office.

> *Andy:* Oooooooooo Mom, look at the toys!

He settled himself on the rug and began to explore the array of play materials kept for such purposes — all of this before his parents were quite in the room. They were following closely behind, however — Mrs. Thomas, breathless, held out her hand, greeted the doctor, introduced herself, and apologized, all simultaneously:

> *Mother:* HelloDr.AndersonI'mCarlasorrywe'relategotheldupintraffiicthisis myhusbandRod . . . andAndy . . . Sayhellotothedoctordearyes aren'tthosenicetoys! Oh! (spilling her purse as she shook hands with the doctor) Isn'tthatthelimithowclumsy!

Mr. Thomas brought up the rear of the procession: he too was breathless, sweeping up after his wife and maneuvering the family group into the office.

They were visually an interesting group. The child was lithe and handsome, wearing new clothes, and looking spic and span. Dr. Tom Jones had said that the parents were both dancers; they looked as though they were ready for a performance of some sort even now. Father was tall and solidly built; he was dressed in a shirt open to the navel. His pants were tucked into knee-length boots, and he was wearing a necklace. Mother, very attractive, had a similar outfit, although her shirt was buttoned. Her makeup was very dramatic; this, together with very wide eyes and a flamboyant hair style, suggested to the doctor the appearance of Raggedy Ann. They were a decidedly interesting family in appearance, and the doctor relaxed, thinking that no matter what happened, this would be fun for him.

Mrs. Thomas completed the retrieval of her purse contents and sat down. Her husband also shook the doctor's hand and took a seat beside his wife. Andy continued to play close by in view of his parents and the interviewer.

> *Doctor:* I spoke with Dr. Jones on the phone; however, I don't have very much of the story. What help would this family like from me?
>
> *Father:* We're not sure if we even have a problem, but we thought . . .
>
> *Mother:* Oh we do, at least *I* do. Andy is just really a handful.
>
> *Doctor:* Explain, Mrs. Thomas.
>
> *Mother:* What do you do, Dr. Anderson, with a child who refuses to stay in

	his seat belt in the car—while you're driving on the middle of the freeway!
Doctor:	(acknowledging the feeling that he heard in her tone of voice) That sounds frightening. How have you handled the situation?
Andy:	(coming over to his mother's chair and putting a toy in her lap) How does this work, Mom?
Mother:	(allowing the interview to be interrupted) It's a puzzle, dear; you put the green piece right in that little slot. No, not like that. Here, I'll show you. There, that's it. Now the red one. Where do you think that goes? Gooooood. Isn't that a fun puzzle? Maybe we could get one like that sometime.
Andy:	(returns to toy shelf and deposits a second item in his mother's lap) Show me this one; show me!
Mother:	All right—why Andy, this is exactly like the one at nursery school . . . You know how that one goes.
Father:	Don't interrupt your mother, son. She and the doctor were talking.
Mother:	He's just so excited by all these toys. You little dickens—are you bringing me another one? Mother's going to run out of lap room.

Discounting the introductory banter as the family entered the room, there had been thus far only twelve lines of dialogue. However, many useful observations were noted.

1. The family was quite lively; their entrance suggested they were also somewhat disorganized.
2. Andy literally led the way in this family, during and *after* their entry into the office.
3. Mother and father were not in agreement regarding even the need for concern, nor were they united in their way of guiding their son.
4. Mother suggested that it was she who felt helpless with her son.
5. Mother allowed and even encouraged Andy to control with interruptions in this situation; she made no attempt to assert her own needs.
6. Father spoke *for* his wife in correcting his son, suggesting that father too saw her as helpless and unable to take care of her own needs in exchanges with Andy.
7. Father was disregarded by both his wife and Andy for his efforts.

There was no single correct way to proceed now. The interviewer could do one of several things. He could encourage mother to set some limits on Andy's interruptions; he could point out her subtle encouragement of Andy's interruptions (through her enthusiasm and interest). He could mention her immediate readiness to drop her own needs and train of thought in the face of Andy's enthusiastic maneuvers. He could challenge father's speaking for his wife and introduce the rule that in the session each person was to speak only for himself/herself. He could ask each parent to share his/her feelings as this family scene was being played out. Or he could ask both parents to talk together about what was happening in the office at the moment.

The doctor did none of these. Perhaps because it was *so* early in the interview, he felt the need for more time to watch their systems unfolding. At any rate he proceeded as follows:

Doctor: You were mentioning difficulty with Andy in the seat belt. . .

Mother: Oh yes, well, it's not just that. He simply won't mind. Is that normal for 4-year-olds? I've heard about the terrible twos, but should it go on this long? It seems as though *everything* is a hassle. Getting dressed in the morning. Rod and I both have to leave very early in the morning for the studio. Andy knows that — it's really a tight schedule in the morning. Getting him to the nursery school and all. He knows how to dress himself pretty well, don't you, honey?

Andy: (sets his jaw and vigorously shakes his head no)

Mother: Well, he does. When he wants, he does it fast — all but the socks and shoes. And I help him with that; I don't mind. I get him up in plenty of time . . . 30 minutes later, I come in and everything is still where I left it, and he's playing on the floor in his pajamas. Doesn't ever do that on Sundays — just weekdays, when he *knows* we have to get going. And I come unglued — there's no doubt about it. Ask Rod — he has to rescue both of us when I blow! That's when he comes in. First of all I have a really short fuse . . . Rod will tell you that! (laughs and slaps her husband's knee)

Father: (smiling) Things do go smoother in the morning if I can get Carla to just either stay cool or stay out of it. *I* don't really have that much trouble with Andy. If she would just. . .

Doctor: (interrupting) This sounds like a message for Carla. Would you tell her that directly now. I'll listen along.

Father: She's heard it before. I'm like a broken record on that one. Isn't that right, hon?

Doctor: Perhaps, but it doesn't sound like you've ever gotten anywhere with it and that must be very frustrating. Do it once again, now.

Father: (turning to his wife) Well, you know, if you would just let me handle Andy's getting dressed in the morning. . .

At this point, having facilitated the start of direct communication between the parents, the doctor had two choices. He could encourage their dialogue and begin work on their communication style with one another. He might ask father, for instance, to leave off pleading and complaining to Carla and to restate his opener in this manner: "Carla, I would like to handle Andy and his getting dressed in the morning." Or he could forgo a focus on communication for now and point out that there seemed to be a united effort in this family to demonstrate that Carla was inadequate and incompetent as a parent. He was about to choose the latter when, true to form, Andy changed the course of the interview. The interviewer had momentarily lost track of him. The child had tired of exploring the toys and eventually meandered to the other side of the room. There he proceeded to strip all the way down to his underpants, looking especially at his mother as he did so. He was smiling. And the doctor noted that his mother returned the smile. In fact she laughed. Mr. Thomas shifted his legs nervously but said nothing about what was happening. He and his wife continued to develop the conversation that the doctor had urged father to initiate. Every now and then mother would turn toward Andy, smile, and then return her gaze to her husband and the interviewer.

An interviewer would feel frustrated were this youngster's provocations viewed solely as interruptions to the flow of the interview and the "adult conversation." They were that, but they were also the child's important contribution to a disclosure of the family system. In short, Andy with his behavior was helping the family to play out their problem in front of the physician. At the moment both parents were talking to one another about Andy's getting dressed in the morning. Their talk was mostly "just words"; however, the child's behavior in the office right now was becoming a far more powerful demonstration of the family dilemma. The problem being both discussed and enacted in the office was this: Andy's clever manipulations stimulated mixed messages (approval and disapproval) from his mother, and mixed messages from his mother stimulated Andy's clever manipulations. The two had developed their own vicious circle. Andy was becoming more and more powerful in his ability to control family situations. Mother as a result was feeling less and less competent in her mothering. The doctor also suspected from what had been said that father augmented the notion of mother's incompetence by entering and being effective is situations where his wife had failed and by criticizing her approaches with Andy.

Hence the interviewer decided to use the situation happening in the family at the moment—in the here and now—to help Mrs. Thomas become effective with her son immediately. Through this process she might also reveal what feelings were immobilizing her with her son. The doctor simply demanded that she take action now, simultaneously helping her to change the dysfunctional aspects of her communication with him. He also decided he would, if it became necessary, keep Mr. Thomas out of it to make sure that he did not rescue her, criticize her, or show her up with his own parenting prowess.

Andy was doing exercises, nude except for his underpants:

Doctor:	(to parents) Tell me what you're feeling right at this moment.
Father:	(shakes his head in exasperation)
Mother:	(whispering as though she didn't want Andy to hear) You want to know what I'm feeling? Huh? I wish the hell that kid would put his clothes back on. I am so embarrassed.
Doctor:	OK, make it happen, Mrs. Thomas (pushing his chair back out of the action).
Mother:	Andy, it's chilly in the doctor's office.
Andy:	I don't care.
Mother:	You might catch a cold.
Andy:	No, I won't.
Mother:	You might (teasing in her voice).
Andy:	I don't care.
Mother:	(turning back to the doctor) See?
Doctor:	Make it happen, now (motioning for her to continue).
Mother:	Andy, wouldn't you like to put your clothes back on?
Andy:	(shakes his head no)
Doctor:	Are you really giving him a choice?
Mother:	Well . . . no, not really.
Doctor:	You want him to get dressed now?
Mother:	Yes, I'm about to boil inside. I've never been so embarrassed.
Doctor:	Well, stop smiling, and make it happen now.
Mother:	Andy, put your clothes on.
Andy:	I don't want to. Can I get a drink?
Mother:	(sputter)
Doctor:	Do whatever you need to do, Mrs. Thomas, to have him get his clothes on *now* . . . if that's what you want.
Mother:	(drops her pleasant expression and gets out of her chair, moving toward Andy and his pile of laundry. She is deadly serious. Her strong voice reflects her feeling and expectations.) I want you to put those clothes on . . . *right now.*

Andy: (starts to cry *and* starts to put on his clothes. His sobbing and stomping increase but do not interfere with his dressing himself right down to his socks, which ordinarily his mother would help him with. He puts those on, too. Finally he stops crying and approaches his parents.) Can I leave my shoes off until we go?

Mother and father both nodded agreement, and Mrs. Thomas fell back into her chair. The whole episode had taken about 15 minutes. Andy played quietly for the rest of the session; he occasionally sat in his mother's or his father's lap. He was not provocative, nor did he interrupt again.

Doctor: I think we need to talk about what just happened. I'm wondering how that experience was for each of you. Mrs. Thomas?

Mother: Hard, really hard. I'm absolutely exhausted. At home it would have been different.

Doctor: In what way?

Mother: I would have walked away from the whole thing, but I might have given him a swat before I did.

Father: Or you would have been screaming at him, and I would have come running.

Doctor: That brings up a point, Mr. Thomas. I was admiring your silence throughout what happened. I was wondering how it was for you to sit and watch but not be involved yourself.

The doctor hoped by a recognition of father's silence to facilitate a sharing of his feelings and expectations regarding what had just taken place.

Father: Very . . . uncomfortable. I guess . . . I guess I was expecting my wife to fail. I think I really was.

Doctor: All right. Again I would like you to say that directly to your wife — with two changes: take the "I guess" out of your statement, and put the whole thing in the present tense.

Father: (turning to his wife and nodding to show that he understands the doctor's directions) Well, hon, that's right; I did expect that you couldn't do it.

Doctor: Good, now once more and put it in the present tense.

Father: (to his wife) I do expect you to fail with Andy!?

Doctor: How does that sound?

Father: It sounds terrible, awful. No, that's not right . . . I don't want her to be a failure with our son.

Doctor: And yet your behavior . . .?

Father: (after a long pause) Yeah, I have been doing that — sort of waiting and predicting that I'll have to bail her . . .

Doctor: (points to Mrs. Thomas)

Father: Predicting that I'll have to bail *you* out with Andy.

Doctor: And is that the way you want it to be?

Father: Hell, no. I don't want to bail her . . . *you* out. I want you to bail yourself out if you need to.

Doctor: What do you say to that, Mrs. Thomas?

Mother: Well, I . . .

Doctor: Say it to your husband, not me.

Mother: I'm not sure I'm up to it. I'd like to, but . . .

Doctor: Hold it . . . sorry to keep interrupting . . . about that word, "but": it has a way of canceling out everything that has just preceded it. Would you in fact like to be able to manage Andy successfully on your own?

Mother: Oh, yes.

Doctor: OK, then begin again: "I would like to, *and* . . ."

Mother: I would like to . . . and . . . I'm scared.

Doctor: Tell your husband, scared of what?

Mother: I'm not sure. But something really clicked in the middle of all that a few minutes ago. When you asked me, Dr. Anderson, if I was giving Andy a choice. Well, I realized that I do that all the time at home. I can hear myself over and over again: "Don't you think you're tired, Andy? . . . Wouldn't you like to finish your soup? . . . Wouldn't you like a nice bath?" Of course he mostly says no . . . and then I'm livid. What do *I* do then? . . . That's when I start screaming usually.

Doctor: So if it's not a choice, don't make it a question. (failing to notice that he had allowed the issue of Mrs. Thomas's fear to slip away)

Mother: Absolutely, now how do I remember that?

Doctor: Now you're trying to trap *me* into seeing you as incompetent. It won't work. I won't buy it. As a matter of fact I think you've been selling yourself short for a long time regarding your talents as a mother.

Mother: (smiles as though she has been caught, nods, and falls silent)

Doctor: Are you clear about what was effective in what you did just now with Andy?

Mother: Well—this changing questions to statements for one thing.

Doctor: And what else?

Mother: Ummmmmmm, getting serious, I think.

Doctor: Right. You let him know that you meant business.

Mother: Uh-huh.

Doctor: How?

Mother: You told me to stop smiling.

Doctor: Had you been aware that you do that *a lot* with Andy?

Mother: What do you mean?

Doctor: Smiling.

Mother: He's so cute . . .

Doctor: Do you see any consequences at smiling at him when he misbehaves and when you want to get something serious across?

Mother: Well, sometimes I just enjoy him — even his antics . . .

Doctor: Are you aware that you let him know that you enjoy his antics and that you are encouraging him? He gets a mixed message from you when your voice and face don't match or when what you want and what you say are two different things. He pays a lot of attention to your smiling encouragement.

Mother: I just find him so delightful — even when he's acting up sometimes. You mean I'm not even supposed to enjoy my child? Well, I don't know . . . and actually I'm not sure that kids, especially as young as Andy, are as perceptive as you are suggesting. Do you think he really watches my facial expressions that closely?

The interview continued for another few minutes; however, it appeared that at least for the moment Mrs. Thomas was not going to buy the doctor's premise about double-level messages. There was obviously still more work to do, and yet the session was almost over. Andy was asleep in his father's lap. The doctor asked if they would like to return. Both parents said yes and volunteered that the session had been very helpful. They made a return appointment. As an extension of their behavior in the interview, the doctor gave each parent an assignment: mother was to concentrate on turning questions into statements with Andy and not to worry about doing anything else differently with him, and father was to focus on developing the ability to stay out of issues between Andy and his mother.

In 2 weeks the family returned. Unfortunately, Andy did not come; he had chickenpox. Mrs. Thomas had called the day before to let the doctor know that Andy was ill. The doctor decided at that time to proceed with the session anyway, since he had some specific threads from the initial visit that he wanted to pick up again, and they could all be pursued without Andy. His pre-interview thoughts about the Thomases were organized in this way:

1. Had each parent been successful in the task assigned? If so, well and good; if not, that issue would need to be discussed.

2. Mother had volunteered that getting Andy to put his clothes on in the office had exhausted her. She also had mentioned that she was

frightened of managing him alone without a rescue from her husband. What was behind all of that?

3. What was standing in the way of her recognizing the very obvious
   double-level messages that she repeatedly offered her son?
4. Aside from father's too available helpfulness, the doctor knew
   very little about him. He wanted to shine a brighter light on Mr.
   Thomas during this second session.

There could have been a number 5 on this list; however, the doctor was
unaware of it at the time and only much later realized that his efforts in
the initial interview to promote direct dialogue between the two parents
had for the most part failed. He had certainly encouraged their talking
to one another. However, a quick review of the previous transcript will
show that no matter what the verbal direction to the parents had been,
the interchange proceeded mostly in a doctor-mother-doctor-mother
sequence. An appropriate fifth concern then might have been: what was
standing in the parents' way of direct communication with one another,
and how could the physician move himself out of their dialogue more
effectively?

Even with these thoughts squarely in his awareness, the interviewer
purposely chose to begin the session by asking the parents to start, thus
giving the family responsibility for bringing up and discussing their own
concerns and indicating that the doctor expected them to develop their
own resources for using the time.

Doctor: How would you like to use this time today?

For a moment, neither spoke. However, they were both looking pleased
and satisfied. Remembering Mrs. Thomas's counterfeit smile of the previous session, the doctor was not sure how to interpret their nonverbal
communication. He waited.

Father: I did it . . . we all did it. (triumphant)
Doctor: Good . . . did what?
Father: Our assignment.
Doctor: Ahhhh. I see. OK, I would like you to talk about your own assign-
            ment, Rod, and Carla will talk about hers.
Father: I was able to stay out of the middle with those two this week. Of
            course it helped that everything was working OK . . . I didn't need
            to come in.
Doctor: How are you feeling about that?
Father: Ummmmmm . . . in a way like 200 pounds is off my back. Oh, sor-

	ry, Carla — you know what I mean. (Both break up with laughter at the metaphor, especially in light of their profession, and that they are dance partners.)
Father:	But I am serious . . . I feel . . .
Doctor:	To your wife, Rod. Say it to her.
Father:	I feel tremendously relieved. I had not realized how much I ran around poised and ready to break up anything out of line between you and Andy.
Mother:	Well, I really depended on you for that. You are a tremendous help. My temper is — well, you know — I flare really quickly. Sometimes it scares me. I think I always have in the back of my head, "Rod will get us cooled down."

The interview was basically going well at this moment. Of course, mother was sloppy in her use of some pronouns (for example, "it," "us"), but the doctor said nothing. For one thing, he was beginning to hear about the success of their assignments, at least from Mr. Thomas. Mother had yet to be heard from on that score. More importantly she was voluntarily returning to the theme of feeling "scared" in encounters with Andy. The doctor had intended to reintroduce that issue if no one else did. Now he wouldn't have to. However, he would make it his responsibility to see that mother's fear, when upset with Andy, didn't get lost this time.

Doctor:	And what if he doesn't?
Mother:	What do you mean?
Doctor:	What do you fear might happen if Rod doesn't rescue you?
Mother:	(long pause and then in a very soft voice) My temper is something fierce . . . (another long pause and then tears)
Father:	(moves for the Kleenex and begins to stuff three into his wife's hand. The doctor shakes his head no, and father stops. The doctor takes the box and puts it down within her easy reach but not in her lap.)

A word of explanation is necessary here. The interviewer's behavior in this instance did not stem from insensitivity, sadistic urges, or the inability to afford Kleenex. One of our consultants in the Child Study Unit, Dr. Alan Leveton, has accurately observed that the "kindly" offer of Kleenex to an individual experiencing sadness and tears often has the effect of drying up that person's tears and driving the accompanying feelings back inside where they remain unavailable for release. It may be that the offerer wants such a drying up because he himself is uncomfortable with the display of such strong feelings. With this family it was another instance of Rod's offering "help" to Carla at a time when "helping" might not be helpful. Providing Kleenex may say, "I see your pain." Unfortunately it may also say, "Stop crying." Realizing this, the doctor preferred not to be too quick with the Kleenex box. It was kept visible and available, and in this way Mrs. Thomas could be in charge of her own flow of tears.

Father: What is it, hon?

Mother: (banging her fist on her knee and continuing to cry softly) I remember how it was with my own father — he had such a mean temper. I hated him. I don't want to do that with Andy, and when he ticks me off, it's right there in a flash . . . I'm so angry I can't stand it. With my own parents it was hit first and talk about it later — except they never talked about it later. It was all so . . . strict. We were never allowed anything, and I mean anything. That house was run like a military school. And the belt was always kept where my brother and I could see it. I used to get *so* angry, but I wouldn't ever let them know. That was the only way I could feel like I won anything — I wouldn't let them — well, actually it was him, my father — I wouldn't let him know how he got to me. And I also decided — by the time I was 13 — that with my own kids it would be different. I wanted them to have spunk, not to feel beaten down . . . I also said I wouldn't treat them like he did us . . . (long sigh and then cries aloud again) *and here I am doing exactly the same!* . . . that's what terrifies me.

Father: You never told me about your dad.

Mother: No — but didn't it seem strange that I never mentioned him much?

Father: Mmmmmmm. I just didn't realize (joins wife in thoughtful silence).

Certainly much had become clearer through mother's breaking down: the origin of her explosive and ready temper seemed obvious. Likewise her double-level messages to Andy were explainable as one method for validating and encouraging his "spunk." It was also understandable now what she feared: that she, like her father, would allow her anger to get out of control and then physically abuse her son. She had unwittingly encouraged spunk in her child to the point that she was now terrified by her own angry reaction to his show of that very behavior with her. It might have been an appropriate step at this point to encourage Mrs. Thomas to complete her "unfinished business" with her father through the use of Gestalt dialogues. Using an empty chair to represent her father, one could ask her to confront "him" with her feelings about him, about his treatment of her, and about the stumbling block that as a result she was now encountering with her own son. The dialogue would then develop from that point, perhaps over considerably more than one session, until she was able to let go of the feelings of anger, sadness, longing surrounding her relationship with her father. Having worked through those feelings of the past, she might then be free to make choices regarding feelings in the present, taking charge of her anger with her son and developing a relationship in the here and now, unhampered by old wounds and past attachments.

The pediatrician chose another direction, setting aside possible Gestalt dialogues for a future session.

Mother: (after the silence she continues) Well, what I didn't say was that these 2 weeks since we saw you have been phenomenal. I did look out for questions to Andy that weren't really questions. And I don't know—something has changed somehow. We just didn't get into all those hassles.

Doctor: And so how are you feeling?

Mother: I guess like Rod . . . relieved. And I don't really understand how it has all happened. I just know that we're—that I am not having the same problems as I was 2 weeks ago. Is it going to last? I keep asking myself.

Doctor: Probably not is my guess. This is probably some sort of temporary change. You all are too good at doing things the old way.

Mother: Doctor, are you being sarcastic? (teasing tone in her voice)

Doctor: I'm just saying, be prepared for things to work around back to the old system.

Father: I hope not.

Doctor: Well, that will be up to you. I would like to see you again.

His prediction of a reversal was not intended to be sarcastic banter. He was aware that reported progress in the family had been very rapid and that sometimes when such is the case an equally rapid return to the previous status quo may occur. The result can be that the family, upon failing, lose confidence in their own ability to change and in the doctor's ability to help them. With his suggestion that a relapse would be very likely, the doctor was cushioning their possible fall and protecting himself as well. If a relapse in fact occurred, they would be prepared, and he would be proved correct. If no relapse occurred, none of that would matter because the family would be enjoying their own steady improvement. He was using Haley's suggestion of encouraging a relapse in order to prevent one. He was, of course, also suggesting with his final comment that they themselves had control and were responsible for their own future behavior.

They were enthusiastic about returning. The entire family was about to leave town for a month, and so the third appointment was set up for shortly after their return.

All three family members attended the third session. They were still very pleased with themselves and with the persistence of change within their family—now over a 6-week period. By and large, Carla was feeling effective and successful with her son. Andy still continued to be provocative at times; everyone agreed that he was very clever in this regard. However, his provocations did not produce the same sequence of behavior as of old, that is, mother did not respond any more by ignoring his provocations or subtly approving of his misbehavior until she could tolerate it no longer, erupting in a rage and bringing her husband into the fray. That sequence had been abandoned. On one or two occasions when the old pattern threatened to return, Rod, hearing bickering between Andy and his mother, simply shouted from wherever he was, "I'm not coming in. Settle it yourselves." That seemed enough to "call the system," and Carla was then able to take the cue and focus on what she herself needed to do to prevent an escalation. She was tremendously pleased to realize that she had control of her own angry feelings and could manage them.

Doctor: I've been somewhat concerned about all that unfinished business with your father.

Mother: I've been concerned about it all my life. But . . .

Doctor: But? . . .

Mother: And . . . and. I think I don't want to get into it right now.

Doctor: That's up to you. What's your objection?

Mother: Maybe sometime but not now. I do have a handle on what to do with Andy—and it's been going OK. Not easy. This is not easy, my setting limits with him. But I'm working on it. And I think I want to leave it there for now.

Doctor: OK by me.

In 4 weeks Carla called to cancel their appointment. Nothing was wrong; in fact things were progressing well enough that she and Rod had decided another appointment was unnecessary. The pediatrician encouraged them to continue the work on their own and said that he would be delighted to see them in the future if they wished. Nine months later Carla called and asked for an appointment.

The parents came in without Andy. They were quick to assure the doctor that their visit was prompted by something quite different than their usual concern from 9 months ago. Setting limits with Andy was going reasonably well for both parents. They no longer described him as a child who "won't mind." This time they were concerned about an incident that had occurred 10 days previous to the visit. Rod had happened upon Andy and another 4-year-old playing "doctor" with one another, undressed. The parents discussed their concerns about how to handle such an episode correctly. They had actually managed the situation quite well with no shaming or blame; both parents had encouraged Andy's questions about his body, and they had responded to the questions accurately and matter-of-factly. Mostly they seemed to be seeking reassurance that exploratory sex play in 4- and 5-year-olds does happen and that they had handled the situation appropriately. The doctor felt he could reassure them on both counts. He never got around to Carla's feelings about her father, and the parents didn't bring the subject up. They ended this session without setting up a return appointment. The doctor did not feel it was necessary.

He did not see the family after that fourth session. He did, however, hear from their referring pediatrician, Dr. Tom Jones, that both Andy and the family were continuing to do well.

Discussion. Therapeutic moves and intent were commented on during the preceding summary itself and will not be repeated here. There are some other discussion points, however.

First of all, work with the Thomas family was brief, four interviews in all, only three of which were devoted to the initial presenting problem. After only four sessions there were many loose ends; the work was somewhat incomplete. Mrs. Thomas's unfinished business with her own father, for instance, was never dealt with directly. Would it return in the future, perhaps around the same issue or a different one, and in some way once again put a stumbling block in Mrs. Thomas's way? The prevailing thought in Gestalt theory would say yes, that this unfinished business will appear again and again for Mrs. Thomas, pushing to the foreground of her behavior until she has completed it. Loose end number 2, it is uncertain whether the issue and impact of double-level messages ever became clear to the family. Was the mother aware of her role in encouraging the undesirable behavior about which she complained? Should that issue have been returned to? Finally, loose end number 3, changes did occur in the family's behavior so rapidly that one could understandably question the permanence of such change. We were taught in medical school that problems such as this are supposed to take longer to work through. Such thoughts might contribute to one's feeling dissatisfied regarding the work done with the Thomas family.

Such uneasy feelings can be balanced by the following: the family came to the pediatrician with a specific problem. That problem disappeared or at least changed enough that the family then felt comfortable handling their business on their own. They indicated that they had received what they came for and that they did not wish to proceed further. In short, they were satisfied. In general an interviewer does well to respect and be comfortable with a family's desire to stop, because respect it or not, the family feeling this way will probably terminate. The doctor's termination with them on good terms is excellent insurance to facilitate their possible return at some future date. If the interviewer suggests that they are running away, avoiding, or acting hastily, the family will then very likely skulk out of the office, angry and guilty; they may not return even when things get worse. Accepting a family's wish to end sessions leaves them in charge of the pace at which they want to face life's problems. The Thomases did return later, and all indications were that they would feel comfortable about returning again should the situation warrant.

Regarding the clarification of double-level messages, it is true these were never definitely dealt with in the sessions. And yet the changes in the family, especially in Mrs. Thomas's increasing effectiveness with Andy, strongly suggest that she did get the message about her discrepant communication and that she also did something about it. This implies that even in the course of defensive nonlistening, patients do sometimes hear what the interviewer is saying.

Concerning loose end number 3 (Does the rapidity with which change occurred render its permanence suspect?), the family did move quickly. They also demonstrated that the changes they produced lasted for 2 weeks, then 4 weeks, and were sustained 9 months later. The last follow-up through Dr. Jones was about 18 months after the family's initial family appointment. As mentioned, at that point the family was apparently functioning well.

Perhaps a final justification for the presence of loose ends is in order.

We have never seen a family in which loose ends have not dangled at termination. There is always the feeling that one hasn't quite gotten this issue on the table, or that problem sufficiently clarified, or that dimension confronted directly. It has not seemed to matter if the work has gone well or badly or if the termination has been the family's idea or the interviewer's. In every instance we have still felt that some unfinished business remained. Such a feeling does not indicate that the interviewer has failed. Rather we have come to accept that as a "given" of the termination process with families. The interviewer's work will stop at some arbitrary point, but clearly the family's work does not.

Concerning another discussion issue, Randall Foster in a 1972 article[5] noted that many parents in his family therapy practice made one striking omission in dealing with their "problem behavior" children. These parents would report to him that they had done "everything" in an effort to change the child's behavior. And it was true, he noted, that they had done a number of things: they punished, spanked, deprived, talked; they threatened reform school, the police, or foster placement; and they promised gifts or money if the child would change his behavior. What was singularly lacking from their lists, however, was the simple fact of telling the child to change. Neither parent said to the child directly and plainly, "Stop it now," or "Do it now." Mrs. Thomas illustrated the omission of such a communication in her approach to the undressed Andy. She used many ploys, all indirect, to entice him to get dressed. Andy did not respond until she gave him the simple command, "I want you to put those clothes on . . . right now!"

Foster's hypothesis is that such a direct communication does not flow from parent to child because the parents have basically come to doubt their child's ability to do what they are requesting. Many of Foster's interventions with children and parents are based then on the following principle: children will do what their parents tell them to do (1) when the parents perceive the child is able to do it, (2) when the child sees himself able to do it, and (3) when the child hears the parents' clear demand to do it.

These three ingredients did develop for the Thomas family in that first interview and were made possible by the inclusion of one additional step. Prior to Mrs. Thomas's successful demand of Andrew, she herself was given a similar command by the pediatrician: "Make it happen now." This command carried the following implication: "I trust your ability, Mrs. Thomas, to make it happen now, or I would not be asking you to do it." We would therefore add one item to the three proposed above by Foster: children will do what their parents tell them to do (1) when the parents perceive the child is able to do it, (2) when the child sees himself able to do it, (3) when the child hears the parents' clear demand to do it, *and* (4) when the parents trust their own abilities to make such a clear demand.

Just as the parent must communicate faith in the child's competence, so too must the interviewer show that he trusts the basic (perhaps untapped) parenting abilities of the mother and father.

The Thomas family was selected for several reasons. Their situation represented a case of brief, successful intervention, through family interviewing, by a pediatrician, for a common pediatric behavioral complaint. In addition they offered an opportunity to demonstrate a large number of the ideas presented earlier in this text. Each of the following concepts, useful in family interviewing, was at least touched upon in work with the Thomas family:

Concept	*Example*
A. Family homeostasis, family system	The family was, for instance, organized around Mr. Thomas's persistent rescue of Andy and his wife from herself. The family balanced itself in this way.
B. Communication style 1. Content and process	There were many examples: most striking was Andy's acting out through silent undressing while the parents were engaged in a verbal dialogue with one another.
2. Functional communication	*Father:* "Hell, no. I don't want to bail her . . . *you* out. I want you to bail yourself out if you need to."
3. Dysfunctional communication	*Father:* "Well, you know, if you would just let me handle Andy's getting dressed in the morning . . ."
a. False assumptions in communication	*Father:* "She's heard it before. I'm like a broken record on that one."
b. Double-level messages	Almost too many to count. Noteworthy was Mrs. Thomas's continuing smile towards Andy as she confided, "I wish the hell that kid would put his clothes back on."
4. Parental validation	The lack of appropriate parental validation for mother in her own

5. Use of pronoun "I"

C. Family structure
  1. Subsystems

  2. Joining through tracking
  3. Restructuring
     a. Actualizing family trans-
        actions
     b. Marking boundaries

     c. Escalating stress
     d. Assigning tasks

     e. Utilizing "symptoms" and
        here and now behavior

     f. Support

D. Repetitive family sequence

growing up was now seriously ham-
pering her validation of her son. Also,
there was little validation of Andy by
his parents in the session when he
would do well.

The parents were encouraged to
use "I need," "I feel," and so on in the
session and directed to talk to one
another rather than about each other.

Mrs. Thomas and Andy had a
fairly well-defined (though conflictual)
subsystem that alternately included (at
home during angry outbursts) and
excluded (in the office when Mr.
Thomas attempted to set limits with
Andy) her husband.

Doctor: "You were mentioning difficulty with Andy in the seat belt . . ."

The interviewer insisted that the
parents talk directly to one another.

The interviewer decided to keep
Mr. Thomas out of the interaction
between his wife and Andy in the
office, thus delineating the boundary
around mother and child so that Mrs.
Thomas might experience success
with her son.

Doctor: "Make it happen now."

Each parent was given a specific
job to work on at home at the close of
the first interview.

Making use of Andy's provocative
undressing rather than considering it
just an interruption.

The interviewer's acknowledgement of feelings of frustration for
both parents. Also the following:
Doctor: "Now you're trying to trap me
into seeing you as incompetent. It
won't work. I won't buy it. As a matter
of fact I think you've been selling
yourself short for a long time regarding your talents as a mother."

Andy provoked mother. Mother
encouraged his provocation. Andy
went too far. Mother exploded. Father

E. Encouraging a relapse in order to prevent one and helping the family to an awareness of its own responsibility in change

F. Unfinished business

G. The stages of an initial interview

H. Four goals of an initial interview

entered. Father took over and calmed the situation. Mother was shown to be a failure. Father left. Andy provoked his mother. And so on.

In response to mother's query, "Will the changes last?", the response: "Probably not is my guess. This is probably some sort of temporary change." Also: "That (the permanence of change) will be up to you."

Mrs. Thomas's relationship with her father in the past.

The session proceeded through the opening stages to a discussion of the family's concerns, to an interactional stage, and to an ending.

First, the interviewer early established that he would be in charge when he said to father: "That sounds like a message for Carla. Would you tell her that directly now." *Second,* he also developed a formulation of the problem (see "family sequence" and "double-level message"). *Third,* family members were touched. The interviewer touched Mrs. Thomas when he recognized her embarrassment with Andy and helped her to act on that and feel successful about herself as a mother. The interviewer touched Mr. Thomas by responding to his obvious discomfort at standing by and watching the scene unfold. Andy's changed behavior in the interview was an indication that he too had been touched. *Fourth,* the family did return.

THE USE OF CONFRONTATION

In this work with the Thomas family and indeed in all the examples presented throughout the book, the use of confrontation with families is obvious. We are in strong agreement with those published reports[1,2,6] that indicate a direct, positive correlation between positive patient change and a high degree of confrontation employed by the therapist. For us, family counseling is an active process in which the interviewer must *do* something (that is, focus and direct) if the family is to change. Passive listening seems to us an extravagant use of time and an inefficient and often ineffectual device, boring for both family and interviewer. However, active confrontation appears to stimulate movement and encourage positive change on the family's part, and it is exciting, never boring.

The confrontation techniques themselves can be one of several varieties. The directive to Mrs. Thomas regarding Andy's putting his clothes back on ("Make it happen now.") was an *encouragement to act.* This sort of confrontation involves the therapist's encouragement of, and faith in, the patient and family to act on their world in some satisfying (to them) manner, specifically discouraging a defeatist, passive stance toward life. A second type, a *confrontation of strength,* was also used with Mrs. Thomas when the interviewer said: "As a matter of fact I think you've been selling yourself short for a long time regarding your talents as a mother." This confrontation focuses on a patient's constructive resources and demonstrated indications of strength.

The third, a *didactic confrontation,* is the variety probably most familiar to physicians. Here the therapist directly clarifies a patient's misinformation or lack of information. In Chapter 3, the therapist didactically confronted Jennifer Maloney's parents when he told them that Mr. Maloney was crucial to the survival of his wife and family, that only he could help to solve this family problem, and that his role was essential. A fourth type of confrontation is termed an *experiential confrontation* and refers to a therapist's commenting on discrepancies that either he or the patient experiences. For instance, a therapist who calls a double-level message in a family member when he notices it is using experiential confrontation. He is also using experiential confrontation when he requests from a family member clarification of unexpressed feelings, as in the following: "My words just now made you look very sad. I don't understand; would you explain?"

By confronting we do not mean the interviewer cavalierly insults family members, or is rude, or walks over their feelings. On the contrary, confrontation of this sort without regard for the patient will probably be counterproductive. Confrontation and regard for the feelings of the family are both necessary. One study, by Mitchell and Berenson,[6] documented that it was not just the use of confrontation that was directly related to positive patient improvement, but that confrontation used by a particular type of therapist, whom they termed a "highly facilitative therapist," most often led to a good outcome for the patient. In their study such a therapist was one who offered to his patients significantly higher levels of the following:

1. Empathy, in which the therapist communicated an accurate understanding of the patient's feelings
2. Positive regard, in which the therapist communicated his deep caring and respect for the patient
3. Genuineness, in which the therapist was freely himself in the relationship with the patient
4. Concreteness, in which the therapist insisted on direct exploration of the patient's specific feelings and experiences, rather than allowing vague, abstract, general discussion

Therapists who rated significantly higher in possessing these four qualities (1) were shown to confront their patients significantly more often than others and (2) were judged to facilitate significantly greater positive change in their patients.

The qualities of accurate empathy, positive regard, genuineness, and concreteness seem to us to be those attributes that encourage a "touching" experience between a therapist and patient. We would agree they are essential qualities for successful work with families, for when all is said and done, good interviewing becomes a process of both touching *and* confronting the family, the therapist balancing each aspect in a way that encourages and supports the family's change.

COMMON FAMILY TYPES

Just as we feel there is no single prototype of the child who won't mind, we also doubt there is one specific type of family surrounding the child with such a chief complaint. In fact the whole concept of family typology, while appealing to consider, has never seemed to work out. It would make family work considerably easier if one could, by looking at a child and his problem, accurately generalize about the family of that child. One could then develop a list: the bedwetter's family, the school phobic's family, the leukemic's family, and so on. It just doesn't work that way; there is no more a typical bedwetter's family than there is a typical bedwetter. Besides we find it offensive to depersonalize children by labeling them as a symptom with the suffix "-ic" or "-er" on the end, for example, a diabetic, an epileptic, a bedwetter. In all likelihood complicated systems such as children and families are just not reducible to such mechanistic conceptualizations.

And yet we have found that in a somewhat different sense, families often do have some common characteristics. Frequently while conducting a family interview, one may observe silently: "I've experienced this family before. Maybe the family's concern was different the other time, but I distinctly recall having faced a similar family system in a previous situation." That realization may be followed by a feeling of elation or despair on the interviewer's part. In any case the commonality linking the two families has to do with how the members of each group are behaving toward one another and toward the interviewer, irrespective of the problem that brought either family into the doctor's office. We have been struck in this way with at least six repetitive family configurations: the enmeshed family (to be discussed in a subsequent chapter), the uproar family, the reasonable family, the silent family, the blaming family, and the intellectualizing family.

The uproar family

The uproar family has been mentioned in Chapter 6 — the Martin family. They are unmistakable and a force to be reckoned with. Quite often their uproar will precede their initial visit with the doctor in the form of frequent phone calls, perhaps from several different family members, several changes of appointment, difficulty with the nurse-receptionist, chaos in the waiting area, and pandemonium in the interview itself. The children seem out of control, moving and talking excessively and in a haphazard, disorganized manner. The parents may sit by silently as the disorganization increases, or they may make frantic but ineffectual attempts to bring order, or they may themselves be out of control. One may assume that the parents of such a family are in some way unwittingly encouraging the disorganized aspects of their children's behavior. In this situation the interviewer's first priority is to establish rules of behavior for his own office. The therapist thus makes room for himself in order to carry on the interview. This task generally takes precedence over any discussion of the chief complaint. Indeed this behavior (a lack of control) is quite often the chief complaint itself. Control measures may range from turning the situation over to the parents for managing, to telling family members to settle down, sit down, be quiet, don't interrupt, talk one at a time, and so on, to actually terminating the interview until order is established. When a therapist feels like a member of a crowd scene in a disaster film, he may be sure that an uproar family has wrapped itself around him and that he has allowed this to happen. Rein-

182   CLINICAL APPLICATION

forcements in the form of a co-therapist can be quite useful with uproar families, since frequently these families benefit from the combined energies of two interviewers.

The reasonable family

Mother: Marvin is such a good boy, really, Doctor. We just don't understand what's been getting into him, do we, dear?

Marvin: (sulks)

Father: We wouldn't want you to think Marvin is always like this. He's shy around strangers. It's all right, son. The doctor is going to help us. Don't be upset.

Mother: Mommy gets upset sometimes too, Marvin — you know, in the middle of the night when you want Mommy to sleep with you. Well, Daddy wakes up too, and he's so busy and tired; he needs his sleep.

Father: It's you I'm worried about, Martha. You can't sleep on that hard mattress of his.

Mother: Nonsense. I can sleep anywhere, Leon.

Father: Well, you certainly don't look very rested in the morning.

Mother: (lip trembling) Leon, I've only missed fixing your breakfast on two occasions.

Father: Now don't get upset, Martha. I wasn't talking about that. Let's not get upset. Nothing is solved by arguing. Actually, Doctor, we're very proud, Martha and I — we don't fight. In fact I don't remember that we've ever had one fight in over 8 years of marriage, have we, dear?

Mother: (blowing her nose) No. Marvin, I'm sure the doctor would like you to sit on that chair like a big boy. Now be reasonable, darling. We're only doing this for your own good.

Father: There must be a reason for Marvin's seeming to need his mother each night. Should we be concerned, or are we just making a mountain out of a molehill? We're willing to do whatever you suggest; you're the doctor.

Just from a communications standpoint, there are many things to note about this family. Both mother and father insist on the use of collective pronouns, "we," "we're," "let's." Father speaks for mother; mother speaks for Marvin and for the doctor as well. The family's collective style is one of avoiding responsibility for one's own thoughts, words, and feelings while at the same time assuming to know the thoughts, words, and feelings of others. Yet they are all so reasonable in their talk. Interviewing Marvin and his family is hard work. Everyone in such a family—often including the identified patient (although in this case, not)—seems nice, fair, reasonable, unemotional, and perpetually looking out for the best interests of others, rather than attending to his/her own needs. The family may be so convincing in its reasonable stance that the interviewer after a time erroneously concludes that the family is a model of "togetherness and understanding." In such a situation, the novice interviewer may then question the need for any sort of family interview or counseling. At other times the family, as Marvin's family demonstrates, will overdo their reasonableness to such an extent that they become almost a caricature of caring and solicitude. These families are particularly prone to turn to the physician as the authoritarian seer, directly asking his advice and vowing to follow his suggestions. They are very reasonable in such requests. Open disagreement or conflict is a missing dimension in their conversation. There is often the feeling by the interviewer of having nothing to grab on to with such a family; they provide no entries for the doctor's intervention. Interviewing the Marvins of this world and their families is hence a very frustrating experience; it closely resembles crossing an expanse of warm tapioca pudding on foot. Failing to find solid footing or substance, one slogs through the hour, hoping in vain to find something hard underfoot on which to stand and dry off.

The specific approach to such a family will, of course, depend on the family and their circumstance. However, some general guidelines may be helpful. We have earlier recommended all of these in interviewing any family. They may be particularly important in helping a seemingly reasonable family to change:

1. Get the family to talk to one another rather than report to the doctor "about" one another. This is especially important with a reasonable family, so that rather than becoming trapped on the receiving end of (and taken in by) reasonable, sensible statements, one may watch how family members use reasonableness with one another.

2. Listen particularly for any hint of interpersonal conflict (it will usually be hidden). Work to encourage its open expression. For example:

Mother: (lip trembling) Leon, I've only missed fixing your breakfast on two occasions.

Father: Now don't get upset, Martha. I wasn't talking about that. Let's not get upset. Nothing is solved by arguing.

Doctor: Leon, would you tell Martha what you see on her face right at this moment.

Father: Well, uh . . . she's a little upset.

Doctor: Ahhh, ask her if you're reading her correctly.

Father: Well, are you?

Mother: (nods) Yes. (then denying her own feelings) But it's nothing. I'm all right now.

Doctor: Not so fast. Your tears are nothing?

Mother: Well . . .

Doctor: Leon, see if you can talk further with Martha: find out what her tears are about.

Do not be dismayed if it does not go this smoothly. After all, such reasonable families are very good at what they do. They have been doing it for a long time. Leon and Martha could easily conspire to defeat the interviewer's suggestions in this way:

Father: Now, don't get upset, Martha. I wasn't talking about that. Let's not get upset. Nothing is solved by arguing.

Doctor: Hold it, Leon. Would you tell Martha what you see on her face at this moment.

Father: (ignoring the doctor's request) I don't think she's really upset. Martha understands that I don't mind cold cereal once in a while.

Mother: (quickly pulling herself together) Leon is really very good in the kitchen.

Doctor: (very confused as to how things slipped from the expression on Martha's face to a discussion of Leon's culinary skills in the short space of 30 seconds) Well . . .

Father: Oh, sure, I can even fix eggs if I have to. But now back to this sleeping problem Marvin is having . . . (removing the focus from himself and back onto Marvin)

The interviewer will simply have to try again. This brings up a point that applies when one is working with any family, not just a reasonable, selfless group. Very often our pediatric residents will exit from an interview, frustrated that they missed this opportunity or that chance to zero in on a specific aspect of the family's system. We are able to reassure them that families are wonderfully obliging in this regard. Since they demonstrate repetitive sequences in their behavior and style of relating, the family members will continue to present their same sequence over and over again, perhaps in a different disguise at times, but the same basic sequence of behavior will come up again and again until the therapist becomes aware of the steps involved. We would be confident in telling the therapist working with Leon and Martha not to worry. There will be numerous future presentations of the same dance step by Leon and Martha: the suggestion of conflict followed by a quick cover-up, indicating that each is denying his own self-needs and feelings. The therapist can then prepare himself to watch for such an event, and when it occurs he may then confront the family with his observation.

3. Concentrate on increasing each family member's use of the pronoun "I." For example:

Doctor: Martha, would you tell Leon what you are feeling at this moment? Start your sentence with "I."

4. Be leery of dispensing quick advice and answers even though the family directly asks for or demands this. As mentioned, their request will seem reasonable, their attentive listening will appear equally reasonable, and they will be most reasonable of all in their eventual disregard or sabotage of the advice given.

The silent family

Silent families are a challenge. Typically the children have vocabularies limited to "I don't know" and "Uh-huh." The mother waits for the doctor's lead, and the father volunteers that "I came because she told me I had to." Opening pleasantries are followed by a deafening silence, and all eyes turn toward the interviewer. Just getting the interview started feels like a Herculean task. Often a pact of silence by the family reflects their collective feeling of fear regarding the interview process. In this situation the interviewer can be helpful by spending time on a discussion of the family's individual and mutual anxiety and their expectations of the doctor, rather than by forging ahead with a premature disclosure of the chief complaint. Such a discussion might be introduced as follows:

Doctor: Before we get down to what problems bring you here, I would like to know what each of you is experiencing as you sit in this office today. Henry, I'll start with you.

or

I am feeling uncomfortable. The family looks very ill at ease. Tell me what worries you about being here today.

or

> I would like each of you to write down two "good" things and two "bad" things that you feel might happen here today.

or

> I tend to feel that my own family concerns are pretty private matters. I wonder if this is a private family, also? If so, maybe we need to talk about that before getting started. I recognize that some family matters may be hard to discuss.

Some families are relatively nonverbal in their interactional style even outside the office. These families will often respond to the assignment of a nonverbal task such as a conjoint family drawing or a family sculpture, both discussed earlier in this text.

Directly challenging a silent member or a silent family itself to get talking about "the problem" usually intensifies the silence and the atmosphere of strained discomfort in the room. The preceding suggestions have the advantage of approaching the family about their fears and expectations in the session rather than encouraging their defensive stance.

The blaming family

In blaming families, someone is always under attack. It may be a child, a parent, or the interviewer:

Mother: Harvey, I said sit up!

Father: She's on him all the time, Doc.

Mother: Well, if you'd be on him a little more, I wouldn't have to. I saw this program on television about a father who . . .

Father: Don't bring television into it, Ethel. That's all you can ever think about.

Harvey: It was a good show. Mom and I . . .

Father: Don't interrupt, Harvey.

Harvey: You never listen to me . . . (sticks his tongue out)

Mother: Harvey, don't talk to your father like that.

Father: Stay out of it, Ethel. I'll handle him. Isn't that right, Doc? When my own kid sasses me, shouldn't I handle it?

Doctor: That is . . .

Father: Geez, I don't know what we're coming here for; it's not helping.

Mother: You're never willing to stick with something for more than 5 minutes. Harvey, I'm not going to tell you again, *sit up!*

This family is only a few insults away from becoming an uproar family. They are escalating into that position from a blaming stance. Something is always someone else's fault. The strategies an interviewer uses in this situation are those that will encourage a focus on their learning to communicate feelings without blame. For instance:

Mother: Well, if you'd be on him a little more, I wouldn't have to. I saw this program on television . . .

Doctor: Hold it, Ethel. That's an important message you just gave your husband. Tell him again, and this time find a way to say it that doesn't blame him.

Mother: (she sputters and indicates that she doesn't know how.)

Doctor: That's a tough spot, having something that important to say and not quite knowing how to say it. What is it that you would like to get across to Mel?

Mother: I don't know . . . I guess that I feel everything is on my shoulders.

Doctor: Ah, then that's what he needs to hear. Tell him that.

Mother: Yeah, why do I have to do it all?

Father: You . . .

Doctor: Hold it. Back up, Ethel. Start your sentence with I feel.

Mother: (after a pause) I feel all the responsibility is mine.

Father: Who asked you to take it all?

Doctor: Mel, is it hard not to answer Ethel with a defense?

Father: Well, she insinuates that I don't do anything.

Doctor: And that leaves you feeling . . .?

Father: I don't know . . . sore, and like she doesn't notice what I am doing.

Doctor: What a dilemma for you both. Ethel, you're feeling overwhelmed, and Mel, you feel unappreciated. There ought to be another way to air those feelings and settle them aside from attacking each other. That must be frustrating for both of you.

Father: It sure doesn't get us anywhere.

The sky looks clear for the first time in the interviewer's struggle. And then:

Mother: Well, if you'd just listen more to what I'm saying . . . you never . . .

Then it's back to go. The interviewer can persist, slow them down again, and continue to urge their expression of feelings other than through attacking and blaming. He needs to be very careful that his interventions are balanced in such a way that individuals in the family do not see him as taking sides in the family struggle. In many ways it amounts to a "gentling" process in which the interviewer slowly helps the family to a realization by experience in the interview that feelings other than blame can be safely exposed and communicated.

The intellectualizing family

The intellectualizing family attempts to beat the doctor at his own game. Doctors are experienced at restricting communication to facts, rational thought, and things of the mind. When a whole family decides to function with one another in this way, the result can be staggering:

> *Mike:* I don't see why I can't stay up until 10.
>
> *Father:* (rather than declaring his own desires on the subject, offers an outside source) I think authorities pretty well agree, Mike, that the sleep a child gets before midnight is the most important.
>
> *Mother:* (siding with her son against her husband) But what about that article I showed you in *Family Circle*? It made a lot of sense to me. It said that a child knows his own sleep needs and will regulate himself.
>
> *Father:* Well, Helen, I hardly think *Family Circle* compares to that piece in the *Scientific American* (again using outside intellectual authority to speak for him and to intimidate others).
>
> *Mother:* The *Family Circle* study *was* done at the Gesell Institute, Arnold. Oh, well, I suppose you're right.
>
> *Mike:* None of the other kids have to go to bed at 9:30.
>
> *Mother:* Other kids don't concern us, Mike. Their parents perhaps aren't as responsible as your father and I.
>
> *Father:* When you have children of your own, son, I think you'll understand what we mean.
>
> *Mike:* I'm the only kid in the ninth grade who can't stay up until at least 10.
>
> *Mother:* Now, that just isn't true. I was talking to Connie Harris's mother, and she . . .
>
> *Mike:* I tell you, I feel like a freak. And besides Connie Harris is in the eighth grade.
>
> *Father:* Think of how much fresher you are each day for school, Mike.
>
> *Mike:* I even get teased about being a baby.
>
> *Mother:* We think you should be able to rise above that, Mike. They probably tease you because they're jealous of your good grades. And if their parents would set some bedtime limits for them, maybe their grades would show it, too. Did you ever think of that?

This family could go on endlessly. The parents have certainly not exhausted their store of good and rational reasons why children should be in bed by 9:30. Whether one agrees with their premise or not, one must concede that something quite important has not occurred thus far. Neither parent has acknowledged his or her own feelings or Mike's. Nor has Mike been given the opportunity to hear the feelings and expectations of his parents. Feelings have simply not been expressed, and for each individual the communication has been a collection of rationalizations supported by authority, a conversation "from the neck up."

In order to crack such a family's intellectualizing style, one needs to help the family members shift to feeling statements. Here the interviewer's responsibility is to pry the family away from their defensive rationalizations with content issues, and direct them toward an understanding of their defensive maneuvers and process. For instance:

Mike: None of the other kids have to go to bed at 9:30.

Mother: Other kids don't concern . . .

Doctor: Stop just a minute. Mike, you say that none of the other kids have to go to bed by 9:30. How does that make you feel?

Mike: I feel like a freak.

Doctor: I would like you to share your *feelings* about that with each of your parents.

Mike: (to his mother) I do. I positively feel like a freak with other kids my age.

Doctor: Virginia, what do you hear in your son's voice and words?

Mother: He just needs . . .

Doctor: No, stop. I want you for this moment to listen to *his feelings* and let him know that you hear him.

Mother: I see that . . . he's upset.

Doctor: Ask him, upset in what way?

Mother: Upset about what, Mike?

Mike: I feel humiliated with the kids at school.

Mother: Now, Mike, that's silly.

Doctor: See if you can listen to his feelings without judging. Were you aware that he was feeling humiliated with his friends?

Mother: Well . . . no; I just thought . . .

Doctor: What feelings are in you, right now, Virginia? Tell Mike.

Mother: Well, I don't think he should feel that way.

Doctor: And yet somehow he does. And what feelings does that trigger off inside you?

Mother: . . . just awful.

Doctor: Tell Mike, starting your sentence with "I feel." I think it is important for you and Mike to share your feelings with one another right

> now, that's all . . . just feelings. Talk together, you two, about what's happening on your insides at this moment.

In this situation, as in all of those previously described, the interviewer must be willing to persist and to repeat his efforts — again, and again, and again. All families, be they uproar, blaming, silent, reasonable, enmeshed, intellectualizing, or anything else, are very practiced and committed to their familiar behavioral style. They will not relinquish it easily, even though that style may be largely responsible for their distress. Fearful of critical judgment from others, they also do not respect their own feelings and needs. Therefore they are unable to express feelings without expecting blame or criticism in return. Helping them develop new and different expectations through new and different experiences in the interviews is the job of the interviewer.

REFERENCES

1. Berenson, B., and others: Level of therapist functioning: types of confrontation, J. Clin. Psychiatry **24:**111, 1968.
2. Bergin, A., and Garfield, S., editors: Handbook of psychotherapy and behavior change, New York, 1961, John Wiley & Sons, Inc.
3. Chess, S., and others: Behavioral individuality in early childhood, New York, 1963, New York University Press.
4. Chess, S., and others: Your child is a person: a psychological approach to parenthood without guilt, New York, 1972, The Viking Press.
5. Foster, R.: Parental communication as a determinant of child behavior, Am. J. Psychotherapy **25:**579, 1971.
6. Mitchell, K., and Berenson, B.: Differential use of confrontation by high and low facilitative therapists, J. Nerv. Ment. Dis. **153:**165, 1971.

CHAPTER 8

Chronic conditions

Mother: You forgot!? Well, you can't forget. That's all there is to it. This is what I'm up against, Doctor. I've told him hundreds of times that this is his only job. I don't ask him to do anything else around the house. I get no support.

Father: Evelyn, I think you're being too hard on the boy. After all, he's only 13.

Mother: (to Frankie) I give up on asking you to do anything anymore!

Frankie: You say that but you won't do it.

Father: Don't speak to your mother that way.

Frankie: Well, why not? . . . You do.

Father: Now, that's about enough out of you, young man.

Mother: Will you get off Frankie's back? That's all the two of you do is fight.

Father: You're a good one to talk.

Mother: Look, Jerome, how are we going to teach this boy to be responsible for himself if he won't do the one job we have asked him to do? *One* of us has to have some expectations for Frankie. And he's certainly not getting any from you.

Father: Like I say, Evelyn. You're too hard. You can't expect the boy to be an adult overnight.

Jerome, Evelyn, and Frankie are involved in a round robin with a familiar topic. We've heard it often, and most readers will recognize the situation either from having witnessed it themselves in a clinical office setting or from having experienced it at some point in their own family chronicles. A family's difficulties around the issue of teaching "responsibility" to the children is a frequently heard refrain—in a home and in a pediatrician's office. This particular family's difficulties with the subject are related to a repeating sequence of behaviors in which the family members have become expert.

191

1. Feeling alone and isolated in her parenting, mother takes a unilateral stand regarding expectations for her son.
2. She feels undermined by her husband and unwittingly sets herself up to be so treated.
3. The son enters with anger, provoking each parent.
4. The parents then attack one another.
5. The son withdraws, unnoticed. The issue of his responsibility falls from view, unresolved.
6. Parental fighting takes precedence, leading to increased feelings of alienation and isolation.
7. Subsequently, mother, feeling alone and isolated in her parenting, will once again take a unilateral stand regarding expectations for her son.

This family could be discussing Frankie's not carrying out the garbage, forgetting to brush his teeth, letting his homework slide, or failing to mow the lawn. The same seven-step sequence would unfold. But they are not discussing these issues. Frankie has chronic renal disease with elements of the nephrotic syndrome. He is currently in relapse, and he has been "forgetting" to take his prednisone. Continued "forgetting" could be, if not fatal, certainly very serious. The stakes then are considerably higher than those of an unkempt front yard or the accumulation of trash under the kitchen sink. Appropriate medical management of Frankie and his renal disease necessitates that he take his prednisone consistently. Since the family's repeating sequence of dysfunctional communication and behavior around responsibility issues stands in the way of Frankie's compliance, appropriate medical management must include attention to, and alteration of, the family's patterns.

We have used Frankie and his family to illustrate that although our clinical emphasis will now change, our focus on the family will remain. For in this chapter we are turning to the child who enters a doctor's care first and foremost because of a presenting physical symptom. This child too lives in a family, and his illness — whether it be cystic fibrosis, a seizure disorder, rheumatoid arthritis, chronic renal disease, diabetes mellitus, congenital heart disease, osteogenesis imperfecta, or epidermolysis bullosa — is very much a family affair. These families also have specific systems, communication patterns, structures, and repetitive sequences of behavior. Their family attributes and the illness of the child are inextricably woven together into one fabric, and a physician responsible for the care of a chronically ill child must pay attention to both the warp and the woof of that piece of cloth.

This does not mean that the clinician must elaborate a new hypothesis for working with the family of a chronically ill child. In our experience the hypotheses that we have previously summarized, regarding how families in general function, hold quite well when it comes to understanding specifically how the members of a family with a chronically ill member interact with one another. Our trainees have occasionally expressed surprise and pleasure after observing us interview, for instance, a family with a teenager suffering from rheumatoid arthritis. Their surprise derived from observing that our clinical approach and intervention strategies had not differed in principle from those utilized in family interviews having to do with "garden variety" behavioral complaints. Their pleasure was apparently in discovering that our stated principles of family function and family interviewing could transcend specific clinical issues and be applied across a wide spectrum of pediatric problems, those "behavioral" *and* those "physical."

PRESENTING THE DIAGNOSIS

One of the most difficult tasks for a physician to perform is telling parents that their child has developed a serious medical condition that the youngster may carry for the rest of his life. The child will *never* be quite the same as he was before the onset of his illness. The specific instances in which such news must be communicated are many: blood dyscrasias (for example, sickle cell anemia, hemophilia), central nervous system disorders (for example, seizures, degenerative processes), congenital and acquired cardiac diseases (for example, pulmonary stenosis, rheumatic heart disease), metabolic disorders (for example, phenylketonuria, diabetes mellitus), chronic infectious processes (for example, cytomegalic inclusion disease, toxoplasmosis), immune disorders (for example, rheumatoid arthritis, allergies, asthma), sensory defects (for example, blindness, deafness), physical defects (for example, ambiguous genitalia, hypothyroidism). In very few of these examples does the disease kill outright or quickly. Generally the patient lives but with substantially altered life experiences, not just for weeks but for years. Dying may take from months to years, and death itself, for some of the conditions listed above, may be a painful, horrendous finale. The family is plunged into a protracted, seemingly unending course along with the ailing child. It is a cruel detour from the mainstream of life for all involved, and frequently the child's physician must be the first to indicate to the child and to the family that such a detour is inevitable. He must say in some fashion, "I'm sorry to tell you that your child has _____." Such a pronouncement is always devastating for the family and may also be for the physician.

In discussing the management of such chronic conditions with our trainees we generally start at the inception of the nightmare for the child and family, when the reality of the diagnosis must be faced and discussed for the first time. For illustration and subsequent discussion we present the following transcript. It reflects the conversation between a pediatric resident, Dr. Elliott, and the family of a child for whom he is caring. What the family knows as this interview begins is that their 20-month-old, only child has not been well for some time. He eats listlessly, has gained weight poorly, and has seemed to have a "bad cold" for the past several weeks. He was hospitalized 2 days before, the cold having progressed into pneumonitis. Tests have been performed; no results have been discussed as yet. The resident knows that the sweat chlorides were highly elevated and that without question the child has fibrocystic disease. Both resident and parents are dreading this meeting.

Doctor: Hi, Mr. and Mrs. Nichols. Let's sit down. Any trouble finding a place to park? No? Well, I'm surprised. The parking situation around here is murder. What's that? Oh, Eddie is doing much better. Have you been in to see him yet? He's still in the tent but breathing quite nicely. He's even been able to take some clear liquids by mouth. I wanted to go over his tests with you.

Mother: He looks so pale, Dr. Elliott.

Father: Jean's been so upset since Eddie was admitted, Doctor. Come on, hon, let's hear what the doctor has to say.

Doctor: Well, she's right. Eddie is pale. However, the vascular system is a very wonderful system. At the moment most of Eddie's problem is in his lungs and with his breathing. His arteries and veins in that area are working overtime, and some of the blood supply normally going out to the skin and giving him good color is now being shunted to his lungs and breathing apparatus.

Mother: He just looks so pale.

Doctor: You musn't worry, Mrs. Nichols. His skin doesn't need his red blood corpuscles now. Red blood cells are the body's main carrier of oxygen. Eddie's skin doesn't need so much oxygen right now, but his vital organs—heart, lungs, brain—do. It is really the body's way of utilizing reserves in an emergency.

Father: You told us yesterday that his blood count was up. Doesn't that mean that he has too much blood somehow?

Doctor: No, Mr. Nichols. That was his white blood count. We all have two kinds of blood cells—well, three if you count platelets—red, white, and platelets. Now Eddie's white count is up above 17,000 — that's because of the infection. But his red cells are if anything a little low, around 2.5 million. I know this must be confusing. Perhaps if I give you some normal figures for white and red counts and draw you a picture of a typical red cell and a typical white cell, that may help you to keep the two straight. (He does and finishes with a flourish, defining the term "differential white blood cell count" and explaining the difference between a neutrophil and a lymphocyte.) Before moving on to some of the other tests that Eddie has had since he came into the hospital, do you have any more questions about his blood?

Mother: So ghastly white, he looks awful. (her anxiety obviously increasing)
Father: Geez, Jean, aren't you listening to what the man's been saying?
Doctor: That's all right, Mr. Nichols. Let's see how else I can explain it . . .

Not surprisingly, finding alternate explanations comes easy to this physician. More's the pity, because not only must the Nichols family endure the stress of their son's serious illness, they must also withstand Dr. Elliott's kindly, well-meaning explanations. And he hasn't even gotten to the diagnosis yet.

The preceding interview need not go so badly. There are some useful guidelines for an interviewer to follow in conducting a session of this sort — one held for the purpose of presenting a diagnosis of serious, chronic illness in a child to that child's parents. We suggest that the doctor: respect the event, share the diagnosis quickly, attend to the feelings of those present, keep medical facts to a minimum, withstand — even encourage — silence, and avoid running away.

Respecting the event

A terrible business will occur with this interview. A lifetime sentence is about to be declared on Eddie Nichols, a child previously assumed to be normal. The physician knows that, and the parents fear it. News of this sort (we wish it could go without saying) is not delivered on the telephone, in the hallway, in the elevator, or in the hospital cafeteria. It is not delivered in a waiting area peopled by other anxious parents, and it is not delivered standing or on the run. The news calls for time, privacy, and a place with as much physical comfort as can be found. We prefer that *both* parents be present, and that perhaps older siblings (depending on the parents' wishes), especially those beyond about 10 years of age, also attend.

Whether or not the patient himself attends this initial interview around the diagnosis seems to depend on many variables, that is, the child's age, his parents' wishes, and the physician's degree of comfort with handling both patient and parents simultaneously during such an event. Many physicians prefer, and appropriately so, to talk first with the parents and designated siblings, excluding the patient. In addition to sharing the diagnosis, the physician may use a portion of this time to help the family plan how and what they will subsequently tell their sick child. A second interview is then held, including the patient with the family. During this time the parents can describe the diagnosis to the child in their own words, using the physician for support and information as the situation warrants. In this way it becomes a personal, family sharing with the doctor present to help out as needed.

All in all, Dr. Elliott has been quite careful with the Nichols family in arranging the interview. Eddie, is, of course, too young to be included; there are no other children. The doctor has asked to see both parents; they are sitting in a quiet, private room off the pediatric ward. He has set aside time for this interview.

Sharing the diagnosis quickly

Here Dr. Elliott has gotten himself and the interview into trouble. As mentioned he *knows* what must be discussed, and the parents *fear* it. The anticipation of that discussion by both physician and parents accounts for the uncomfortable, awkward, and off-the-subject dialogue reported previously. Each of the three persons has entered the room feeling alone and silently thinking a different refrain:

> *Doctor:* Your son has a terrible, terrible disease for which there is no cure. Why do I have to be the one to tell you this news?
>
> *Mother:* My son is going to die, I know it. That's what his paleness means — he looks like a ghost. And that's what those tests are going to show. I don't want to hear about them — and yet I do. I can't even think clearly.
>
> *Father:* My wife is so embarrassing in her upset state. What will that man think of us? I'll have to stay very calm. And what is wrong with our son? It must be bad. Do I really want to know about Eddie's tests?

Since very little of this is explicitly stated, the ground is prepared for a conversation that takes on an "as if" quality, coming across as something of an enactment. Mrs. Nichols talks about "pale"; for her it is a metaphor about death. Death is unmentionable; "pale" is not. The physician cannot know this, of course; she hasn't told him. But he might assume that any parent in this interview situation, Mrs. Nichols included, is terrified. Such feelings require noticing and acknowledging. However, neither Dr. Elliott nor Mr. Nichols attends to the mother's feelings or behavior (process); each instead responds to her words (content). Mr. Nichols at first gently chides his wife for her preoccupation with their son's pale appearance; he becomes more openly critical of her with time. The doctor, albeit in good faith and ostensibly "listening" to his patient, chooses to focus on Mrs. Nichols's words rather than her feelings in a somewhat different way. He launches into an inappropriate discussion of the causes of pallor in acute illness. He may be medically correct, but he has failed to remember that medical exposition is not the reason for holding this interview. Further delay in achieving his purpose, that of relaying bad news—even in the name of caring concern and "helping parents to understand"—becomes a cruel prolongation of their pain that stems from having to cope with the unknown. Little of a positive nature is accomplished by the physician's stalling or holding off in the delivery of bad news. For many parents the longer the doctor delays, the greater their fears become. The enormity of their child's medical condition becomes directly proportional to the time required for disclosure. ("It must be really bad, if he's taking this long to tell us.")

Of course in the specific interview preceding, the doctor's stalling is unknowingly encouraged and reinforced by Mrs. Nichols's inability to express her fear. Detailed talk about blood cells forestalls approaching the larger issue that she dreads. Even in this situation we would encourage the interviewer to move quickly into a discussion of the diagnosis with the parents. The unapproachable must be approached, and if need be, the doctor must lead the family there. If the diagnosis is known and if the interview is being held for the purpose of relaying that information, a reasonably rapid declaration is important.

Attending to the feelings of those present

In certain respects this type of interview differs not at all from any other family interview. The interviewer has a responsibility to touch, through acknowledgement, the feelings that are spoken, shown, or suggested by each family member. As mentioned, it was Dr. Elliott's failure to acknowledge Mrs. Nichols's worry and fear that precipitated his lengthy and unnecessary blood cell discourse, delaying a discussion of the diagnosis. How might he have proceeded differently? The following is one possibility.

Doctor: (finishing his opening, as stated previously) I wanted to go over his tests with you.

Mother: He looks so pale, Dr. Elliott.

Father: Jean's been so upset since Eddie was admitted, Doctor. Come on, hon, let's hear what the doctor has to say.

Doctor: Actually you both look pretty worried. And I've been pretty concerned myself. What's most worrisome to you about Eddie's looking pale?

Mother: Oh, I don't know. He just looks so sick, so awfully sick.

Doctor: He has been—very ill. It's been a nightmare for you, I'm sure. Have there been times when you wondered if he was going to make it?

Mother: (nods yes)

Father: Don't worry about us, Doc. What about Eddie? You said you had some tests back.

Doctor: I do. I would like you to know that I am concerned about both of you as well as Eddie. The first thing I want you both to hear is that Eddie is not going to die. His pneumonia is under control.

Both parents express relief.

Doctor: (continuing) Eddie is going to get over this pneumonia, but our tests show that the reason for his pneumonia is very serious. Eddie has a condition called cystic fibrosis.

Here the doctor is juggling two transactions simultaneously—leading the parents quickly to the business at hand (the diagnosis) while inserting and thus legitimizing attention to feelings during the process, both the family's and his own. The simultaneity is important. Occasionally one of our trainees will ignore this aspect in his zeal to put into practice his newly learned concepts regarding the discussion of feelings with parents and patients. Recognizing the importance of "feelings" and excited that he now has some techniques for encouraging patients to talk about emotions, the resident may pay such close attention to feelings, to the exclusion of all else, that the following occurs:

Doctor: Before we get down to the business at hand, Eddie's condition, I need to know how each of you is feeling.

Mother: We want to know about Eddie, Doctor.

Father: Yes, have you gotten his tests back yet?

Doctor: In just a minute, Mr. Nichols. You look really worried.

Father: Damn right, I'm worried. Neither Jean nor I have slept in 3 days. This business is hell.

Doctor: I'm sure it's been hard. You sound angry, too. I think we need to talk about that a little bit.

Father: Hell's bells, man—I don't want to talk about my anger. I want to know what's wrong with my son. What do you have to tell us?

Doctor: I can understand your rage, Mr. Nichols. And there's probably a lot more. Just let it out . . . get it off your chest.

Father: Do you have the results or not?

Doctor: It's important for me to understand your feelings first. I *am* going to be talking to you about Eddie's tests in just a minute. What are you feeling at the moment, Mrs. Nichols?

Mother: Well, I . . .

Father: (sputter, fume)

To be sure, this interviewer is persistent; he is also delaying a discussion of the diagnosis, not through medical exposition this time but through his dogged determination to "get feelings on the table." In so doing he, like the earlier Dr. Elliott, has lost sight of the purpose of his interview. The session is not being conducted primarily to explore, discuss, or work with parental feelings. The family has not come for psychotherapy. They have come for concise, understandable, diagnostic information regarding their child. Hence it is information, delivered with an awareness and acknowledgement of the parents' feelings, that must be afforded to them. Information alone won't do; neither will the exclusive and forced focus on feelings described previously. Either used in isolation transforms the experience into a caricature of reality.

Keeping medical facts to a minimum

Returning to Dr. Elliott and Eddie Nichols's parents, the reader will remember that we left that interview scene with the doctor saying, "Eddie is going to get over this pneumonia, but our tests show the reason for his pneumonia is very serious. Eddie has a condition called cystic fibrosis." Now of course the interview is not terminated with this thunderbolt. But in some sense the session has ended for the family. Quite often families have reported to us that once the diagnosis of a serious, chronic illness was verbalized to them—directly and explicitly—all subsequent talk and discussion coalesced into an amalgamated blur. It was as though the mind could not move beyond the enormity of the words: cystic fibrosis, diabetes, renal failure, or whatever. This phenomenon has been described by parents even with little medical expertise and with scant knowledge of the specific disease involved. For most, it is simply clear that a serious condition of some kind exists in their child, leave alone the details, and in the moment of that recognition a (protective) barrier descends, preventing the assimilation or integration of additional medical facts. This is not to say that individuals in such a state fall silent. On the contrary, most parents inundate the doctor at this point with a multitude of questions, all important, some unanswerable. It may go something like this:

> *Doctor:*   Eddie has cystic fibrosis.

There is a pause. Both parents are visibly shaken. Mr. Nichols speaks first.

> *Father:*   What does that mean? Where did he get it? I've heard of it, but I don't know anything about it.
>
> *Mother:*   It's that awful lung disease, Harvey. Remember that family down the street in Petaluma — their two boys?
>
> *Father:*   Eddie's not like them. They were much older . . . and, and they were like . . . invalids. I don't even think they could get out of bed. Eddie's not like that. Before this pneumonia he was fine.
>
> *Mother:*   What does it mean, Dr. Elliott? What do we do now? Is there some treatment Eddie has to have? Isn't there some medicine? (she begins to cry)
>
> *Doctor:*   Well, that is . . .
>
> *Father:*   What my wife is trying to ask is how do we get him over it? Can they do operations for this sort of thing? He is going to get over it?
>
> *Doctor:*   He *is* going to recover from this bout of pneumonia. But the difficult news that I must tell you is that he will very likely continue to have difficulties with recurrent lung infections.
>
> *Mother:*   For how long?
>
> *Doctor:*   Probably for the rest of his life.
>
> *Mother:*   (crushed) Why?
>
> *Doctor:*   For an answer to that, I need to talk with you in some detail about cystic fibrosis, what it is, and what we can do about it.

The doctor may proceed at this point with a discussion of cystic fibrosis, or he may not. If he does continue, he would do well to understand that much of what he says, though it is correct and important, will probably not be understood or remembered by either parent. The prior announcement was simply too staggering. Hence we have sometimes found it simpler and more advantageous to acknowledge the blow directly, rather than proceeding with questions and answers.

Doctor: I do need to talk with you in some detail about cystic fibrosis. At the moment I am aware that I have just hit you with very serious news about Eddie. And I wonder if you can hear much more in the way of information right now.

Mother: I feel numb.

Father: (shakes his head and wipes his eye)

Doctor: (after purposely allowing a significant silence to intervene) You are going to have a thousand questions. You've already asked me several that are extremely important. I would like to answer all of them as well as possible. Yet you are both really stunned. Let me give you some time for that. Just hearing what I've said so far is enough for anyone to withstand. I would like to meet with you again at a time convenient for you, later this afternoon or tonight, and we can begin to go over your questions one by one. How would that be for you?

Mother: I can't think, yet I have a million questions.

Father: Is he . . . is he . . . ever (with tears) going to come home from the hospital?

Doctor: (sensing father's fears) Absolutely. What are you frightened of, Mr. Nichols?

Father: That he's going to die here in the hospital.

Doctor: (placing his hand on Mr. Nichols's arm) I thought so. Eddie *is* going to recover from this pneumonia, and I feel certain that he will be home with you in just a few more days. Do you believe me?

Father: I don't know. I don't know anything. (He breaks down completely. He and his wife cry and comfort one another. The doctor does *not* leave immediately.)

We would support Dr. Elliott's decision to avoid being led into a detailed discussion of prognosis, possible complications, the use of specific medications and therapies, the purchasing of specialized equipment, genetic implications, and etiology *at this time.* Every one of these aspects must be explored with the family at some point, but we question such an exploration so hard on the heels of the diagnostic announcement. This is a very crucial spot in an interview of this sort. The parents are often desperate and insistent in their questioning, and most physicians are far more comfortable and skilled at answering questions, discussing disease parameters, drawing diagrams, and quoting statistics than they are at tolerating the grief, anger, and despair that surfaces or threatens to surface under a controlled veneer of persistent parental questioning. Some questions, of course, must be answered, but only a few; the rest can be tackled in subsequent interviews. We suggest this because the two — persistently questioning parents and persistently answering physician — can work together, resulting in an interview that is medically sophisticated and humanly a disaster. Following such a session the parents may come away feeling overwhelmed by the news and alienated by the doctor's "clinical and unfeeling" approach. All too often the physician may come away feeling incorrectly that he has done a good job. After all, he answered every question and sounded impressive in his knowledge to boot. If in addition he congratulates himself that for no question was he reduced to responding "I don't know," one may be sure the interview was not well done. For then the need to preserve the myth of medical omniscience took precedence over human tragedy.

Withstanding — even encouraging — silence

Silence in interviews is often underutilized, particularly in this type of interview. Too frequently silence is viewed as awkward, as a sign that the interview isn't going well, as something to overcome. We have observed sessions in which both family and doctor have behaved as though they were in a contest with one another to see who could fill up the silent spaces in the interview faster. That is unfortunate, because silence, adroitly used, can be quite helpful.

Upon the delivery of bad news to a set of parents or a family, one need not rush in with accompanying facts, words of solace, or explanations. One might just as readily encourage silence to allow a momentary turning inward for each family member, so that he or she can pay attention to the feelings welling up inside. For the flood of feelings in each individual will stand in the way of attentive listening to subsequent issues in the interview. Encouraging silence is a way of giving permission for each family member to recognize his own feelings and emotions. It is one method for the interviewer to communicate: "I expect that this news is a hard blow, that you are in a sense reeling from it. I consider you and your feelings important enough that I will keep still and not rush past your emotions with words and talk." Dr. Elliott illustrated the judicious use of silence well at another time in another clinical situation:

> *Doctor:* Yes, it is serious. It's hemophilia.
> *Mother:* (gasps and then buries her head in her hands)
> *Father:* But, doctor, how could it . . .
> *Doctor:* (placing his hand on the father's shoulder) For just a moment I feel that there needs to be quiet here. Each of you, for a brief time, just

stay with your thoughts and feelings. (He maintains the silence for more than 3 minutes and then reopens the conversation.) Mrs. Trombetta, share with me and your husband what's happening inside, right now.

Mother: (sobbing) It seems so unfair. First Edgar and now John—both our sons. I can't bear that.

Father: (takes his wife's hand. They talk comfortingly to one another.)

In this situation the use of silence to permit a focus on feelings prevented the start of a question and answer sequence between father and the doctor. In the place of such a sequence, mutual support between mother and father was facilitated and set the stage for continuing movement in that direction. This beginning process of mutual support between spouses, although not always achieved in actuality, needs to continue for optimal management of any child with a chronic illness.

Avoiding running away

It is expected that not only the parent but every physician anticipating the type of interview under consideration will enter it with strong approach-avoidance feelings. His own handling of these feelings is crucial and can be quite variable. He may, for instance, accede to the avoidance literally, by canceling the session, by asking another member of the medical team to do the job, or by attempting the interview over the telephone with perhaps only one parent. Such literal avoidance is certainly regrettable. Other less glaring but equally effective maneuvers to avoid the encounter exist. A doctor may figuratively avoid, while literally attending, by conducting the interview in a detached manner that ignores the family's feelings, by the use of too much and too complicated medical explanation, by the presentation of too hopeful a picture, or by a quick presentation of the diagnosis and then a rapid "ducking out" with the excuse that "an emergency has come up." In each instance what is being avoided, of course, is the doctor's acknowledgement of deep feelings—the family's and his own. That impulse to put distance between oneself and painful emotions is understandable. Yet no more important emergency exists than that which confronts the physician in this interview setting: the emergency of two parents potentially overwhelmed by information that the doctor has just delivered. We would urge the physician, having done so, to "screw his courage to the sticking-place" and not flee the scene (unless the family asks to be alone), staying instead for a while to offer strength and support through his presence, even his *silent* presence.

SUBSEQUENT ISSUES FOR THE FAMILY

Steinhauer and colleagues[2] have said that the family of a child with chronic illness initially comes to the physician with specific questions in mind:

1. What's the matter?
2. What caused the condition?
3. What can the physician do to help?
4. What can the parents do to help?
5. How long will the condition last?
6. Will the child be completely cured?

We would agree that a family asks such questions of the physician. It seems to us that the family also has in mind their own set of idealized answers, even before the physician is consulted.

Questions	Hoped-for answer
1. What's the matter?	Nothing serious
2. What caused the condition?	No one, certainly not the parents
3. What can the physician do to help?	Everything necessary
4. What can the parents do to help?	Everything necessary
5. How long will the condition last?	Almost no time at all
6. Will the child be completely cured?	Yes, of course

Trouble arises for the family when they must hear the physician respond with different answers, often considerably less ideal, to the questions posed. If the doctor must instead communicate that the child's condition is serious, that it was genetically transmitted, that medicine has little to offer, that the parents are essentially powerless to change the situation, that the illness is going to be lifelong, or that there is no cure, it is likely that family dilemmas around certain aspects of the child's illness will arise. For those situations in which not just one, but *all* of the above answers must be given, the presence of real family stress is not only likely, it is a certainty. Such family dilemmas and stress may quite appropriately call for a family approach and the use of conjoint family interviews.

GRIEVING

The preceding, of course, is just the beginning. Family members will move away eventually from the moment of diagnosis, some rapidly, some slowly, only to be faced with a vast array of questions, problems, and unexpected events in their lives. Circumstances will vary from case to case. However, for nearly every such family there is one task that each member needs to complete. It is one the doctor–family interviewer would do well always to anticipate and one in which he may be able to offer the family assistance. The task is that of grieving. In a subsequent chapter we will be discussing grieving and its stages and characteristics in some detail, particularly regarding the family of a dying child. To be sure, for many chronic conditions death is not in the picture, and for many others it is only remotely lurking, many years away. Then why do we suggest that for chronic conditions each family member needs to go through a similar grieving process? Regarding chronically ill children, the staggering fact is not that the child will die but that he or she will live—very differently than originally envisioned by parents or child. Irrevocably and unalterably, the child's life is changed and with it often that of the parents and siblings as well. It is then the loss of the "normal" child together with all the family's hopes and dreams surrounding the (now broken) promise of that child's growth and future that each must mourn. Such mourning is appropriate. It is a way of saying good-bye to an ideal no longer possible. It is also important. Often the circumstances of a child's chronic illness will require substantial alterations in the family's mode and pattern. A refusal to let go of the old hopes and plans may stand in the parents' way, preventing them from facing the present, perhaps rendering them unable to help their child cope with his illness and his changed existence in the here and now. Such a situation arose in the family to be described next. The Morenos illustrate painfully well the dilemmas often facing the family of a child with a chronic handicap, demonstrating especially that when the necessity of mourning is not appreciated and is denied in chronic illness, a family can get itself into serious trouble.

The Moreno family

Kathy Moreno had diabetes. It had been discovered 2 years ago when she was 10 years old. Now 12 and in the sixth grade, she had been doing reasonably well with regard to diabetic control until perhaps 6 months ago. Recently, however, ketoacidosis had cropped up several times, on two occasions necessitating brief hospitalizations. At home she still had not progressed to the point of administering her own insulin, although clearly she was competent enough to do so, and dietary management remained almost exclusively in her mother's hands. On this particular visit her pediatrician was seeing her for something other than diabetes, or so he thought. Because of mother's concerns on the telephone, the doctor had asked the whole family for an interview. The family consisted of Ray Moreno, 31, a city police officer, his wife Ann, 28, a clerk in a local department store, and their two children, Kathy, the identified patient, and Lee, a 2½-year-old boy. Lee did not attend the interview; his mother had left him with a sitter at home.

The family entered the office in a single bolus, mother tightly grasping 12-year-old Kathy with one hand and then swinging her into a chair as if she were a much younger child, not letting go until the girl was firmly established in her seat. Mother motioned with a nod of her head the chair in which she wished her husband to sit. He did so immediately and then slouched and began picking at his nails. The picture was that of a very controlling, very busy, very exasperated mother with two errant children on her hands, a preteen and an adolescent (that is, Mr. Moreno). No one looked very happy. Mother sat down in such a way that father and Kathy were lined up facing her. She was alone.

After initial introductions and a brief social interchange, the doctor asked how he might help this family. Mrs. Moreno unleashed an angry storm:

> *Mother:* Stealing: That's what it is, stealing! Now don't look away, Kathy. There's no other word for it. I don't understand it. We give her everything—it's not as though she's wanting for anything. Am I wrong, well, am I? That man there (indicating her husband) works the equivalent of two jobs, and I work, too. We do it for just that reason, so that our children and our family can have the things they want. And this is the thanks we get. Stealing . . . I can't believe it, in my own family!
>
> *Doctor:* You're *really* upset, Mrs. Moreno.
>
> *Mother:* Well, that's something that I can't tolerate for 1 minute, dishonesty. We've worked so hard for our kids, and . . . and . . . (her words trail off).
>
> *Doctor:* And what?
>
> *Mother:* Oh, I don't know. I'm sure part of this right now is pressure from his family (again pointing to her husband).
>
> *Father:* Well, that's always there, Ann. We always have to deal with that. That's not new.
>
> *Mother:* We always have to deal with it? What's this "we"? I'm the one, Ray. I'm the one who has to manage your parents. You know that, and I do, too.

So much was happening and so fast that the pediatrician was in danger of being inundated by mother's flood of feeling. The chief complaint was Kathy's stealing, and yet that concern was quickly becoming supplanted by some sort of family difficulty with another generation, that of father's parents. A quick glance at Kathy decided the direction for the pediatrician conducting the interview. She was looking increasingly frightened, embarrassed, and worried to him. Thus the doctor chose to move to her:

Doctor:	Kathy, it's pretty hard, I imagine, to be sitting here right now.
Kathy:	Uh-huh.
Doctor:	What are you feeling?
Kathy:	(very glum) Mom's right. It is stealing. (She looks up briefly at her father.)
Father:	It's all right, Kathy. That's what we're here for. We have to talk about it.
Mother:	You'd better believe it. And tell him *all* about it while you're at it. Tell him everything you've been doing.
Father:	I don't think anything is served by that sort of thing, Ann.
Mother:	Look, Ray. I'm the one who had to face some of *your* co-workers at *our* front door and explain to them how come *my* daughter has been stealing. I don't understand why you're not more embarrassed about it. It was the most humiliating experience I have ever had.
Doctor:	And the hurt of that humiliation is still with you.
Mother:	Doctor, I don't think I will ever forget it. Ever.
Doctor:	And it's so big that you find it hard to forgive Kathy right now.
Mother:	Well . . .
Doctor:	You still have too much anger inside?
Mother:	Oh, I am still *furious.* I know it's probably wrong, but . . .
Doctor:	Just a minute. I can understand that if you are still feeling so angry, then forgiveness seems some way off just now. You know, you don't have to apologize for your anger. You were placed in an embarrassing position.
Mother:	I was. Indeed I was.
Doctor:	I understand. For a minute I would like to talk a little more to Kathy about what's been going on.

By taking the time to validate mother's feelings and communicate that she had a right to her anger, the pediatrician "touched" Mrs. Moreno. She almost visibly de-bristled at this point, became silent, and allowed the doctor to continue with her daughter.

> *Doctor:*   Kathy, even though it's hard to talk about, I need to know—what have you been stealing?
> *Kathy:*   (almost inaudibly) Money.

Kathy then explained that she had been stealing as much as $10, usually from her mother's purse and occasionally from her aunt. Ten days before, she had entered a friend's house while the family was out and had taken $20 from that family's piggy bank. It was that incident that brought the police and eventually the scene that mother had earlier described, during which she had to face some of her husband's fellow police officers and account for her daughter's behavior.

> *Doctor:*   (since Kathy seemed quite willing to discuss the whole business) Tell me what you do with the money.
> *Mother:*   (breaking her laudatory silence) Sweets! Sweets! Sweets! This child has the worst sweet tooth you ever saw. She can spend $10 on candy bars alone and then go back a day later and buy a box of cupcakes! And of course she's not supposed to have much of that at all nowadays. But that's where all the money has gone. And her urine, of course, is always 4+ these days. Now tell the truth, Kathy, isn't that so?
> *Kathy:*   (nods her head in agreement)
> *Mother:*   And I've been over that and over it. I don't know why she can't understand how that wrecks her diet and how damaging sweets are for someone with diabetes. Maybe she'll listen to you. She sure doesn't to me.
> *Father:*   Kathy just won't consider the seriousness of her condition, Doctor. I thought those two hospitalizations might even be good—a way of showing her what can happen. But nothing seems to make any difference. She almost seems to be defying us now around this diabetes thing.
> *Doctor:*   So both you and your wife are feeling exasperated on that score.
> *Father:*   Absolutely. But, well, it probably isn't as much a problem for me. I'm not there as much as the wife. She's the one who has to find the candy wrapper under the bed and all of that.
> *Mother:*   You can say that again. I've preached at her until I'm blue in the face. And him (pointing to her husband), he's never home for the bad times. He can't understand why I get so upset. And I tell him, "Ray, if you were only home . . ."
> *Doctor:*   Well, I would like you and your husband to talk to Kathy now about those things you'd like her to know and remember about her diabetes.
> *Mother:*   But, I've . . .

Doctor:	Already done it 27 times? I'm sure you have. I would like you to do it once more, this time in front of me, and now I will help you get your message across.
Mother:	I hardly know where to start.
Father:	Well, I tell her. . .
Doctor:	Tell her now.
Father:	Like I've told you, Kathy . . . having diabetes is nothing to be ashamed of. You are normal, completely normal, and there's nothing to be embarrassed about. Haven't we always tried to tell her, Ann, that she is normal?
Mother:	Absolutely, Why, most of her friends don't even know she has it. I don't think they have to know anything about it. You just have to watch what you eat and when they ask you about it, just tell them that you think diet is important for everyone's health. And it is, you know. You wouldn't be lying to them. There's no reason why you can't do everything all other kids do, anything at all. You just have to be careful about certain foods. The fact that you take insulin is nobody else's business. As far as anyone else is concerned, you are completely normal. We haven't even told Ray's parents — your own grandparents, Kathy — that you have diabetes. And they don't suspect a thing. So you see how normal you are — your own grandparents don't even realize.

Mrs. Moreno then explained that the reason they had not disclosed Kathy's diabetes to her husband's parents was to save them certain worry. Mr. Moreno's father had been a diabetic for 25 years, with serious complications — failing eyesight and most recently the amputation of his right foot. Kathy visibly blanched at the mention of the amputation. So did the pediatrician. He also noted silently that Mrs. Moreno frequently referred to her in-laws as she talked and always with an edge of icy exasperation in her voice. The doctor filed this observation away for possible use in the future.

Certainly many themes, some repetitive, were beginning to appear to him: the obvious connection between the presenting complaint of stealing and Kathy's illness, diabetes; the continuing "presence" of paternal grandparents in mother's thoughts and words; mother's exasperation with father's too frequent absences from family crises; and the persistent determination of both parents to have Kathy viewed as "normal." All of these seemed important. Were they related, and if so, how? At the moment the mixed messages around "normality" were repetitive and were being delivered with tremendous intensity and flair. Listening to the double-level messages, Kathy could and probably did hear the following contradiction: having diabetes is normal—but let's keep it a secret. The pediatrician decided to pursue this discrepancy with the family and help them understand the confusing messages they were giving to their daughter.

> *Doctor:* (to both parents) You use the word "normal" often in describing Kathy and her diabetes. She does have diabetes. Is that, strictly speaking, normal?
>
> *Mother:* (a little shocked) I don't know what you mean. We have worked very hard in these past 2 years to make Kathy understand that she is no different than any other child.
>
> *Doctor:* Yet isn't she different?
>
> *Mother:* Well, not really. I mean, that is . . . ˉ she just has a type of medical problem. But that shouldn't stand in her way. We have never wanted it to interfere with her leading a perfectly normal life. And that's what we've tried to tell her.
>
> *Doctor:* I hear you. I'm beginning to wonder, Mrs. Moreno, if you haven't been working *too* hard at telling her that. (pause) Kathy, what's it like for you to have diabetes?
>
> *Kathy:* Awful. I just hate it.
>
> *Mother:* Well, it wouldn't be so bad if you'd just follow a few simple rules.
>
> *Doctor:* Wait, Mrs. Moreno. Kathy, I want you to think of all the worst parts of having diabetes, all the things you hate most. Wait—don't tell me—just think about all of them for few moments. Make a list in your head.
>
> *Mother:* (while Kathy is looking very thoughtful and obviously mentally composing her list) Doctor, do you think it is wise to discuss such negative things in front of Kathy? We have tried so hard to have her see the positive side.
>
> *Doctor:* You deserve a lot of credit for encouraging her positive attitude. Facing the negative side of her illness is not easy, not for Kathy nor for you as parents. But I think it will need to be faced, by Kathy and by you, if she is to cope adequately with diabetes for the rest of her life.
>
> *Mother:* (falls silent)
>
> *Doctor:* (when Kathy indicates that she has formulated her list) All right. Now I would like you to tell your mother and father all the things you hate about having diabetes. First tell your mother. But before you begin, turn your chair so that you and your mom are facing one another and be very sure that you are looking at one another. You must catch her eyes. Take her hand as well.

Kathy: (holding her mother's hand) I *hate* not being able to eat what I want, especially sweet things . . . I *hate* shots and testing my urine . . . I don't like . . . (at this point her voice cracks and she is close to tears) having always to be so careful . . . of everything.

The doctor noticed that Mrs. Moreno had tears streaming down her cheeks as she looked intently at Kathy, listening to her words. Mr. Moreno's eyes also were teary.

Doctor: Tell your mother, Kathy, that there are many times when you don't *feel normal.*

Kathy: (now openly crying) I don't—I never feel normal! Yet you and Daddy are always saying that. If I'm so normal, how come I can't eat sugar? How come those shots—every day? How come the hospital? How come this bracelet?

All the previously displayed bitterness and anger left Mrs. Moreno's face. In its place was an expression of profound sorrow. She reached out and took her daughter's other hand.

Mother: I'm going to tell you something I've never said, Kathy. I hate it, too, all of it. From the first day that you got sick and the doctor said it was diabetes—I never went back to see that man, ever again. That's why we switched doctors—it wasn't anything that he did really. It was just that he was the one who gave us the news, and I could never forgive him for that. He dashed my hopes and dreams for you, and all I could see was your grandfather with his lifetime of problems. I was determined that I would prove him wrong— your life would *not* change. Your father went along with me, and I decided then and there that you would be treated absolutely normally, so that nothing for you would be different. And . . . and (now sobbing) it's all a mess.

It was no wonder then, as father had said, that "Kathy just won't consider the seriousness of her condition." Both parents, clinging to their own dreams of a "normal" Kathy, refused to acknowledge to themselves the seriousness of her condition, and through this denial they communicated to Kathy dangerous messages that she too could deny facing the reality of her condition. And yet when she followed their lead and joined in their denial, she was always scolded for her behavior, and she sometimes became ill. This was discussed in the session, and Kathy declared that she felt she could never win. If she talked about her illness, particularly if she complained, she had noticed that both parents, especially her mother, would fly into a rage, berating her for feeling sorry for herself and not acting "adult." A lecture about her "normality" would follow. If she then took the lecture seriously, considered herself normal, and disregarded her diabetes, that brought its own problems: ketoacidosis and more lectures, this time about irresponsibility.

Clearly, until both parents had come to accept the reality of Kathy's diabetes, she would continue to be on the receiving end of very confusing messages regarding what her own approach to her illness should appropriately be. Thus the doctor decided to encourage the parents to own, perhaps for the first time, their own negative feelings around the issue. If they could come to consider that diabetes with all its ramifications was real, an "above the table" topic, then perhaps their daughter would no longer have to sneak and steal regarding her medical condition. They would have to drop their denial and relinquish their dream that nothing serious had happened to their daughter. That wish for a normal child would have to vanish so that new, more appropriate, plans might develop.

Kathy and her mother were still holding hands; more importantly, they were listening to one another. It was no longer an assault situation; instead they were effectively sharing feelings with one another.

Doctor: Mrs. Moreno, put your own tears into words now, so that Kathy can understand what you are feeling.

Mother: I . . . I . . . I . . . feel so stupid, crying like this. It isn't like me at all.

Doctor: I agree, it's not like you. Your tears have been a missing, but very important, element. (then to Kathy) Were you aware that your mother had such deep feelings regarding your diabetes?

Kathy: (indicates no) She just always seems mad.

Doctor: So perhaps, Mrs. Moreno, it's important that Kathy understand that you feel more than anger about her diabetes. Wait a minute. No "perhaps" about it . . . it is important. Tell her now what you are feeling inside.

Mother: I feel . . . as though we've been in a nightmare for 2 years, Kathy. I keep waiting for it to end, and it doesn't. I ache for you . . . and even sometimes I . . . (She doesn't finish.)

Doctor: Keep going, Mrs. Moreno.

Mother: I can't . . . it's so selfish.

Doctor: Your "self" is very important and deserves to be heard.

Mother: Sometimes I feel sorry for . . . me. But what right have I to feel that way? She's the one who has it, not me. Anyway that's what I tell myself.

Doctor:	You can't give yourself permission to feel sad, angry, and cheated that your daughter became ill?
Mother:	I shouldn't. No.
Doctor:	Where in the world did you get that idea?
Mother:	(returning to her bitter tone of voice) Ask him. (She points to Ray.)

The session had become one of those in which the interviewer found himself peeling off succeeding layers of the onion. The outermost layer was stealing, which became stealing sweets, which became Kathy's denial of her illness, which became mother's denial of Kathy's illness, which became father's . . . but until this moment the doctor hadn't gotten to father. And the omission was beginning to trouble him. However, it now seemed inevitable, with mother's last remark, that Mr. Moreno's role in the unfolding drama would be revealed. That left only his own parents still in the wings. The pediatrician had not forgotten them either. All in good time, he hoped, but, as he looked at the clock, probably not in this session — there were only 10 minutes left.

Doctor:	It sounds like something that the two of you need to talk about, rather than Mr. Moreno and I.
Mother:	(feeling hopeless) It's no use.

There was a long silence, eventually broken by Mr. Moreno.

Father:	What my wife is referring to . . .
Doctor:	Say it directly to her, Mr. Moreno.
Father:	What you mean is . . .
Mother:	What I mean is I'm not supposed to complain, and you know it. You and your precious parents. Sometimes I feel like I married three people — you and your mother and father. So I don't complain. I make it a point.
Father:	No, not in words you don't.
Mother:	What's that supposed to mean?
Father:	No matter what I say, you jump down my throat . . . like right now.
Mother:	(beginning to cry again) What am I supposed to do, Ray? What am I supposed to do? I'm not supposed to complain about Kathy because "that would worry your parents and they have enough to worry about already." Or you tell me that the guilt would just kill your father if he ever found out that his disease had been passed on. Or you tell me that I'm the strong one, that your parents count on me to be a rock, that they depend on me for everything. But what about me, Ray, who can I depend on? Who's my rock? When

> does my time come? (There is a profound silence as Mrs. Moreno sobs.)
>
> *Doctor:* Be her rock, right now.
>
> *Father:* Er . . . that is, uh . . .
>
> *Doctor:* Comfort your wife.

The pediatrician was thus suggesting several changes in this family's accustomed structure. Mother, not Kathy, was moved openly into the position of "needing." Kathy was shifted to the periphery of the action, an unusual and probably welcome position for her. And father was encouraged to be the strong, competent force in the trio at this time of his wife's need. Implied in the pediatrician's command was that father had that capability and could do the job.

He did. Rising from his chair he moved to his wife and put his arms around her, holding her close and saying in words that even the pediatrician couldn't improve on: "It's all right. I'm here." He no longer looked or acted like a chastised teenager; he seemed a man.

The final 10 minutes of the interview had passed, but they had been put to good use. An additional 5 or 10 minutes was spent drying tears, commenting on what had just taken place, and making plans to meet again in 2 weeks' time. The parents both looked drained. They left with father still keeping his arm around his wife. Kathy looked relieved.

The Moreno family did return in 2 weeks. The work was certainly not finished. Considerable time was spent in five succeeding sessions on having Mr. Moreno make some choices between his present family and his parents. With much support he began to separate somewhat from his parents, taking a stand in favor of his wife and children. In similar fashion, Mrs. Moreno needed continuing encouragement to step down from her previous controlling position of "strength"—the one in which she viewed herself as always capable, always strong, no matter what the demands. Although she had complained bitterly of being placed in that position by others, she nonetheless kept herself there and gave it up grudgingly at first. However, as Mr. Moreno began at home to attend increasingly to the unmet needs of his wife, she became less tight-lipped and bitter and more willing to accept from others. Even Kathy noted the change. As for Kathy, there were no succeeding instances of stealing. At the time of this writing, 2 years later, there has been only one episode of ketoacidosis in the interim. It was caused by an intercurrent infection and was unrelated to any dietary indiscretion.

Discussion. Adhering to a rigid style of denial, this family had developed no avenues for discussion of the child's disease. Any "difference" attributable to the disease was simply not allowed. Consequently Kathy, as is often the case with youngsters with chronic diseases, came to feel ashamed of her condition and isolated, certain that she was in some major way a disappointment to her parents. The Morenos needed to grieve the calamity of Kathy's diabetes, face it realistically, and move on. They did that. Of course the work was not quite that simple, involving as it did several issues spread through three generations of the family. Nonetheless the completion of that bit of business allowed Kathy to develop a more realistic appraisal of her situation with diabetes. This in turn permitted her and the family a more open, healthier coping style for the vicissitudes of her medical problem. Helping the family to grieve, face the reality of diabetes, and put aside old unworkable dreams was facilitated by the pediatrician's attention to and alteration of family structure, communication pattern, sequence, and system. The family performed magnificently in supporting our view that chronic illness is often an important family affair. Appropriate medical treatment thus meant inclusion of the family in that treatment process.

A family with a chronically ill child must face many other issues, aside from grieving their loss. These issues to which we refer were well elucidated in an article by Chancellor and Luben,[1] which outlined the coping problems of families having a child with cystic fibrosis. While the authors limited themselves to this particular patient population, they seemed to describe accurately the major dilemmas facing most families with a chronically ill child, regardless of the specific condition. In our experience with such families, major dilemmas and concerns have centered in the following areas.

Isolation. Many families have reported that their child's illness has rendered them alienated and distant from situations and people outside the immediate family. Energies once devoted to the maintenance of social relationships away from the family are diverted inward toward the ill child and his needs and toward managing the grief reaction of each family member as the reality of the diagnosis becomes felt. Facing the diagnosis of serious, perhaps lifelong, illness in a family member brings inescapable feelings of anger, guilt, and frustration. Preoccupied with such feelings, parents, the ill child, and often siblings may tend to withdraw from outside contacts, and former relationships may then fall away. The chronic sorrow in family members engendered by the fact of the child's illness is also uncomfortable for outsiders to be around, and former friends may stay away "out of consideration" or because "I just don't know what to say anymore." This, of course, only compounds the problem; not only are family members pulling inward, their social contacts are pulling away as well. The family may need to discuss these feelings with a physician. Along with acknowledging their predicament, he may be helpful in assisting the family to resolve this issue, putting them in touch with other families in the same situation and encouraging their participation in parent groups or any environment in which the family can begin to feel less cut off from the rest of the world.

Discipline. With inevitably heightened feelings of sadness, fear, guilt, and anger, parents of a chronically ill child almost always find their discipline notions in disarray. On the one hand, they worry about the child's ability to tolerate the frustrations inevitable with consistent limit setting, and on the other hand, they fear "crippling" their child with over-indulgence and permissive behavior on their part. The danger, of course, lies in parents' overreacting at either end of the spectrum. Parents who fear that the child will use his illness to manipulate and exploit may become overzealous in their determination to set limits and enforce discipline. They and the child then become caught up in a battle over rules far more rigorous than they had previously experienced. Conversely some parents, particularly those in whom guilt has taken a serious foothold, will find themselves immobilized when it comes to setting even appropriate and expected limits with the ill child. Concerned primarily with the child's vulnerability and "not wanting to make the situation worse," these parents abdicate any position of responsible authority with the child. Even for parents not represented by either extreme, the subject of discipline for their sick child and his siblings—what, when, and how much—is a perpetually arising dilemma. It often requires discussion with the doctor.

Family relationships. Very often when a child becomes seriously and chronically ill, the machinery of the family stops. Previous routines and activities are curtailed, and the focus falls exclusively on the sick child. This can become particularly difficult for well siblings who suddenly and permanently find their lives altered and restricted for reasons that seemingly have little to do with them directly. Parents are no longer as available, and even when available, they seem different—perhaps short-tempered and irascible, preoccupied with worry about the sick family member. Since they may experience their parents' lack of contact without necessarily understanding the reasons behind it, siblings may begin to conjecture on their own. They may surmise, inaccurately, that they are no longer loved or considered important by the parents.

In addition the family's mobility may be curtailed, especially if the sick child can't be left for extended periods or requires special equipment to go along on outings, or if certain environments are found to be hazardous for the child's precarious state of health, and so forth.

Parents may not only be finding less time for their well children; each may also feel it necessary to forgo adult time alone with the other spouse, becoming so caught up in the care of the ill child that the care and feeding of their own marital relationship is allowed to be seriously neglected. One parent may single-handedly take on the child's illness as a "career" to the exclusion of all other relationships, interests, and people. Anyone other than the child and his disease may be considered an irrelevant interruption, and "anyone" may include the spouse. Communication difficulties between husband and wife are then inevitable. As a matter of fact, communication difficulties arise among all family members in such a situation. Feelings are everywhere, but often they are those that are considered "unspeakable" so that each family member begins contributing to the development of a "conspiracy of silence." When one is feeling angry, ashamed, guilty, selfish, jealous, neglected, vengeful, sad, despairing— and when one is feeling those things toward or because of a very ill child who never asked to get sick in the first place—then one often swallows those feelings as well as possible and tries to get on with life. The sad culmination of this decision is that each family member walks around with a burdensome load of uncomfortable feelings and no place to discharge them. This was certainly well-illustrated by the Moreno family.

Financial burdens. For many families with a chronically ill child, especially if hospitalizations and medical equipment are required, the financial responsibility can be staggering. In those families experiencing significant guilt around the issue of the child's illness, this may be a taboo topic for discussion, since, "how, with Mary so ill, can we possibly allow ourselves to worry about how much it is all costing?" Such an attitude, while lofty and humanitarian, can be tragic. Extended hospitalization these days can completely wipe out a family's financial worth. To prevent this from happening, parents must be realistic from the outset about their own economic ability and limits. A physician can be helpful in encouraging a family to face this issue directly, rather than as something that is shameful and needs hiding. Financial difficulties can also contribute to the problems of isolation and the difficulties in family relationships stated earlier. Less money is available for trips, for family activities, for getting out and away. And of course siblings may then complain that "we don't ever get to go skiing anymore, not since Mary got sick," for which they could conceivably receive a tongue-lashing from a parent who is already feeling regretful about that very fact.

Misunderstandings. Medical jargon and terminology are especially troublesome for the families of chronically ill children. Since the child's condition is very often lifelong and will clearly necessitate the active participation of the parents and perhaps even siblings in the ongoing care required, unnecessarily complex and obfuscating terms used by the medical staff are just one more frustrating hassle for the family members to put up with. Families continue to request that explanations from physicians be more simple and understandable. It is a reasonable request, since medical simplicity and clarity can only enhance a parent's understanding and care for his own child.

Parents' emotional concerns. Parents with a chronically ill child worry. They fret about the physical appearance of the child. They suffer from the "thoughtless" comments others make to and about their sick child. They ask themselves and each other how to cope with such problems. They worry about having more children. Having seen the disease previously in a childhood friend or a neighbor's child may cause them to worry that their child will have the same dreadful course and outcome as in the remembered case. Parents wonder if they are "giving enough" to the sick child and to his siblings. They worry about the sick child's emotional state, his anxieties, unspoken worries, feelings of inferiority, and so on. They especially worry about their role in helping the child with these problems. They will often need considerable help from the doctor with these and other worries.

Hope for a cure. Even for parents who accept head-on the hard facts of a particular illness and its course and prognosis, a kernel of hope still remains, hope that a cure will be found in their child's lifetime. It is quite often an irrational, highly improbable hope. Nonetheless it is essential, facilitating the withstanding of a difficult present and allowing for some, even limited, planning. As one parent stated, regarding her teenager with systemic lupus erythematosus: "You can't live thinking they're going to die every minute. You do that at first. Then you learn to live for their life, not for their death." Hope for an eventual cure is an important factor in nourishing day-to-day hopes, fostering the pursuit of limited goals such as getting the child to school for a full day or having him obtain his driver's license, successfully manage one overnight trip away from home, and so forth. Hope springs from other sources as well. Some parents derive hope and satisfaction from fully acknowledging the child's condition and moving on from there to help the child find a meaningful daily existence in his permanently altered life situation.

Parental guilt regarding transmission. Even for those diseases not clearly transmitted genetically, parental guilt over "having given this to my child" is a prominent issue. The physician would do well to assume this feeling is present in *every* parent of a child with chronic illness, even if not stated directly by one parent or the other. Quite often it is not verbalized directly; the shame and guilt are hidden but present nonetheless. Unfortunately, the form of a medical history does much to activate these feelings in parents. Even before a diagnosis is made, when parents know only that something is seriously wrong with their child, they are subjected to a medical history during which the physician, doing his thorough job, asks in detail about a positive family history for this or that dread disease and about the details of conception, pregnancy, and delivery. One conclusion is inescapable for many parents: "He is looking for the cause of my child's condition in something I have passed on or something I did to my child." To be sure, even without this line of questioning, parental guilt would still be present in many situations. It is, however, unfortunate that one aspect of traditional and accepted medical practice seems destined to augment such an uncomfortable feeling in parents. The physician can help in this topic by bringing parental feelings out into the open for discussion rather than leaving them hidden and unspoken. Parental guilt, particularly in diseases that are transmitted genetically, will not vanish with one discussion and some reassurances from the physician. Alleviation of such feelings will require considerable time, from months to years; the physician can initiate the process. He should also be willing to persist and to recognize that the family's resolution of guilt requires a process extending over much time.

Fear of death. Just as parental guilt regarding transmission is present in situations where it has no business appearing, likewise the fear of death seems to be ubiquitous in families of chronically ill children, even in situations where the disease is not particularly fatal. Hence it is also useful with this issue—the fear of death—to assume that it is present in every situation, even when not verbalized. This is often the most taboo topic of all, and the conspiracy of silence mentioned earlier can be particularly upheld around this fear. One may also assume that if the fear is alive in one family member, it is probably felt at some level by every family member, even though it has never been discussed. That means that if a parent is fearful of the child's death, in all likelihood the child himself is aware of a similar, though perhaps less specific, dread—even though the fear may be completely ungrounded. These fears may need to be discussed with the family by the physician. In so doing, that "conspiracy of silence" around a family's reactions to death and dying can be avoided.

Treatment regimen. A family's focus on this issue depends to a large extent on the specific condition. Families of a child with cystic fibrosis, for instance, can become absolutely preoccupied with the working of mist tents, compressors, motors, and nebulizers. For families facing other diseases, for example, seizures, the focus can be much simpler, limited to a single medication or combination of drugs. In either case the family is actively engaged in the treatment process of their sick child, and so engaged they will have a multitude of questions. Again the issue of medical terminology and explanations arises. Family members need to know what to do and how to do it. Their feelings regarding specific treatment approaches also need to be considered. For without (1) parental understanding and (2) parental acceptance of the prescribed treatments, the best planned regimen will fail.

Another aspect of the treatment regimen deserves mention. Depending on the age of the child, it is extremely helpful to have him participate in his own care so that he develops a sense of responsibility and competence in the management of his condition. Occasionally in an effort to "protect their children," parents thwart such participation by the sick youngster, taking on themselves the total responsibility for his care. This is particularly true when one parent adopts the child's illness as a career, as mentioned previously. Such a trend, excluding the child from any responsibility toward maintenance of his own health, must be interrupted. This situation may often be handled well in the context of a family interview.

Actually for all of these issues judicious family intervention by the physician may be essential at times. Taking the issues mentioned in turn, we would recommend a family interview and approach, often (not always) including the ill child, for situations in which a family member has said:

"We feel so alone; there's no one to talk to about this problem."
(isolation)

"He just won't stay in his tent, and you said it was essential."
  (discipline)
"We just never get out anymore; no babysitter could do the job."
  (family relationships)
"There's just never any money anymore to do things."
  (financial burdens)
"I don't know how we're supposed to do that. And also, what in hell
  does phlebotomy mean? Isn't that some sort of illegal brain operation?"
  (misunderstandings)
"She just seems to be giving up, Doctor."
  (parents' emotional concerns)
"Sometimes I think I just can't hope any longer. It's been so long."
  (hope for a cure)
"I read that article about diethylstilbesterol, Doctor. Just what could
  that mean for Mary's situation? I took that medication, you know."
  (parental guilt about transmission)
"He's been having trouble breathing at night but wouldn't tell us for
  days. He said he didn't want us to worry."
  (fear of death)
"Harvey seems awfully young to be giving himself his own shots. Are
  you sure he's ready to do that, Doctor?"
  (treatment regimen)

In family interviews surrounding these complaints we would explore
in exactly the same fashion as illustrated elsewhere in this book the
family's communication style, structure, system, and sequences of behavior. Meeting with the family together would afford an unparalleled
opportunity to evaluate and assist in the family components of a child's
chronic condition. One could, for instance, observe a family's level of
acceptance and understanding of their child's illness or help a family
with their grief reaction. One could certainly evaluate the involvement
of siblings and their feelings regarding family life changes. One might
be able to clarify misunderstandings surrounding the medical management of the child. One could help the family to broach formerly unspeakable topics, from death, to anger, to exhaustion. One could begin
to foster a mutual support network among family members. And one
could provide emotional support when the family flags and feels done
in by the mean trick life has played. When a child suffers a chronic
illness, it is a family matter. Attention must be paid.

REFERENCES

1. Chancellor, B., and Luben, H.: Conferences with parents of children with cystic fibrosis, Social Casework **53:**140, 1972.
2. Steinhauer, P., and others: Psychological aspects of chronic illness, Pediatr. Clin. North Am. **21:**825, 1974.

CHAPTER 9

In the hospital

Most of the clinical examples shared thus far have been family interviews with pediatric outpatients. We have also often utilized family interviews in our work with hospitalized children. Family interviews on our own pediatric ward have happened to revolve most often around some issue of a child's chronic medical condition. More than anything else this fact probably reflects the character of our particular pediatric inpatient service at the University of California. Because the hospital functions as a referral center for northern California and beyond, the patient population of the pediatric ward consists primarily of critically ill children with serious, complicated, and often chronic conditions. In this regard our facility is probably similar to many other university teaching hospitals throughout the United States. To illustrate the character of our patient population in the hospital, we offer the following list. It represents conditions for which family interviews were conducted by one of the authors (B.A.) during a randomly selected 4-month period:

Chronic headaches
Ulcerative colitis
Multiple and varied psychosomatic complaints
Nephrotic syndrome
Cystic fibrosis
Failure to thrive
Hypothyroidism
Hypoglycemia
Tuberous sclerosis
Microcephaly with mental retardation
Achondroplasia
Chronic abdominal pain

Chronic vomiting

Psychomotor seizures

Acute glomerulonephritis

Gilles de la Tourette's syndrome

Anorexia nervosa

Family interviewing by the pediatrician has proven a useful clinical tool in situations such as these. We assume that it would be used equally well in pediatric inpatient settings elsewhere where the character of the patient population might include a larger number of acute, shorter term conditions.

Family interviews with pediatric inpatients can serve a variety of purposes. Our pediatric staff has used them for:

1. Clarification of a diagnostic dilemma
2. Helping the pediatric staff to understand (and therefore work more effectively with) a family's in-hospital behavior
3. Initiation of ongoing family counseling when this has been indicated
4. Sharing with the family diagnostic findings and therapeutic plans concerning a sick child
5. Providing support to a family that has requested or demonstrated their need for help
6. Preparing a child and family for a proposed surgical procedure on the child

CLARIFICATION OF A DIAGNOSTIC DILEMMA

Family interview consultations for hospitalized children have been most frequently requested by our pediatric ward staff for one particular purpose: assistance in reaching a diagnosis concerning a child and his unexplained, confusing symptoms. A single diagnostic session with the family can be useful in this regard, and it can be incorporated into an inpatient diagnostic assessment just as readily as the other, more traditional, studies of X-ray films, blood chemistries, and so on. A diagnostic family interview is an invaluable tool, especially when there is concern for the presence of behavioral components that are affecting the child's health. Since we have most often used family interviews with inpatients in this area of diagnostic assessment, the clinical illustration we have chosen to demonstrate the utilization of family interviews with hospitalized children will be drawn from one of these experiences, in which the pediatric ward staff asked our help in arriving at a diagnosis concerning the severe headaches of Jason Douglas, age 12½.

The Douglas family

Jason had had headaches since he was 6 years old, almost as long as he could remember. They were severe, occurring as often as twice a month and sometimes lasting for an entire day. They were so painful that Jason would be disabled essentially for the duration of an attack, forced to stay in bed and remain as motionless as possible. Analgesics had little effect. His parents had never felt that he was malingering or "putting on." He was always genuinely upset when an attack appeared, hating to curtail his many activities. In school he had always been a hard worker and straight A student. He was active and talented in sports. Boy Scouts took considerable time, and he was very involved in the youth program of his church. He was immensely popular with other children, and his parents described him as "almost a model child . . . just a totally normal, delightful boy."

Father was a banker; mother was a housewife. The family lived in a well-to-do suburb of a large Texas city. Extensive medical evaluations had been done at a university medical center there on several occasions. He was seen first as an outpatient and then subsequently hospitalized for further studies. Laboratory evaluations and detailed physical examinations failed to disclose any medical reason for this youngster's continuing severe bouts of headache. Still the parents continued to search for an answer. They changed doctors, had Jason undergo extensive allergy testing, altered his diet, and read voluminously on the subject of pediatric neurology and the causes of head pain in children. Nothing, however, caused his symptoms to disappear or even subside. Finally they took the advice of Mrs. Douglas's brother. This man, living in the San Francisco area, had on several occasions urged them to consider seeing a particular pediatric neurologist at the University of California Medical Center. After some deliberation, the Douglas family packed up, moved in temporarily with their relatives in San Francisco, and made arrangements for Jason's hospitalization and his evaluation by the pediatric neurologist recommended to them.

By the time Jason had been in the hospital for 7 days, only one or two of his laboratory tests were still incomplete. Those diagnostic efforts that had returned yielded no new findings, nor did they suggest a diagnosis.

Many disease entities had been ruled out, but then, those same diseases had been ruled out previously when Jason first underwent study and tests in Texas. The ward staff was feeling frustrated, and in this feeling they joined the Douglas family. Jason and his parents had now traveled almost a thousand miles. New answers regarding his headaches did not appear to be forthcoming.

The Child Study Unit was requested to hold a diagnostic family interview. The pediatric resident explained to the family that a discussion with all of them was a part of Jason's total diagnostic evaluation and that the discussion would be led by a pediatrician who specialized in helping families of children with puzzling diagnostic problems.

"Just as long as we're not seeing a psychiatrist," was father's reply. He indicated that doctors in Texas had suggested that Jason's difficulty "might be emotional"; both parents had considered that patently absurd. A previous consultation with a child psychiatrist in Texas, after complete testing by a child psychologist, had confirmed the parents' view. According to Mrs. Douglas, these consultants had declared that Jason did not have psychological problems. "And so we really prefer not to go through that again," she concluded. "It would be such a waste."

The resident agreed that he would not want to duplicate that study either. He explained that this interview would be somewhat different, especially since it would include Jason together with his parents and since a pediatrician would be in charge. Reluctantly the family agreed. A suitable time was arranged.

Performing the first (and sometimes only) diagnostic interview with the family of a hospitalized child is in many ways similar to performing any sort of initial family interview. Such initial encounters with a family were discussed in Chapter 6. There are, however, some unique, additional, previously unmentioned features to consider when the initial interview is to be, as in this case, a single episode for diagnostic purposes, concerning a child who is hospitalized for a medical condition of some kind.

First of all, our experience in working with hospitalized children has been that resistance to the idea of participating in a family interview is high among family members, more so than we usually encounter in the majority of similar outpatient experiences. Winning the family over to a family view and facilitating their support rather than their anxious reluctance requires considerable work by the interviewer. Such feelings of anxious reluctance in the family probably derive from a variety of sources. Family members are already anxious, frightened, and under stress because of the hospitalization itself, an experience decidedly outside the norm for most families. Also, hospitalization usually signifies the seriousness of a child's condition. That the child's hospitalization is on a pediatric floor underscores the belief that concerns about the child are "medical." For many parents then, the hospitalization denotes that their child (1) is seriously ill and (2) has a medical condition. Being asked to participate in a "family interview" does not seem to fit with that scheme, sounding somehow too "psychological." For many families their inner question becomes, "Are they trying to say that we have psychological problems?"—an understandably unsettling query. Superimposed on that, particularly for those situations in which the child's complaint is psychosomatic, may be the family's long-standing apprehension and adamant denial (prominent long before hospitalization ever occurred) that psychological issues are involved. This apprehension and denial can further feed a family's reluctance to enter the unknown and (to them) "dangerous" environment of a family interview.

The reluctance of the Douglas family was therefore not surprising. We have come to expect this with pediatric ward consultations for family interviews. Approaching such a family calls for a delicate touch, with considerable sensitivity for and acknowledgement of family apprehensions. How the subject is introduced even before the interview takes place is quite important. On our own pediatric inpatient service this introduction and preparation is usually done by the pediatric resident. We have observed that he may help some families and the family interviewer as well by mentioning that the interview will be conducted by a pediatrician—since, however inappropriate in this day and age, there is still considerable reluctance to be interviewed by a psychiatrist, especially when the stated problem is felt to be "physical." He may also state that a thorough evaluation of the child involves a discussion with his family, that this procedure is considered an integral part of the patient's hospitalization. It may be useful, especially if a good relationship has been established with the child and the family, to mention that he himself and/or the child's nurse will attend the interview. Explaining the role of the interviewer as one who specializes in helping families of children with confusing diagnostic problems, or those with chronic illnesses, or families with hospitalized children, and so on, may be more comfortable for the family than hearing that the interviewer "will explore emotional aspects of Jason's illness."

If there are siblings at home, the family may ask why those members must also attend. The individual preparing the family may state that obviously the patient's medical condition has had an impact on the entire family and that everyone's input during this one family meeting may be useful. Nonetheless, acknowledging the inconvenience of assembling all family members when this means missing school, leaving work, traveling distances, and so forth is certainly indicated.

An additional feature of this type of interview deserves comment. That is its solitary nature. In our discussion of the four goals of an initial family interview, the final goal mentioned was that of ensuring the family's return. This is often not an option with family interviews on pediatric wards such as ours. The family has frequently come from hundreds of miles away, hospitalization is short, and the patient's time is filled with a multitude of other tests and procedures. More than one family interview in such instances may not be practical, nor is a follow-up visit after discharge. Hence the time frame may be considerably different for a single consultation interview than it would be were the family embarking on the first of several subsequent interviews. This fact is frequently at odds with the family's heightened apprehension about the interview, mentioned previously. They enter the session with considerable fear and anxiety about the process; this calls for a gentle, *slow* pace to the interview. Yet it may be the interviewer's only opportunity to meet with the family. Therefore the interviewer's goals in this type of initial interview become:

1. Establishing that he will be in charge of the interview
2. Working quickly to establish a diagnostic formulation
3. Making the interview a "touching" experience for every family member
4. Making recommendations for follow-up and further care
5. Facilitating the family's acceptance of treatment recommendations

This is a tall order for one interview, and sometimes it frankly isn't possible. Goals 4 and 5 especially may require subsequent interviews, particularly if one is suggesting to the family ongoing counseling of some type to take place in a community many hundreds of miles away. And yet there are times when the entire process can be accomplished in one interview, as with the Douglas family.

Their interview was held in a conference room off the pediatric ward. Besides Jason, both his parents, and the interviewer, the pediatric resident also attended. The family was an attractive group. Jason was dressed in his pajamas but even so gave the appearance of being prepared and organized for any event. The doctor had never seen a child in pajamas who looked so fully dressed. He mirrored his parents in this regard. There was not a trace of casualness in their dress or manner. The family looked positively "squeaky clean." Father was first into the interview room, taking the lead by introducing himself and the rest of the family. Next was Mrs. Douglas; she was equally forthright in her approach and very correct. Clothes for both adults were tailored, stylish, and impeccable.

Jason was last into the room. He shook everyone's hand and took a seat between his parents. The family was exceedingly polite. They also looked quite nervous. A brief period of social talk about the hospital, their trip, finding their way around San Francisco, and so on did not change that look. The interviewer moved quickly into the subject at hand.

Doctor:	This business of Jason's headaches has really been a long-term problem. I imagine that you must all be feeling very frustrated by this time.
Jason and Father:	(nod vigorous agreement)
Mother:	We're almost used to it, aren't we, Jason—it's been going on for so long.
Doctor:	I would like to spend some time today discussing the problem with you. It has certainly dominated this family's life for the past several years.
Father:	Six years, Doctor.
Mother:	I don't think it's been that long.
Father:	Oh yes, it has. Jason was in the first grade. It was the year we lived in St. Louis.
Mother:	Well, you can't really count that, Merrill. Jason was having allergies at that time. It wasn't until a year or so later that the headaches, as they are now, came on. Isn't that right, son?
Jason:	I . . . I think so. I'm not sure.
Mother:	I'm certain it is. You just don't remember. Well, anyway it's a small point. What were you asking us, Doctor?

The family had indirectly already said much about themselves. The need for properness, decorum, and control was abundantly displayed in their appearance and manner. Father and son seemed willing to acknowledge feelings of frustration in their situation. However, Mrs. Douglas seemed to sidestep feelings of any sort. Furthermore, she had suggested so far with her controlling behavior that she considered her version of things the proper one, correcting her husband and speaking for her son. Jason meekly complied, knuckling under to her control.

The family continued to talk for a while about Jason's symptom itself, about all his past experiences with doctors and hospitals, and about the chronicity of the problem. Although the doctor was filing away preliminary observations regarding how family members behaved with one another and with him, he kept the conversation directed toward a discussion of Jason's medical complaint and all that the family had experienced together since the trouble began several years ago. Children's chronic headaches, those not caused by a space-occupying lesion or some other dread disease, have often in our experience been associated with a considerable reluctance on the child's part to show anger and with vigorous, unspoken family rules forbidding its direct expression. Aware of this, the doctor was therefore particularly mindful of the theme of anger in this family, watching for its appearance or its conspicuous absence. He had even opened the session with an invitation for them to acknowledge possible frustration. Mrs. Douglas, as noted, was admitting to no such feeling. Her husband and son did, but they were having difficulty so far getting a word in edgewise. All of this was very tentative, but the interviewer found himself waiting for the opportunity to introduce a discussion of the subject of anger and its expression in the family.

As the discussion continued, Mr. and Mrs. Douglas began praising Jason, telling of all his activities and many accomplishments. The picture was that of a bright, talented, athletic, gregarious young man who never complained and had his 12½-year-old world by the tail. They were very proud of him. Once again the doctor offered them the opportunity to declare angry feelings about the subject of Jason's disabling headaches.

Doctor:	How maddening for all of you to have Jason's busy life and many accomplishments so frequently interrupted by his headaches.
Father:	Yes, sometimes I feel . . .
Jason:	If only . . .
Mother:	(quickly) We just do the best we can. Jason is the greatest little patient in the world. Wouldn't you say that, Merrill? (then without waiting for an answer) He is absolutely a wonder, Doctor. There are times I can tell the pain is really getting to him. But not one

complaint out of him . . . ever. (She reaches over and pats her son's knee.)

The pediatrician noted for the second time that abortive attempts to acknowledge frustration by Mr. Douglas and his son were quickly swept away by Mrs. Douglas in a controlling gesture that each time minimized the existence of frustration and praised silent adaptability and denial as the desired way to cope.

Doctor: Jason, you were saying, "If only . . ." Finish that sentence.
Jason: If only . . . if only we knew what was causing them.
Father: You can say that again. This whole business has gotten very old. And no one seems to have any answers, or at least any correct answers.
Doctor: What answers have you had from doctors along the way? How have they explained Jason's headaches?

Mr. Douglas then listed all the diagnoses that had at one time or another been included in, then ruled out of, Jason's differential diagnosis: brain tumor, migraine, seizure equivalent, cerebrovascular abnormality, allergies, sinusitis, and so forth.

Doctor: None of those has turned out to be the case with Jason. And the whole business just keeps dragging on. That must be tremendously aggravating. Generally when a family is confronted with such a continuing question — and no answer — everyone begins to have his own ideas about what might be going on, logical or illogical, rational or irrational. Now, I realize you don't know what's been causing Jason's difficulty, or you wouldn't be here now. But I would like each of you to share with me what you've occasionally *thought* might be causing his headaches over the years, as you've tried to make sense out of this business. I'll start with you, Jason. You've been experiencing these headaches for a long time. What have you yourself thought might be causing them? Your answer may be quite different from what the doctors have told you. But that's all right. I am interested in your own ideas about this situation.
Jason: Well . . . (he hesitates for a considerable period of time)
Doctor: Even your wildest thoughts. What in the world could be behind these headaches?

The interviewer was not expecting the answer given, but he was instantly grateful.

Jason: (becoming very somber) Sometimes I think I worry too much.

> *Mother:*   Worry? Why Jason, whatever do you have to worry about? That's nonsense.

Once again Mrs. Douglas was attempting to cover over feelings in a family member through the use of denial and imposition of her own view.

> *Doctor:*   What do you see on your son's face right now, Mrs. Douglas?
> *Mother:*   Nervous, he's just a little nervous about his meeting today. That's all.
> *Doctor:*   Ummm, is that what you're feeling, Jason?
> *Jason:*   Yes, I guess so.

Again some of Jason's feelings seemed to be going underground, covered by a surface layer of agreement with his mother. The doctor was also concerned that he might have lost the moment for making contact with Jason around the issue of "worry."

> *Mother:*   Jason and I have a very special relationship, Doctor. I usually know what's going on with him. I can tell when he's upset; he shares everything with me. I have always encouraged him to be completely open with me. Isn't that right, Jason? Don't we tell one another our problems? I guess I would know if you had any sort of worries. (then turning to the doctor) But you know, this boy is amazing. No matter what he has to do, he doesn't complain. Jason is the eternal optimist.
> *Doctor:*   Ask him if he ever has some private inside worries.
> *Mother:*   You don't, do you son?

Her question so phrased was a disguised command, ordering him to reply "Of course not." Yet in spite of her wording, which clearly and subtly communicated the answer she hoped for, Jason spoke up.

> *Jason:*   Sometimes I do.
> *Mother:*   But they're not anything serious. (She uses a period, not a question mark, in her voice.)
> *Doctor:*   Wait, ask him instead to share his worries with you.
> *Mother:*   Well, of course, that's what I always want you to do. You know that.
> *Doctor:*   Ask him to, now.
> *Mother:*   What is it Jason? Tell me.
> *Jason:*   Sometimes . . . I worry . . . about the kids at school.
> *Father:*   What do you mean?
> *Jason:*   I don't think they respect me.
> *Mother:*   Jason, darling, don't be silly. They all look up to you.
> *Doctor:*   Ask him instead, Mrs. Douglas, what leads him to feel as he does.
> *Mother:*   Well?

At each turn Mrs. Douglas was there with a disclaimer for Jason's feelings, insisting ostensibly through "reassurance" that he didn't or shouldn't have the feelings he was attempting to share. If Jason were to open up in this session, the doctor realized he would have to continue to encourage Mrs. Douglas to *ask* her son questions, rather than allowing her to close him down by declaring her own version of his feelings.

Jason responded to his mother with a story about his best friend, Mark. The two of them were apparently very much alike, the "popular" boys in the class and in the entire school for that matter. Both he and Mark were candidates for the school's prestigious annual citizenship award. Mark won the prize, not Jason. Tears welled up in Jason's eyes as he now spoke.

Jason: I am happy that he won it. Really, I am. He deserved it. And besides he's my best friend. But now all the kids seem to pick *him* for their teams and stuff; they don't seem to respect me anymore . . . and . . . Mark, he doesn't seem as nice as he used to be. I know he really deserved that award; he should have gotten it, but . . . . (Falling silent he pounds his fist gently on the arm of the chair; he continues to have tears in his eyes and is obviously exerting effort so as not to cry outright.)

Doctor: What feelings do you see in your son right now, Mrs. Douglas?

Mother: (avoids answering the question) I remember this whole business, Jason. I was so proud of how you handled that situation, when Mark won the award instead of you. Remember, you didn't let it bother you at all. Remember that I told you that?

Doctor: (aware that mother has avoided facing her son's feelings) What do you see on his face?

Mother: (does not answer verbally but shakes her head indicating that words will not come, appears very sad, and looks directly into her son's eyes)

It was a moment when the two of them made real contact with one another. There was silence in the room. The doctor noted that Mr. Douglas had been listening and looking intently throughout this whole interchange, although he had said little. The doctor turned to him.

Doctor: How about you, Mr. Douglas? What do you see going on with your son right now?

Father: I see a great deal of sadness and anger. I had no idea that he was so upset.

Doctor: Check that out with him. Find out if you are reading him correctly.

Father: Am I?
Jason: (nods yes)
Doctor: See if you can find out what his feelings are about.
Father: I know.
Doctor: But don't assume. Ask him.
Father: I don't think he'll tell me. He's embarrassed.

Now, using somewhat different but equally effective means, father — not mother — was cutting off Jason's sharing of feelings. By making assumptions about the child's feeling state (for instance, "I know," and "he's embarrassed") he was discouraging Jason's own disclosure. His prediction ("I don't think he'll tell me") was also a form of disguised command, a message that Jason could easily hear as: "Don't tell me." Both parents in subtle and repetitive ways were thus indirectly discouraging any openness Jason might venture regarding the expression of serious thought and feeling.

Doctor: Ask him anyway.
Father: You are embarrassed, aren't you. (like his wife, using subtle wording to program a preferred answer)
Jason: (looking down, no answer)
Doctor: Mr. Douglas, try this one: "Jason, tell me about your anger."
Father: (laughs) OK, tell me about your anger.
Jason: I don't know . . . if . . . I thought . . . (finally) I wish that I won.
Father: Is that what you're angry about?
Jason: (nods yes) Mostly at myself.
Doctor: And partly at Mark, too?
Jason: I shouldn't be, but . . .
Father: You are.
Jason: A little.
Doctor: Tell your father, "I *am* angry at myself and at Mark about that award."
Jason: (to his father) I do feel a little mad mostly at myself that I didn't win . . . some too at Mark.

The doctor noted that Jason needed to soften and qualify his feelings in the statement of his anger. Nonetheless it was a beginning for him, and the doctor did not comment or interrupt.

Father: (He is obviously touched by what is taking place.) This is all very hard. I guess I see things differently than my wife. For me, Jason is not one to show his feelings. That's why I am amazed right now. I had no idea. I never know when he's mad. In fact I didn't think he got mad. And he certainly doesn't come to me with what's on his mind. We have *never* actually talked like this before. And I've never been really clear about what's going on inside with Jason. He's just always been very good-natured.

Mother: (having composed herself and returning to her former stance) Actually none of us, I guess you would have to say, ever gets really angry, Doctor. There's so much anger in the world . . . and we really don't need to have anger for one another. We can almost always settle things without getting mad.

Doctor: I see. Yet when Jason gets angry, sad, upset — as we all do — *as Jason is right now* — I wonder then, how he is able to show you his feelings? How can he let you know? Can he let you see?

Father: Well, I certainly see what he's feeling about this Mark situation right now. (pause) Now I'm thinking: is it that Jason generally doesn't show his feelings, or is it perhaps that I haven't been looking?

Doctor: Ask him.

Father: (turning to his son) Well, I'm ashamed to say that I know I haven't been looking very much, but . . . how about it, son, do you keep things inside?

Jason: Most of the time.

Father: Why, Jason, why?

Jason: (after a silence) I can't talk to either you or Mom. (voice cracking) I don't want to worry you or make you not proud . . . of me.

Father: (says nothing and continues to look with concern toward his son)

Doctor: What are you experiencing right now, Mr. Douglas?

Father: Well, now I'm remembering all sorts of things . . . like last summer.

Father then described how the previous summer had been particularly difficult for the family. In addition to headaches, Jason developed severe "rectal spasms" (with diarrhea, cramps, and weight loss) before going off to summer camp. He continued:

Father: What was that all about, Jason? How many other things are you doing to please us or not to worry us? Did you want to go to camp . . . for yourself . . . or for us? I remember I couldn't figure it out at the time.

Mother: Now, Merrill, really . . .

Father: Don't interrupt, Dorothy. We need to talk about that, son.

Jason: It . . . it was sort of a combination . . . I knew you wanted me to go, and I did, too . . . sort of, but . . .

Father: But what?

> *Jason:* (becoming tearful again, but holds the tears back) I was worried about getting headaches there, but I knew you had paid all that money for me to go.

The doctor now noted that it was mother who was looking on silently. Even though she was remaining reasonably controlled, she appeared moved by her son's words. She looked very touched. He noted happily that she was not rushing in to disavow Jason's feelings. She was tolerating the boy's disclosures both for him and for herself. Eventually she broke the silence.

> *Mother:* (sadly) I wish you had told us these things.
> *Jason:* I couldn't . . . (long pause) You don't listen.
> *Doctor:* Is there a part of you that would like your parents to listen?
> *Jason:* Sure.
> *Doctor:* I would like you to tell them that now, each one of them.
> *Jason:* Huh?
> *Doctor:* Go ahead, say it to each of them, here. Say this sentence to each of your parents: "I would like you to listen to my feelings."

Jason complied with the doctor's request. His mother responded with a meaningful, assenting nod of her head and no words. Mr. Douglas said, "I want to do that, Jason" and squeezed his son's hand.

The doctor asked the family to discuss what they had learned about themselves in this session. Both parents acknowledged feeling deeply touched by their conversation with their son, realizing with regret that there had been too little genuine openness between him and them. Jason felt both relieved and guilty — relieved at sharing and guilty that he had somehow disappointed his parents. The doctor shared his thought that the family — everyone in the family — needed help in "uncorking" their feelings with one another. They all agreed. Mrs. Douglas then voiced a fear that also sounded somewhat like a threat:

> *Mother:* That (uncorking) could be dangerous if I ever started that! (bitter laugh)

She allowed a trace of anger to flash across her face and looked directly at her husband. Father turned his gaze away. However, the doctor made no comment. Enough had taken place in this hour; little time was left, and it seemed wrong to open up more issues that could not be completed in this session. The interviewer saw the interchange as just one more in-dication that ongoing counseling work was long overdue and that each family member would need to learn how to communicate feelings in an open, functional manner.

He proceeded instead to the brass tacks of finding a resource for counseling in the family's home community, no small task since they were in San Francisco discussing the possibility of finding help in Texas. He suggested that some of the work should include them as a family group; hence, he was definitely recommending family therapy. However, he knew of absolutely no resources for them in Texas. Fortunately, Mr. Douglas had some connection with the university medical center near their home. He was even aware of a specific family therapist in the department of psychiatry there. To the doctor's surprise (since Mr. Douglas had originally said he hoped the interviewer wasn't a psychiatrist) father declared that he would be most willing to follow through with that department toward a referral for family therapy.

Interestingly enough, the family did not ask any more questions about Jason's headaches. After the interview the doctor reviewed his work with the pediatric resident and Jason's pediatric neurologist. The few remaining medical test results were returned the next day; they were completely normal. A final conference was held the day of discharge with Jason, his parents, and the pediatric neurology staff. The pediatrician-interviewer was unable to attend. Both staff and family agreed that Jason's headaches now seemed related to "stress and worry." Mr. Douglas had by this time already made contact with the intended family therapist in Texas, and an initial appointment was waiting for them on their return home.

A brief note came to the interviewer from Mr. Douglas about 8 months after the family's initial interview. He wanted to say that Jason's headaches were less frequent now, although he still had an occasional attack; there had been two episodes in the 8-month period since hospitalization. Mr. and Mrs. Douglas were now in marital therapy. Jason did not attend the sessions at present. Father closed by thanking the doctor for pointing the family in a "new direction."

HELPING THE PEDIATRIC STAFF
WITH A FAMILY'S BEHAVIOR

Most pediatric wards are busy places with a hectic pace and a significant number of stresses, not just for the sick child and his family but for the staff caring for that sick child as well. Nurses, doctors, social workers, recreational therapists, aides, clerks, housekeeping staff, and others must continuously work closely with one another, often in crisis-ridden situations. They must also encounter children and families in all varieties. The patient and his parents, of course, bring their own stresses to the hospitalization; it is a formidable event for all concerned. And when understandably stressed staff must work with an understandably stressed family, the resulting chemistry is sometimes less than ideal and often not understandable at all, to one, the other, or both. When this happens, mutual frustration, alienation, and distrust develops, none of which is conducive to helping the sick child.

In such circumstances a family interview can sometimes be advantageous, particularly if it can help an offended medical staff to become "curious rather than furious" with a family.[8] Providing some insights into the purpose and origin of a family's particularly troublesome behavior may assist the staff in transcending their feelings of irritation and anger and allow them to interact more effectively with the family. Providing these insights can sometimes be accomplished through the judicious use of a family interview that includes selected pediatric staff members as participant observers.

For instance, Tracy DeMartino, age 4, was seriously ill with chronic renal disease, renal failure, and hypertension. Around-the-clock medications, injections, fluids, and treatments were required. Her father was with her constantly, and he was particularly adamant about being present during the administration of any medications. Since our pediatric ward had for some time provided living-in arrangements for parents, the staff was used to the presence of parents and expected them to stick around, particularly with a child of this age. But there was something different about Mr. DeMartino's stay. The staff felt that it was not so much that he wanted to reassure, support, and comfort his daughter as that he distrusted the staff. Of course, they were offended and intimidated, feeling that they were being watched and largely disapproved of by this man. With time, no one was eager to be assigned Tracy as a patient. Her care was a dreaded experience for nurses, house staff, and particularly medical students, who felt father's disapproval most keenly. For instance, the following interchange took place between father and a fourth year medical student around the subject of a proposed venipuncture:

Student: Hello, Mr. DeMartino. I'm Robert Garfield. I'm working with Dr. Carter to take care of Tracy.

Father: What is that syringe for?

Student: Tracy has to have a little blood test.

Father: I haven't seen you before. Are you new on the case?

Student: Well . . . Tracy has been my patient since Tuesday. I came on the service two days ago.

Father: Well, how come I haven't seen you?

Student: (by now on the defensive and feeling very intimidated) Well, we've had a lot of conferences, and it took some time also to get oriented to the ward and that sort of thing.

Father: Well, where is Dr. Carter? He's supposed to be the one in charge.

Student: He's on rounds right now.

Father: Well, exactly what kind of doctor are you? Are you an intern or are you a real doctor?

Student: I'm a doctor in training, a medical student.

Father: Well, I'm not going to allow any of that. There is to be no practicing on my daughter. I don't know what this blood test is, but Dr. Carter is going to do it if anyone is. He's in charge. You tell him I want to talk to him.

Student: I don't think he can be interrupted . . .

Father: There will be *no* blood test. (He draws the curtains around his daughter's bed.)

After several similar episodes between father and various members of the ward staff, a family interview was held with the parents and Tracy present. Besides the interviewer (a pediatrician with training in family interviewing), a nurse and medical student also attended. In the course of the discussion Mr. DeMartino told of his own father's death in a hospital in Italy 3 years previously, from an inadvertent administration of the wrong medication. He had not told any of the staff of this incident. His behavior now became understandable to the staff.

Things became considerably easier after that. Mr. DeMartino continued to watch closely; now the staff encouraged him and even went to find him in the waiting area if by chance he had left Tracy's bedside and a treatment were about to take place.

INITIATION OF ONGOING FAMILY COUNSELING

Had Jason Douglas, the child with the headaches described previously, lived in the San Francisco area, we would have suggested that the family enter family therapy with us, and the first interview on the pediatric ward would have been the initiation of that process. Many families hospitalized on our pediatric ward do not live far away; for these families the inpatient family interview can be a logical introduction to continuing work with us on an outpatient basis. One of our pediatric residents has referred to this as the "get-them-into-treatment" interview, and while there is something slightly offensive about that phrase, it is true that one needs to lead a family to accept a referral for ongoing counseling assistance. Some will accept the recommendation easily, some with difficulty, and some not at all. A family interview while the child is hospitalized can be used for the purpose of introducing and, if all goes well, facilitating a family's acceptance of the referral. The crisis of hospitalization itself has often been helpful in rendering a family agreeable to ongoing counseling. In such cases the anxiety surrounding the event of hospitalization may mobilize the family to act on their particular set of difficulties, and they look favorably on the suggestion of continuing family work.

Even if the opportunity is not present to extend the initial inpatient family interview into ongoing sessions with the same interviewer, one can use this interview, as we did with Jason and his family, to suggest that continuing family counseling take place elsewhere. This, of course, requires that the interviewer have some knowledge of available resources both locally and at some distance. We are reasonably well-informed about family counseling facilities in the northern California area and have generally been able to recommend resources to families living in this area. Texas is another story for us, and we were relieved that Mr. Douglas was able to effect his own referral for the family. Therefore we recommend that one learn not only *how* to make a referral for ongoing family therapy, but also *to whom* one can refer in one's own locale.

SHARING DIAGNOSTIC FINDINGS

Sharing diagnostic findings has already been discussed in some detail in the preceding chapter. Eddie Nichols was an inpatient with cystic fibrosis. His situation was used to illustrate that in sharing initial diagnostic news with families, one must respect the event, share the diagnosis quickly, attend to the feelings of those present, keep medical facts to a minimum, withstand silence, and avoid running away. We recommend these as useful rules for the interviewer to remember in any encounter with a family concerning diagnostic and/or therapeutic considerations. Our suggestion that medical facts be kept to a minimum should not be construed as meaning that we feel patients and families should be kept in the dark regarding medical information. On the contrary, we feel that the more open a medical staff can be with a family regarding medical information, the more family members will feel that they are participating in the care of their child. Such a sharing can do much to lessen a family's anxiety and feelings of helplessness. However, we also caution that medical information be shared at a pace such that the family can assimilate the news being delivered. Too much and too detailed information given too quickly can be simply overwhelming for troubled families, and in this instance anxiety mounts rather than diminishes.

PROVIDING SUPPORT TO A FAMILY

Had we extended the story of Eddie Nichols, his cystic fibrosis, and his family into subsequent interviews, the category of providing support would already be familiar to the reader. As time went on, Eddie and his parents required considerable support from the medical staff, first with simply accepting the diagnosis and subsequently with all sorts of issues, particularly the use of medical equipment and the almost overwhelming feelings of isolation that each parent disclosed during a subsequent hospitalization for Eddie. Those issues were explored and discussed in succeeding family interviews with a pediatrician. We have utilized inpatient family interviews in many similar situations, during times when families have specifically requested some assistance in coping with their child's medical problems and chronic condition.

PREPARING FOR SURGERY

The necessity for adequate preparation of a child who is to be hospitalized for any reason is certainly well-recognized. The subject has received significant attention in the literature for many years.[6,9,11,13,14] This preparation is generally initiated prior to a child's actual hospitalization. We consider such prehospitalization preparation extremely important. However, that preparation is not the purpose of our discussion in this section. One aspect of preparation for hospitalization very often takes place after the child has been admitted, and it is this aspect that we have often addressed through the use of family interviews and that we will discuss here. We refer to the preparation of a child for some sort of surgical procedure. This subject has also received considerable attention in the literature.[1,2,5,7,10,12]

Increased awareness of the psychosocial needs of children by parents and health professionals has diminished the frequency with which inappropriate or damaging statements are made to a child concerning an upcoming operation. It is mercifully rare now, for instance, that a child is prepared for a tonsillectomy and adenoidectomy by a reassurance that he is going to a nice place where he will be able to eat lots of ice cream. And parents no longer, as they once did, bring their children to our pediatric ward having told them only that, "Mommy and Daddy are going to take you on a trip to San Francisco where we will take you to the zoo" (leaving out the fact that a bilateral inguinal hernioplasty and 4 days in the hospital will follow that trip to the San Francisco Zoo). These examples today sound laughable and ludicrous; they once were commonplace and accepted practice. Unfortunately they have not totally settled into disuse — almost, but not quite.

Nowadays it is recognized that children require truthful preparation for anticipated surgical procedures. Children, just like everyone else, cope better with the known than with the unknown. To deny that pain lies ahead when in fact it does, only contributes to a child's sense of betrayal and distrust. Anticipatory talk about what will take place can mobilize a child's anxiety in a useful manner, allowing him to disclose his worries and discharge some of them, and can also provide an entree for the delivery of emotional support and strength by those around him. A ghoulish preoccupation with blood and mayhem is not called for, but rather a sensitive, accurate, somewhat matter-of-fact prediction of what lies in store for the child, together with reassurance about the child's most pressing fears. For children under the age of about 4, separation from important loved ones, that is, mother and father, is an almost universal terror.[3, 4] Aside from an explanation of the operation itself, a child this age needs particular reassurance that his parents will be with him as much as possible and that he will not be abandoned, either before, during, or after the surgery. For children this age and older, the fear of separation gradually becomes supplanted by one equally terrifying: the fear of mutilation and pain.[7] This child, too, requires honest reassurance in addition to an explanation of the operation. Depending on the circumstances, such reassurance may mean that one can say to the child that neither of these eventualities will occur. For others it may mean acknowledging that pain will happen but that it will be bearable and will go away, that medicine will be available to make the pain go away, that there will be no scar, or that the incision will heal without a trace.

Almost always lurking in the background with children, particularly between the ages of 3 and 7, is the notion that "this whole operation and hospitalization thing" is some sort of punishment for the child's real or imagined misdeeds.[15] Reassurance on this score is universally indicated. Wishing that one could place one's younger brother in the trash compactor and undergoing surgery for strabismus are *not* related, and children need to hear explicitly that surgery is not punishment for "evil" thoughts or acts.

Many of a child's apprehensions around hospitalization and surgery are thus connected to family and to family relationship issues of trust, abandonment, separation, and punishment. It makes sense that the family should be involved in the child's preparation for the surgical event, and a family interview can be quite helpful in assisting family members to (1) prepare themselves and (2) plan the preparation that they wish to carry out with their own child. Preparation of the child by the family members themselves seems in many ways a much more appropriate maneuver than preparation by a stranger, even a kindly, knowledgeable stranger. For such family preparation to take place, however, requires that the family is knowledgeable enough—and prepared enough—to do the job well. In this sphere we have utilized family interviews for surgical preparation of children, helping family members decide what, when, and how they will tell their child about an upcoming operation. The Baxters were one such family.

The Baxter family

Michael Baxter was 5 years old. Four months before he had had surgery on his left eye for a malignant growth of the orbit. The eye did not have to be removed. Neurosurgeons were cautiously optimistic that all of the tumor had been excised; they could not be certain. Surgery was followed by 6 weeks of radiation therapy, during which time Michael was an outpatient. Until 2 days prior to this present admission, Michael was doing well and gradually returning to relatively normal routines, even kindergarten. Then quite suddenly signs and symptoms of tumor growth reappeared: proptosis, discoloration, decreasing visual acuity, and some soft tissue swelling around the affected area. Michael was immediately hospitalized for further evaluation. Neurosurgical and ophthalmologic opinions agreed on both the problem and on the treatment required. Michael's tumor, a rhabdomyosarcoma, known to be highly malignant, fast-growing, and invasive, had spread throughout his left eye; the left orbit would quickly have to be surgically removed. The parents were informed of this on a Wednesday; surgery was scheduled for Friday morning. Panic understandably ensued. They were to have less than 2 days to prepare their son for a truly horrible event, an event incidentally that he had worried about several months before when the first surgical procedure was performed. He had been told at that time that his eye would not be removed. Now he would have his worst fears confirmed. Mr. and Mrs. Baxter turned to the ward social worker whom they knew well and whom Michael trusted and asked for help in preparing their son. She in turn, feeling equally stunned by the enormity of such a task, asked for assistance from pediatricians in the Child Study Unit regarding this family's crisis.

It seems likely that all of the staff felt overwhelmed by the problem, because after discussing matters briefly with Mrs. Winter, the social worker, a decision was made to handle the situation "by committee" in an interview attended by a pediatrician from the Child Study Unit, Michael's nurse, the social worker, and Mr. and Mrs. Baxter. Michael would not be included in this initial family session.

The parents, in their mid-40's, arrived on time for the interview. Their other two children, both teenagers, were in school and did not attend the session. In retrospect they certainly could have participated and would have been welcome. The two parents and three staff members sat around a conference table. Mr. and Mrs. Baxter looked very upset. Mother was visibly agitated, doing most of the talking, smoking constantly; her hands trembled. She was striving to look controlled and collected, but it wasn't working. Her husband's discomfort was much more subdued. He looked sad and frightened. He remained quiet and nonverbal for extended stretches throughout the session.

Perhaps a word should be said about the appearance of the staff as well. Not one of them looked eager for this interview to take place; all were feeling somewhat overwhelmed by the subject matter and looked very worried. Like the parents, the staff was experiencing considerable turmoil over how in the world one tells a child that his eye is about to be removed. The pediatrician spoke for the others when he began:

> *Doctor:*   This is an awful business. Let's see, how can we get started?
> *Mother:*   I just don't know what to tell him . . . I just don't know.

Sensing that both parents were ready to jump out of their skins with worry and fear, the doctor made an effort to slow things down at the start by asking the parents first for particular details of Michael's illness, for the sequence of events leading up to the present crisis, and for the parents' understanding of Michael's condition. It afforded an opportunity to find out not just about Michael's tumor, but about the parents, their coping styles, and their present feelings as well.

Mrs. Baxter clearly took the lead in this family. She was articulate. She was also the central coordinating figure for Michael and his illness. It was she who talked most often and most directly with the neurosurgery staff. It was she who sat by Michael's bed for most of his previous and present hospital stays. It was she who had explained his previous procedure to him—and quite well, incidentally. It was she who carried messages to the other children regarding Michael's progress and changing condition. And it was she who continued to run the household at home as well as spend 8 to 10 hours a day at the hospital. She appeared to possess basic good sense in helping her son deal with what had been a very difficult problem. The latest turn of events, however, seemed like just too much, hard on the heels of just too much else. She said she was nearing the end of her rope. Preparing her son for the removal of his eye was beyond her skill. She was lost.

Mr. Baxter, as mentioned, was often quiet. He initiated little verbal activity on his own and seemed to prefer that his wife remain in charge. He worked hard, long hours in his own business and came straight to the hospital after work, not even stopping off at home. He would remain for the evening with Michael, relieving his wife of her bedside vigil. She would then leave the hospital, going home to take care of the rest of their family. The parents, during this hospitalization as during the first, were seeing very little of one another except to trade places. Considerably less articulate than his wife, Mr. Baxter gave the impression of being quietly overwhelmed by an event that he could not fully comprehend. He was handling the situation by doing what he did best: working hard and staying out of the way.

As the interview progressed, the pediatrician asked how and what Michael was to be told.

> *Mother:* Well, I just think Michael has to know about his eye surgery before the operation. But how? How?
>
> *Doctor:* What ways of telling him have come to your own mind as you've thought it through?
>
> *Mother:* (with an anxious laugh) Absolutely nothing comes. I haven't the least idea of how to go about it, and that's what we're ask-

ing your advice about. Any suggestions would be appreciated. I just stop completely whenever I think about actually doing it. (pause) And Walt here doesn't think we should tell him anything.

Doctor: What *are* your thoughts about this business, Mr. Baxter?

Father: Well, I'm not sure, really.

Doctor: You have some doubts, it sounds like.

Father: My own thoughts about it, Doctor — if you want me to be very honest — I feel we shouldn't tell the boy until after the operation. I think we ought to get him through this first of all and then take our time telling him about it. Now that's the way I see it, maybe you can change my mind, I dunno, but that's where I stand.

Doctor: What would be your objection to telling him before the surgery?

Father: I know he's worried, and I don't want him to worry more and get really upset before the operation. I guess that's it — I don't want to worry and upset him.

Nurse: My concern, Mr. Baxter, is how will Michael react when he wakes up from the surgery and finds his left eye gone? I worry that *then* he will really be upset.

Father: I hadn't thought of that, really. That's a point.

Nurse: I've been able to be very honest with Michael ever since he first got sick. I don't want him to learn that he can't trust me to tell him the truth now.

Social worker: He's been so worried off and on about losing the eye. And we've always up until now been able to reassure him that they were not going to remove it. He trusts what we've all said — you, his parents, and us, the staff. I feel that not telling him something would be a betrayal of that trust.

Father: You're right. And yet . . . I don't want to upset him.

Social worker: I can understand your concern. Trouble is, I see no way for him *not* to be upset. This whole subject is very upsetting, very . . . for all of us as well. If we explain things ahead of time, you're right . . . he is going to be upset.

Nurse: And if we wait until after the operation he will feel upset . . . and betrayed.

Father: Yeah.

Mother: Oh, Walt. We must tell him. I feel that strongly — as strongly as I've ever felt anything. But I don't know how or what.

Father: (after a silence) I do agree with you, Marge. He has to know something. I don't think I can do it, though.

The pediatrician was struck with an unusual, fine quality about this interview as it was proceeding. The magnitude of the event had drawn everyone into the conversation. It was not so much an "interview" in the formal sense of the word as a mutual sharing of feelings and opinions by all the participants. Staff and family were sharing their feelings; each was listening to the other. The spirit was very much one of, "How can we all work together to help this youngster?" The pediatrician began to feel somewhat relieved. The active participation by both nurse and social worker meant that he could count on others to help during the course of this very difficult interview.

Doctor: So then who will be doing the telling?

Mother: (with a touch of resignation in her voice) I will.

Doctor: That's a big job for just one person. How did that fall to you alone?

Mother: (not looking at her husband) I most often get the tough jobs with the kids. That's just the way it seems to work in our family.

Doctor: Do you want it to be that way?

Mother: (after a long pause) Yes, I think I do . . . for this. I must.

Doctor: It's very important for you that you be the one to prepare Michael?

Mother: Extremely. I've handled things so far. I'm not going to back down now.

Doctor: And how is that for you, Mr. Baxter?

Father: OK . . . I think. I don't believe I could do it myself. That would be too hard.

Doctor: Do you want to be there when your wife speaks to him?

Father: Yes, I will be there. I'm not sure that I will say anything, but I will be there.

Doctor: And is that acceptable for you, Mrs. Baxter?

Mother: Yeah, that's how I imagined it would go.

Doctor: That's what you imagined. What is unclear is, do you want it that way or another way?

Mother: Well, when you get right down to it, I don't want it *any* way. But if Michael is to be told, then I want to be the one to do it.

Doctor: OK. I respect your courage.

Mother: (says nothing, but permits her eyes to fill with tears)

Doctor: What will you say?

Mother: Oh, oh . . . oh, as I was saying, I just don't have any ideas. I'm lost.

It seemed somehow inappropriate to stop at his point, having armed Mrs. Baxter with courage but no words to use with her son. The interview group had already demonstrated their ability to provide mutual support for one another. The pediatrician decided to capitalize on this spirit of mutual helping to develop the next segment of the interview: how and what the child was to be told.

Mother: Actually, I do know what I would tell him at first. That I can do, even though it means telling him about his eye. It's what comes after . . .

Doctor: Do it right now. Something as important as this deserves a dry run or two. Tell me, as though you were talking to Michael himself, about the operation.

Mrs. Baxter at first protested that she felt silly "in front of all these people"; but then she quickly settled into serious thought, planning concretely the words she would use with her son.

Mother: I would say to him that . . .

Doctor: I will be Michael. Say it to me directly.

Mother: Michael . . . you know you have gotten very sick again. The doctors have decided that you must have an operation. Remember we said that you might have to have a second operation? Well, you do. But this time it is more serious . . . they are going to have to take out your eye . . . (She breaks off and is visibly shaken. So is everyone else in the room.)

Doctor: What is it?

Mother: (brief sob) I can get that far every time. I've already done it in my head many times. It's what follows that I can't handle. I don't know what to do with all the questions I'm sure he will have. I don't even know what they will be. But the thought of his questions frightens me.

Doctor: Perhaps the group here can give you some help with that. You've done a beautiful job so far. Rest for a minute, Mrs. Baxter, while I talk to the others. (turning to the other participants) All right. For just a few minutes I would like each of you to put yourself in Michael's shoes. That means that you are 5 years old, that you know you have had one operation on your eye, and that for some reason your mom says you are going to have another, but this time the doctor is going to have to remove your eye itself. I would like each of you, in this position, to think of one question that comes to mind. You may make it the most frightening question you can imagine. (turning back to mother) Mrs. Baxter, it seems to me that what you need most right now is some practice in fielding the questions you dread hearing from Michael. So I am going to have each person here in turn face you—as Michael—and he or she will ask a question Michael might ask. Just respond with whatever comes to mind. Should you get stuck, one of us may have an idea to help you. One important thing to keep in mind: for the kinds of questions you will hear, there are most likely no single, correct answers. Everyone in the room would probably respond differently to the same question. It is mostly a matter of style. For the moment, just rely on your own very good style with your own son. You will be all right . . . . Are you ready?

Mother: (indicates yes)

Asking family members to practice or rehearse in the face of catastrophic expectations is a useful device. The doctor's strategy here was developed with several purposes in mind. Mrs. Baxter appeared to be blocked by the thought of approaching the "unapproachable" and being asked the "unanswerable." Perhaps by utilizing the supportive, safe environment of the present interview situation, he could allow her to practice, moving beyond the impasse she imposed on herself through her own catastrophic expectations. He also hoped, by encouraging her to experience being on the receiving end of very difficult questions from "simulated Michaels" and surviving that experience, to put her in touch with her capabilities and strengths for handling the actual situation, rather than allowing her to continue to focus on her self-doubts. If need be, after this initial role play he was also prepared to have the roles reversed in the proposed simulation. That is, he could have Mrs. Baxter take the role of her son. She, as Michael, could then ask someone else in the room, playing the role of Mrs. Baxter, those terrible questions that she herself dreaded to face. Having her first play herself would help her organize her approaches and put her in touch with her strengths. Having her play Michael would allow her to verbalize those questions that she herself most feared and would also allow her to pick up hints from others as to how one might respond to the specific awesome queries. Having her experience both of these roles might be necessary in preparing her for the actual job ahead. The doctor asked her to begin by playing herself.

The nurse, playing Michael, faced Mrs. Baxter:

Nurse: Mommy, is it going to hurt?
Mother: During the operation? No, you will be sound asleep and it will not hurt. When you wake up afterward and come back to your room, I will be right there with you. It may hurt then; you may be sore.

Nurse:	Will I be sore a lot?
Mother:	I don't know, Michael. I hope not. The nurses and I can help you by giving you medicine to make the pain go away. And I will stay right there with you.
Doctor:	(to mother) How is it going for you so far?
Mother:	This one I can handle, I believe. I did before when he had the first operation.
Doctor:	Good. You're doing great as far as I'm concerned. If you feel comfortable with that one, let's move on to another question. How about you, Mr. Baxter. Be Michael for a moment and ask your question.
Father:	(turning to his wife after some thought) What will it feel like, Mom?
Mother:	How do you mean, Michael?
Father:	When they do the operation.
Mother:	You still worried about hurting?
Father:	Yeah.
Mother:	Michael, tell me what you remember about the first operation.
Father:	It didn't hurt. I don't remember much. I was asleep, you said.
Mother:	That's right. This one will be like that too . . . Are you scared?
Father:	(indicates yes)
Mother:	(stepping out of role) I think at this point I would just hold him and comfort him. Not talk, necessarily.
Social worker:	Great. That's just what he would need at that point. I would hold him, too.
Doctor:	(turning to social worker) What would be your question, Mary, if you were Michael?
Social worker:	What will I look like, Mom?
Mother:	Ohhhhh, now that's getting into something really tough.
Doctor:	Do it. Answer your son (communicating his faith in her ability to take the next step).
Mother:	When you come back from the operation, you will have a bandage over your eye. Underneath your eye will look closed, that's all.
Social worker:	Is it going to look all cut?
Mother:	No, Michael. The doctor says not. (again coming out of her role) I know what he will ask next, and I think this is the one I've been dreading.
Doctor:	Say it.
Mother:	Michael will want to know if there is going to be a big hole in his face. (She breaks down. Aside from that there is silence.)

> *Doctor:* (after the period of silence and after Mrs. Baxter composes herself) Answer him.
>
> *Mother:* Well, no, Michael. There isn't going to be a big hole. Everything will look all right on your face except that your eye will look closed. No, honey, there isn't going to be a big hole. Have you been worried about that? (leaving her role) That's how I understand it — that the surgery is not going to be disfiguring. They are not planning to take out any bone or change the shape of his face?

Since she seemed to be asking for reassurance, the nurse spoke up and agreed that this was her understanding as well, that Michael's face would not be changed. Undoubtedly mother's own fear of this eventuality made answering that question so difficult for her. The group discussed this, and she appeared relieved to have verbalized her fear and to have had reassurance that the fear was ungrounded. She also felt more comfortable now about approaching Michael regarding the subject. The pediatrician continued:

> *Doctor:* I have one further question as Michael.
>
> *Mother:* Yes?
>
> *Doctor:* Mom, after the operation, am I going to be able to see?
>
> *Mother:* Yes, of course, honey. People can see with one eye just about as well as with two eyes. You will be able to see . . . (leaving her role) and then I would love him again.

The doctor shortly brought the role playing to a close. His goal had been accomplished: Mrs. Baxter had a sense of what to do and how. She seemed eminently capable. He then asked each person in the group to share with Mrs. Baxter some way in which he or she had felt touched by the mother's approaches to her child. Everyone in turn, including Mr. Baxter, could acknowledge feeling moved by her caring and impressed by her savvy and courage in the various encounters. These comments in themselves provided an extremely touching moment in the session. A discussion was then held as to how mother wanted to arrange telling her son. Did she, for instance, want anyone there besides her husband? How could the staff assist? And so forth. She decided that, if Mr. Baxter were agreeable, she wanted the preparation talk to be a private time, involving just the three family members. Her husband agreed, and the interview concluded shortly thereafter.

Later that afternoon Michael was told of his upcoming surgery, as planned. The parents reported to the social worker afterward that things went reasonably well. They felt able to be open and honest in their own comments. Michael cried, and then they all cried together. Both parents remarked to Mrs. Winter that the "practice session," as they called it, had been tremendously helpful in preparing them for the job that had to be done.

Tragically Michael's surgery, although itself successful, was unable to save his life. He died less than a year later with extensive metastases. Dealing with this even more difficult phenomenon — death in children — will be discussed in the following chapter.

REFERENCES

1. Adams, M., and Berman, D.: The hospital through a child's eyes, Children **12:**102, 1965.
2. Bergmann, T., and Freud, A.: Children in the hospital, New York, 1966, International Universities Press.
3. Bowlby, J.: Grief and mourning in infancy and early childhood, Psychoanal. Study Child **15:**9, 1960.
4. Bowlby, J.: Attachment and loss: Vol. 1. Attachment, New York, 1969, Basic Books, Inc., Publishers.
5. Davenport, J., and Werry, J.: The effect of general anesthesia, surgery, and hospitalization upon the behavior of children, Am. J. Orthopsychiatry **40:**806, 1970.
6. Gofman, H., and others: The child's emotional response to hospitalization, Am. J. Dis. Child. **93:**157, 1957.
7. Kenny, T.: The hospitalized child, Pediatr. Clin. North Am. **22:**583, 1975.
8. Leveton, A.: Personal communication, 1971.
9. Mason, E.: The hospitalized child — his emotional needs, N. Engl. J. Med. **272:**405, 1965.
10. Mattson, A.: Long term physical illness and psychosocial adaptation, Pediatrics **50:**801, 1972.
11. Plank, E.: Working with children in hospitals, Cleveland, 1962, Case Western Reserve University Press.
12. Prugh, D., and others: Study of the emotional reactions of children and families to hospitalization and illness, Am. J. Orthopsychiatry **23:**70, 1953.
13. Spitz, R.: Hospitalism, Psychoanal. Study Child **1:**53, 1945.
14. Vernon, D., and others: The psychological responses of children to hospitalization and illness, Springfield, Ill., 1965, Charles C Thomas, Publisher, Inc.
15. Wolff, S.: Children under stress, London, 1969, Alan Lane, Penguin Books, Ltd.

CHAPTER 10

Fatal illness

In some ways it is artificial to consider a discussion of fatal illness as separate from one concerning simply serious chronic conditions of a disabling nature. Too often in pediatrics the latter is tragically transformed into the former. To be sure, many chronic illnesses do not necessarily spell a fatal outcome for the pediatric patient. Diabetes mellitus, some convulsive disorders, and asthma are three very common examples. Conversely there are even situations in which a fatal event is not preceded by much in the way of preliminary illness, sudden infant death and accidents being two such examples. For the most part, however, physicians are dealing with death in children as the final event in a youngster's lingering illness of long standing, as in the case of solid tumors, leukemia, and degenerative central nervous system disorders. Therefore a separate chapter on fatal illness in children seems justified.

ELISABETH KÜBLER-ROSS

The writings of Dr. Elisabeth Kübler-Ross,[4] a Swiss psychiatrist now living and working in the United States, have been very helpful in our approaches to the dying pediatric patient and his family and in our teaching of pediatric trainees. Kübler-Ross is currently recognized as a leading clinician and author regarding death and dying. In her work she has noted that terminally ill individuals generally proceed through five different stages from the moment of diagnosis until death. Furthermore, other family members appear to go through these same five stages as well. We would add from our own experiences that a physician often confronts each of these stages, not just in the family but also within himself as he becomes involved in the care of a particular dying patient.

253

Kübler-Ross's work, upon which these five stages are based, was done primarily with dying adults. However, she is convinced that children experience these stages as well. Hence the five stages seem to be experienced by child, parents, siblings, and physician alike, although no two individuals may be experiencing the same stage at quite the same time. The embarkation upon the first of these stages is usually stimulated by the physician at the moment he discloses the diagnosis.

Stage one: denial

Anticipatory mourning begins for parents immediately upon hearing that their child has a disease that is ultimately fatal. In addition to the shock and confusion of the moment, very often a parent screams (inwardly at least): "No, not my child! It can't be true!" This protective denial of the facts is almost universally present among parents, in Kübler-Ross's experience. It may last a few seconds, or it may persist for weeks and months. We have also noted that it seems to wax and wane with both patients and family members, disappearing after the initial shock and then transiently reappearing at intervals throughout the course of the illness. Initially denial is most commonly revealed through the parents' seeming inability to hear the facts presented, even when they are presented logically and well. Precisely for this reason, we urge physicians not to deluge family or patient with abundant medical facts at first. The very normal and to-be-expected stage of denial simply prevents their assimilation of detailed information regarding the child's illness and treatment plans.

Families may also express their denial by seeking other medical opinions and "doctor shopping." A physician may be of considerable assistance to the family by concluding that this is a statement of the family's need for protective denial rather than a comment on the doctor's competence or incompetence. In this way second opinions may not only be tolerated but, appropriately, encouraged by the initial doctor. Angry defensiveness on the doctor's part when a second opinion is requested is certainly contraindicated and can only serve to make a family feel guilty "for having insulted the doctor," an unnecessary addition to their other already overwhelming emotions of the moment.

With time, denial may take other forms as well; particularly if it becomes prolonged and develops into an accustomed pattern for viewing the child's illness. Parents in such circumstances may insist that their child not be told anything of his diagnosis nor any details of his care.

They may decide to isolate him more and more from peers and relatives and indeed from any circumstances outside the immediate household for fear that someone will slip and tell the child of his disease. They may encourage his absence from school for the same reason. Denial of this sort may be considered by the physician in a different light than the temporary denial expressed and shown initially as the family copes with the diagnosis. Temporary denial is just that, a transitory protective coping mechanism that sets the stage for Kübler-Ross's second stage of anticipatory mourning, anger. This temporary denial is to be expected among family members. Chronic denial, on the other hand, denial as a way of life, may actually hinder the proper care of a fatally ill child by increasing his sense of isolation and fostering the development of serious communication difficulties among family members, since no one can speak the truth. Families in this bind need help in dropping their rigid refusal, so they may cope more realistically with their child and his illness. (For an example of how family interviewing can be used to diminish a family's chronic denial of their child's condition, see Chapter 8 and the case discussion of the Moreno family.)

The child, too, may participate in subterfuge through denial in his own efforts to ward off the inevitable, particularly if he is aware that other family members are caught up in the same defense. The child then begins to model his behavior accordingly, playing his own game of "No, not me. It can't be happening to me." He may refuse to acknowledge that he is sick and needs to stay in bed; he may refuse to discuss his illness with anyone. He may resist medications and treatments vigorously, not just through fear of pain but also because it is one way of protesting that he is not really ill or in need of the therapy being offered. We have observed that if parents, either spontaneously or with help, can pass through their own stage of denial, they are then usually able to help their child move beyond his refusal to acknowledge the disease. A child's persistent denial over the course of his illness generally indicates that his behavior is being unwittingly, or even explicitly, encouraged by one or both parents.

As a rule, physicians and other health personnel caring for the sick child can handle this stage, denial, adequately within themselves. Although they may wish irrationally to dismiss the reality of the diagnosis with denial, most often they do not. Instead, some of the other stages that Kübler-Ross describes more often furnish exquisite difficulty for the medical staff. These will be described subsequently.

Stage two: anger

For most families the stage of denial is short-lived. All too soon there is a crushing realization that the diagnosis is not a mistake. The cry, "No, not my child!" becomes instead, "Why my child?" And with this second cry, strong feelings of anger and frustration are understandably unleashed. Such feelings may be directed at the physician, at the hospital, at the nurses, at one another, at other family members, at the hospital food, at God, and even (although usually in secret) at the sick child. The feelings need not be rational, nor are they necessarily justified. Simultaneously, expressions of anger and outrage may be shown by the patient himself, often through demanding, critical, difficult outbursts. He too rails, "Why me?" It is an extremely difficult stage for those providing treatment and support, first because the family and patient may be just plain unpleasant to deal with, and second because the health professionals themselves are often having their own struggles with this particular stage in the care of the dying child. For they may also be exclaiming inwardly and angrily: "Why me?"

The roots of a physician's anger vis-à-vis the dying pediatric patient are many. For a good many pediatricians, their choice of this subspecialty as a career was in some part determined by the basically optimistic nature of pediatric practice. Children are generally associated with vitality, energy, health, growth, and beginnings. One who elects to care for children as a career often chooses pediatrics for its emphasis on, and preoccupation with, these very qualities. A fatally ill child erases this emphasis for a time. Caring for this child requires the pediatrician to confront instead lethargy, enervation, illness, failure of growth, and a premature ending. For some it can be an enraging turnaround, one the pediatrician had largely hoped to avoid by his choice of career. And yet children do die. Physicians can become angry at having to face this unalterable fact. The death of a child often, if not always, seems unfair, a betrayal. Death and a pediatric ward never seem to fit somehow. The impropriety of death's presence among children is for many doctors a significant contributor to their feelings of outrage and frustration when a child becomes fatally ill.

In addition, physicians have unfortunately been conditioned to view a patient's death as a personal failure and an indication of their own limitations and ultimate helplessness. Helplessness is an uncomfortable experience for anyone, but many doctors seem to find the feeling not only uncomfortable but intolerable. Undoubtedly this has stemmed in part from long years of medical training spent with a single-minded focus on helping patients get well. What has been overlooked in medical training, of course, is that death is a part of life. A physician can assist patients to face their dying as well as he can assist them in their living. Were those two tasks to be accepted by the physician as having equal importance, *both* requiring his attention and care, then any sense of personal failure at a patient's death would vanish, for the doctor would have done what was required—for the event of living and for the event of dying. For too many physicians, acknowledging the reality of a child's death is still difficult. For these individuals a child's death unfortunately remains a crushing personal defeat, an exposure of the physician's limits and basic helplessness. Such reactions in the doctor can lead to additional feelings of anger and outrage at being so exposed.

Finally there is the almost universal experience of having to confront one's own mortality and eventual death when confronted by the event in another human being. Physicians are not exempt from this experience. Depending on the individual doctor's relationship with his own destiny and death, the confrontation can be accepted reasonably well or experienced with extreme discomfort. If the latter occurs, the physician may well feel anger at having to face such an anxiety-provoking situation.

Varying combinations of the above sources of physicians' anger may be present for a given individual. As a result, many physicians approach the care of a fatally ill child with a decidedly ambivalent mix of emotions. On the one hand, the doctor has been trained to, and wants to, aid and comfort the patient. On the other, for any or all of the reasons stated previously, he also wants very much to withdraw, move away from the dying child, from the situation, from death. Rothenberg[7] cites this basic conflict between two powerful, normal, but antithetical emotional forces as the core struggle for a health care worker faced with a dying patient. How the conflict is resolved will determine in large part the success with which effective comprehensive care is delivered.

This may become particularly apparent during this second stage of anticipatory mourning (anger). With the family and/or the patient demonstrating angry, difficult behavior, the physician who is saddled with his own uncomfortable supply of frustration and anger will be less than effective in dealing with the family's sense of outrage. He may have little or no energy for helping them express and discharge their feelings. Such a discharge, however, is essential for individuals to move from this stage to subsequent stages proposed by Kübler-Ross. A brief clinical illustration will demonstrate how difficulties can arise when both family and physician are burdened with angry reactions to the fact of a child's illness.

Joe Van Sant, age 5, had leukemia. The planned treatment regimen had so far been unsuccessful in inducing a remission, and each day the laboratory reported a more dismal peripheral blood picture. He was not only not getting well, he was apparently getting worse. The staff had been feeling very puzzled and frustrated by Joe's course. Most children in Joe's situation had begun a remission by this time. Joe, when acutely ill as now, was testy; his parents, in the staff's eyes, were testy all the time. Dr. Ferguson, the pediatric resident, entered Joe's room and was somewhat dismayed to find both parents at the bedside. He had hoped they were having coffee. He greeted them and also said hi to Joe.

> *Doctor:* I'm going to have to draw a little blood, Joe.
> *Joe:* (sniffling) Why?
> *Mother:* Dr. Ferguson. They took blood from Joe at 7:30 this morning. What is *this* one for?
> *Doctor:* It's one more blood test that couldn't be done with what was sent down earlier.
> *Father:* Well, couldn't you have thought of that then? I do not understand why Joe has to have so many shots. Why couldn't it have been done earlier?

Dr. Ferguson's thought was: "It's because he's getting so much worse that we had to add this test. Get off my back, man. I'm trying to help your child. Besides, it wasn't my idea. The attending physician suggested it." Aloud, however, he said:

> *Doctor:* Mr. Van Sant, why don't you and your wife step out while I draw this sample?
> *Father:* Not on your life. You people come in here and think you can do anything to my son at any time. I won't allow it.
> *Doctor:* Let's be reasonable.
> *Mother:* Reasonable! Reasonable! About what? This kid is like a human pincushion. Around this ward no one seems organized. People just keep coming at Joe all day long. I don't know how you doctors think he's supposed to get any rest.
> *Doctor:* Look, I'm not some kind of ghoul, no matter what you think. Now are you going to let me draw this blood or not?

Neither parent makes a move.

Doctor: I insist that you leave the room so that I can draw this blood. You are not the only parents on this floor with a sick child. I have many other much more important things to do. You know, Joe's hospitalization would go a lot more smoothly if you were both a little more cooperative.

Joe, of course, watching all of this, was coming unglued and joined his parents, protesting loudly that he didn't want any needles. The scene was a shambles. It could have proceeded somewhat differently. For example:

Doctor: I'm going to have to draw a little blood, Joe.

Joe: (sniffling) Why?

Mother: Dr. Ferguson. They took blood from Joe at 7:30 this morning. What is *this* one for?

Doctor: You're angry. What is it?

Father: Damn right, we're angry. He had to have three different needles this morning. They couldn't hit the vein. We just told him now that there would be no more today. What is this?

Doctor: I've put you in a terrible position. I'm sorry. There was no way for you to know. As a matter of fact I didn't know either until 30 minutes ago that this test would have to be run. I'm angry myself. I had thought Joe was all set for today, that he wouldn't have to be bothered. And then I find that *I'm* the one who has to bother him.

Father: Well, why don't you people get together and plan things a little better?

Doctor: I think I would be angry in your shoes also.

Mother: Our shoes? What do you know about being in our shoes? What does anyone else know?

Doctor: What's the most difficult part of having to stand by with Joe so sick?

Mother: All of it, all of it . . . everything.

Doctor: It seems overwhelming?

Father: It sure does.

Doctor: It's hard for me too. I'm very fond of Joe.

Rather than sparring and exchanging angry blows with the family, this second Dr. Ferguson took a different direction with the family. He quickly moved to an acknowledgement of the parents' feelings and delivered a message that such feelings were appropriate. The parents continued for a time to express their frustration, and then, since they knew they had been heard, they were able to move on, leaving anger behind for the moment and softening in their encounter with the physician. Dr. Ferguson number one gave the parents no choice but to act out their anger, with potentially disastrous results for the care of the patient. This physician was too bound up in his own anger to tolerate hearing the parents' plight. Dr. Ferguson number two listened. His ability to do so and to support the parents indicated that he had recognized his own feelings of anger. Most importantly he was acknowledging his feelings—first to himself—and then also he was willing to share his anger openly with the family. Discharging his own feelings in this way allowed him the capacity to listen and acknowledge those of the parents.

Stage three: bargaining

Kübler-Ross feels anger gives way at some point to a coping mechanism that helps the patient and the family sustain day-to-day life for a time in the face of impending death. They bargain—with fate, God, the doctors, one another. The bargaining can take many forms. Some parents develop a secret pact: "If we can get him to Disneyland this summer for that trip he's wanted for so long, then we will be ready to face his death." Others hope to make a different kind of exchange: "Maybe my increased activity with the American Cancer Society will somehow buy some time for Annie. Don't ask me how. I just know that I have to do it." Still others ask God for a reprieve, offering to commit some important part of their own life to God in return for 6 more months of health for the child. Physicians also bargain, from a very personal standpoint: "Don't let him go sour the night that I am on, please." And so forth. Generally the bargaining period is rather short-lived. The disease progresses inexorably in its course and bargaining is no longer feasible. In its place comes another stage, depression.

Stage four: depression

For most individuals and their families, the reality of what is to be eventually comes to be faced. Bargaining no longer seems to work; the encouragement and reassurance of others loses its effectiveness. Both patient and family begin the painful process of separating from one another; they begin to grieve and in so doing encounter feelings of sadness and depression, emotions that they were able to stave off during the earlier stages of denial, anger, and bargaining. Now these feelings are unopposed, and both patient and/or family members may become very sad. In Kübler-Ross's view this sadness is a perfectly normal phenomenon for the situation and should be encouraged—not discouraged—by those attending the child and family. In this respect she suggests an approach that many have not generally followed with the dying patient. Usually health professionals make it their business to cheer up patients and families, suggesting that at all costs depression and the expression of sadness are to be avoided until the moment of death. Kübler-Ross sees the situation quite differently; she says that without the opportunity to acknowledge, express openly, and experience sadness over time, neither a dying patient nor the patient's family will be able to master this feeling or move beyond it to the fifth and final stage of acceptance.

The proscription by the medical profession against allowing dying patients and their families to experience and display feelings of depression is unfortunate but understandable. Sadness is often viewed with no more ease than is anger by doctors and others, and for the same reasons cited previously, not the least of which is that a physician must acknowledge his own sadness when he confronts depression in a dying patient or a patient's family. If he is uncomfortable with acknowledgement of his own sad feelings regarding death, he will surely be uncomfortable when faced with the sadness of another. To relieve this discomfort such a physician may work hard to minimize, disallow, or forestall the manifestation of depression in his patients. As the unfortunate result of such a forestalling, necessary grieving on the patient's or family's part is short-circuited and allowed to develop incompleted, unclosed. Under these circumstances acceptance of death will not, according to Kübler-Ross, take place.

Stage five: acceptance

Kübler-Ross feels that if the previous four stages are attended to, allowed to develop, occur, and be resolved for the patient and for his family, the dying patient may be able to reach a final stage of acceptance as death draws very near. Acceptance refers to the feelings that "death is approaching now, and it is all right." Kübler-Ross makes a distinction between acceptance and resignation. Resignation suggests the continuing presence of anger, while acceptance contains no rancor or bitterness. Certainly we have seen many parents and siblings who have expressed, finally, their acceptance of the child's impending death after a chronic disease process has plunged them all into each of the four stages listed above. But except in the case of older adolescents, we have not seen children who have reached (or perhaps expressed is a better word) an acceptance of death as Kübler-Ross conceives it — a peaceful readiness for what is to come.

A child's acceptance of death will be influenced not only by his completion of Kübler-Ross's four previous stages but also significantly by the child's understanding of death. Children can't accept death until they understand what it is. Such conceptual understanding is heavily age-dependent. Studies since the early 1940's[1] have documented that children at different ages have very different concepts of, and reactions to, death.

Below the age of approximately 3 or 4 years, children treat death largely with indifference. It has little impact on them except as it relates to separation. Separation, of course, is the paramount fear for this age group. And certainly the death of a parent is felt by a child of this age but apparently most acutely because the death produces a separation between the child and a loved one. Conceptualizing his own death probably does not occur for the child at this age and certainly does not cause him much preoccupation and worry. His own fatal or serious illness can still be very worrisome for the child under 4. He can clearly perceive that something serious is happening to him, as mirrored in the faces and actions of those around him, and the separation that may inevitably occur at times during the course of his illness can give him considerable distress. Children in this age group therefore need reassurance and protection not from death but from separation during their illness.

By about the age of 5, children may become intensely interested in death, incorporating it into their play and talk. From this time until approximately age 8, death for children is often fascinating and invested with magical qualities. They may consider it reversible; it is frequently viewed as a punishment for wrongdoing, as a judgment from God. Its finality is not appreciated. For some children between 4 and 8, death is not particularly frightening. Children of this age, indeed of any age as mentioned, are incredibly adept at picking up on the cues of those around them, however. Hence a dying child in this age category may carry some confusing thoughts—his own magical, fantastic, and even optimistic notions about death and his observance of the obvious fact that parents and the hospital staff are very upset, very angry, and very sad. If the child feels that the adults are so upset that he can't even bring the subject up, or if his parents have decided that no discussions regarding the child's condition are to be had with him, the child must attempt in isolation to integrate his fantasies with his observations. He can become very confused and troubled in the process, finding himself without avenues for clarification. Asking such children somewhat open-ended questions like

1. What do you think is the matter?
2. How did you get sick in the first place?
3. What do you think is going to happen?
4. Your mom looks worried. I wonder what that's about? What are your ideas?
5. No, I don't know about heaven. What do you think it will be like?

can lead to startling answers and provide an opportunity for the child to express his confusion and his worries. The fears of a child of this age are most often concerned with the "route" to death, that is, pain and mutilation, rather than with death itself. It is not a question of *whether* to talk to children about their condition but rather *how*. Fears about pain and fantasies about death can and should be explored with them. This is discussed in more detail in a later section of this chapter.

After the age of about 8, children begin to drop their magical concepts surrounding death. It comes to be considered more realistically, and certainly by age 9, most children have a rational concept of death as a very final, often tragic event. When a loved one dies, children of this age mourn the event as an adult would. Their own death likewise becomes an understandable although perhaps still frightening concept.

FAMILY INTERVIEWS IN FATAL ILLNESS

A physician who takes on the care of a child with a fatal illness consequently takes on the responsibility for administering medication *and* for assisting the child and his family to cope with each of the five stages proposed by Kübler-Ross and with a multitude of other issues as well, as described accurately by Binger and colleagues.[2] The doctor's assistance will span four separate time periods. At some point in each of these periods, family and individual interviewing may be indicated and useful. The four time periods are:

1. The period of diagnosis
2. The middle period of the disease
3. The terminal event of death
4. The period following death

The period of diagnosis

Helping the family hear and accept the diagnosis of a fatal illness requires no different approaches by a family interviewer than those used to help the family hear and accept the diagnosis of a serious, nonfatal condition in their child. We have already discussed is some detail the sharing of a serious diagnosis through family interviews. Similarly, we would recommend that in presenting the diagnosis of a fatal reticulum cell sarcoma, a physician proceed just as outlined with the family of Eddie Nichols (the youngster with cystic fibrosis mentioned in Chapter 8). A meeting between family members and the doctor to hear that their child has a fatal sarcoma also requires that the doctor respect the event, share the diagnosis quickly, attend to the feelings of those present, keep medical facts to a minimum, withstand silence, and resist running away. The same issues are at stake in this initial moment of diagnosis whether the disease is definitely fatal, possibly fatal, or not fatal, just lifelong.

The middle period of the disease

There are few differences between the middle phase of a fatal illness and the middle phase of a serious but nonfatal illness. In either case the family must settle down to "living with the disease" — finding some way to cope with all the changes introduced into their individual and family lives. The time span will, of course, vary from situation to situation. Certain highly malignant and rapid-growing tumors for which treatment is ineffectual at best may provide only a few weeks. Some families indicate that they actually prefer such a rapid course if the disease has to occur at all. However, most are outraged, feeling cheated by the lack of time and unprepared for a rapid downhill course, the precipitous death of their child, and loss. They have had insufficient time to work through more than one or two, if that many, of the stages proposed by Kübler-Ross. When death is so rapid, quickly following the diagnosis with almost no significant illness interval before death, a family may have time to experience only being stunned into denial and perhaps feeling paralyzed with rage. Grieving is hardly begun, much less completed. For these individuals the period following the child's death may be particularly difficult, and extensive individual and family work may be required to facilitate the family members' mourning, a process they are forced to begin, topsy-turvy, *after* the child's death, not before.

This precipitous course is not always the case. In fact, regarding childhood fatal illness, it is not often the case. Most diseases that kill children have a middle period of indeterminate length. It is a time with its own excruciating pain coming from a multitide of directions for the family. Nonetheless such a middle period does have one saving grace; it allows some families to begin and even complete anticipatory mourning so that acceptance of the child's death is occasionally realized. During this middle period, Kübler-Ross's stages of anger, bargaining, and depression are most often encountered and worked through. Also during this period, in just day-to-day living, the family must confront and manage those same themes (discussed in Chapter 8) faced by the family of a child with a lifelong chronic illness:

Isolation
Discipline
Family relationships
Financial burdens
Medical misunderstandings
Parents' emotional concerns
Hope for a cure
Parental guilt regarding transmission
Fear of death
Involvement in the treatment regimen

Judicious family interviewing and intervention may be indicated for any one of these. In the following example, George Nelson and his family needed some help during the middle period of his illness. Help was offered through the utilization of family and individual interviews.

THE NELSON FAMILY

In October of his ninth year George Nelson suddenly developed dizziness and an unsteady gait. Immediate hospitalization, studies, and quick neurosurgical intervention verified the diagnosis of medulloblastoma. The tumor was removed—totally, the surgeon felt; no metastases were seen. However, tumor cells were found in the cerebrospinal fluid, a bad omen. Following surgery and beginning convalescence, George was started on a treatment regimen of first, radiation therapy and then, chemotherapy. George's prognosis was generally believed to be very grim—not hopeless, but grim.

However, since George continued to do well clinically, evidencing no sign of progression, the medical staff became especially reluctant to make any prognostic statements to the boy or his family. According to statistics he should not be doing well; actually he should be going downhill. The fact that George was not following the predicted pattern meant that there was no certainty as an anchor, not even the awful certainty of death. He had an illness that was supposed to be fatal, but he clearly wasn't dying, at least not at the moment. It was a situation in which all bets were off. No one was sure whether to pursue hope or begin grieving. Life took on a frustratingly suspended tone for George and his family. Their only certainty seemed to be the unknown.

For the next 2 years life continued in this way. Hospitalizations and treatment were very expensive. The family went into debt, and in fact their entire existence seemed to wrap itself around George and his brain tumor. His nonsurgical treatment rolled on inexorably. Some of the effects were not pleasant. He quickly lost all his hair and was forced to wear a cap. The outpatient treatments caused him nausea and pain. Worst of all, according to George, he was regularly forced to miss 1 or even 2 days of school when a treatment was given. It was a long drive from home to the hospital and back again, the treatment itself took considerable time, and then there were the inevitable aftereffects. All of this put him out of commission for sometimes several days. In addition every 6 weeks he was required to come into the hospital to stay for a few days for periodic follow-up studies. For any trip to the hospital or clinic, of course, a parent was required to drive George and stay with him. Since both parents worked full-time, that meant that one or the other had to miss an entire day of work. George's 13-year-old brother, Russell, saw less and less of his parents and George. He didn't mind not seeing George; the two boys didn't get along. They seemed to fight constantly, especially since George had become sick 2 years ago.

Approximately 2 years after his initial surgery, George started becoming very "difficult"—abrasive and uncooperative, particularly for medical procedures that were a necessary part of his outpatient treatment. A lumbar puncture precipitated a tremendous commotion. George exploded with tears, anger, hysterics, and physical flailing about, refusing to permit the procedure to take place. The staff had always viewed him as a very bright, reasonable, and cooperative youngster. They were shocked and puzzled by his behavior, as were his parents. The neurosurgeon who had worked steadily with the Nelson family over the years suggested that they seek counseling help. He arranged for George and his family to be seen by one of the pediatricians in the Child Study Unit. An initial interview including all family members was held.

As the interview began, George sat somewhat apart from his family. The other three family members were grouped together with Russell between his parents. George, for all that had happened to him, looked vigorous and well except for mild pallor and his ever-present cap. More than anything else this family looked tired and depressed. The air was very heavy in the interview room. The father began:

Father: We just don't know what's going on. Recently George seems to fall apart over trivial things and this isn't like him at all. He won't tell us what's the matter.

Mother: I tell him he's being unfair—to the doctors, to us, to everyone who has worked so hard to help him through this.

George: They're right. I don't know what it is myself. It's not that I *won't* tell. It just seems that the least little thing gets me upset.

Russell: You can say that again.

George: Oh shut up, big mouth!

Russell: You gonna make me?

Mother: Stop it, both of you. This is another thing. Goes on all the time. I just don't know what to do with either of them. Come on—George, stop glaring at your brother.

George: Me! See, that's always what happens. It's not fair.

Russell: Talk about fair, why don't you?

Father: What's that supposed to mean, Russell?

Russell: Oh nothing. Nothing.

Mother: I'm so tired of all this bickering.

Obviously this was not a family the doctor would have trouble getting to interact with one another. On the contrary, he might have trouble keeping them quiet, but he did not feel the need for that yet. He had done little more than greet them and exchange some introductory small talk; however, they themselves were off and running. As they continued it gave the pediatrician time to form some impressions regarding the group and each family member. They were articulate and well-educated. Their dress suggested Bay Area suburbs. For his 11 years George was very bright, well-spoken, and forthright; his brother was equally so. Mother was attractive and at the same time looked the most haggard, worn, and especially sad. She worked in a bank. Father was a high school swimming coach. Of the boys, George was the student. Even major neurosurgery had not dimmed his ability nor his enthusiasm for learning and academic accomplishment. Russell seemed just a little less successful in school. Both boys were exceptional athletes. Since the surgery, however, George had definitely fallen behind his brother, no longer finding the physical energy or stamina to keep up as he had previously done. Russell had the athletic edge now. However, regardless of which boy had the advantage in which realm, they certainly saw themselves in open competition with one another.

As the family continued to discuss the problem of bickering between the boys, the parents began to bicker over how to handle the bickering.

Mother: Sometimes I just want to throw up my hands and say "forget it."

Father: I think you exaggerate, Gail. They're just boys.

Mother: I don't think "just boys" run around actually hurting one another. You've seen them, Max. Well, sometimes you have.

Father: It's not as bad as you think, I keep trying to tell you.

Mother: And I keep trying to tell you that you don't see what I do. Between meets and Boy Scouts, you aren't around them as much as I am. You don't know.

Father: Well, you'll just have to handle it yourself at those times.

Mother: Why does it always have to be left up to me? That's not fair.

Father: Look, I can only do so much. Besides, I'm the one who drives George over to the clinic all the time. What's fair about that? I do it, and I don't ask you to do it.

Mother: Right. Well, I'm not exactly loafing, you know.

Father: Who said you were loafing? Geez, how do we get started on this all the time? Well, let's not argue here. We can do that at home (laugh).

There was a general tone of irritation, no matter who spoke or what the subject. Nothing seemed to be going right for anyone in this family. George himself was the last to be heard from.

George: Well, look, if it's such a pain to take me to the hospital, forget it. I certainly don't want to go. Just leave me home.

Father: Don't be idiotic, George. And don't be smart-mouthed.

George: Well, I'm not being smart-mouthed. I mean it. Every time I go over there, to the hospital, I get about a week behind in school. They give us too much homework in the first place, and then when I tell the teachers ahead of time that I am going to have to be absent, they won't even give me my assignments ahead so that I can be working on them. Then I get behind. That's not fair.

Father: It isn't really. We've tried to explain George's situation to the school, and they don't handle it very well, except for one or two teachers. School is very important for George, and it really bothers him if he doesn't get A's. It doesn't seem quite fair somehow that they won't help him particularly to keep up with the work. It's not his fault that he has to be absent.

Everyone in the family was expressing irritation and outrage at "unfairness." Mother felt that George was being unfair in his unreasonable behavior during a lumbar puncture. George felt that his mother was being unfair to him when she intervened in an argument between him and Russell. Russell acknowledged his own strong feelings about "fair" and then quickly backed off. Mother felt that it was unfair that she was so often required single-handedly to manage the boys at home. Father felt that his trips to the hospital with George were an unfair burden. And finally George felt that school was treating him unfairly regarding expectations for school work. Quite obviously no one felt fairly treated in this family. No wonder; this family had experienced little that was fair for over 2 solid years, and the result seemed to be individual and collective outrage at injustice.

The interview was providing an excellent example of something family interviewing trainees in the Child Study Unit have been long taught: families are extremely obliging. They will continue to express their major conflict over and over again, this way and that way, until the interviewer hears. This family was fairly screaming theirs at the doctor. No matter what the specific subject under discussion, the bare bones of their message was "Unfair! Unfair!" Well, they wouldn't need to continue. He had heard it at last. He came right to the point.

Doctor: *Unfairness* is the issue, isn't it?

Mother: (bit her lip and looked on the verge of tears. She said nothing.)

Father: Now what do you mean?

Doctor: I was just putting myself in your shoes and realizing that this whole business of George's illness and so forth has been tremendously unfair for all of you, for George and for all of you.

Mother: (No longer on the verge of tears, she was crying outright.) It just goes on and on. And nobody can tell us anything definite.

Doctor: And that must be enraging for you to have to live with.

Mother: (nods her head yes)

Doctor: You must have each experienced tremendous feelings of "It's not fair." Am I right?

They all agreed. The tumor itself, the unknown prognosis, the noncommittal medical staff, the disruption of family life, the painful treatments, the expenses, the side effects, the total absorption in worry and fear—all these and more the family acknowledged as unjust and enraging.

Doctor: Have you been able to discuss these things openly with one another? Is it OK to complain?

George sadly shook his head no. Now no one spoke. Their silence told the doctor that such an open discussion had not taken place. He talked with them further. No one in the family had felt he or she had a right openly to own such feelings. It seemed somehow selfish and shameful to expect fairness for oneself. And yet to hear someone else complain was extremely irritating (for instance, "What right does he have to complain? Look what I'm having to put up with.")

Doctor: As far as I'm concerned each of you has a right to be feeling tremendous outrage. Life has not treated any of you fairly for some time.

There was silence in the room. The doctor felt that each individual was turning inward. He hoped that each was considering his/her own feelings of righteous indignation and the possibility that such feelings were not shameful or needing to be hidden.

Doctor: I would like each of you to do something right now. George's disease has been extremely unfair—maybe for every one of you in a different way. I would like each of you to share aloud one way in which you have felt cheated or that things are unfair. (The doctor fell silent and gave them time to formulate their thoughts.)

Doctor: How about you, George? What's most unfair?

George: I don't know. School, I guess, right now. That really bugs me that I get so behind with work, and it's not my fault. I don't understand why the teachers can't get more organized and plan my work ahead of time. They always know about a week ahead.

Doctor: (surmising that school was only the tip of the iceberg) And what else strikes you as unfair about your brain tumor? What makes you really angry about it?

George: That I ever got it in the first place—that it had to happen to me. No one knows why.

Doctor: I agree, that is unfair, very unfair. Must make you furious.

For some reason the interviewer felt there was much more that George was not saying; he seemed reluctant to continue. He wondered if the boy's reluctance had to do with the presence of other family members and decided at this point that he wanted to see him alone at some time in the future. He did not mention this plan until the close of the interview.

Instead, after he acknowledged George's fury, the doctor continued around the circle, eliciting "unfair" feelings from the rest of the group.

Doctor: Russell?

Russell: (after a long pause) I don't get to spend time with my dad much anymore.

Doctor: And you would like to?

Russell: Sure.

Doctor: What stands in the way?

Russell: I don't know. He seems more busy. . . and mad a lot of the time. We just don't do things together much.

Father: (apologetically) Actually, Russ, that's very close to what I was going to say too. I resent that nothing seems to happen together for us much anymore. We're all so busy doing what needs to be done that there doesn't seem to be time for one another. I would like to do things with you, too.

They talked about "maybe" going to a movie over the weekend, just the two of them. It was an interchange during which they made emotional contact with one another. When they had finished their discussion, mother was the last to comment about unfairness:

Mother: What's unfair? Well, I'm exhausted, I'll tell you that. I don't even have time to clean my house anymore. Now that may seem like a small thing to you, but my house is very important to me. What I wouldn't give for just plain old ordinary housework, time to do the grocery shopping. It seems unfair that I'm doing the shopping on Sunday nights or weeknights. I don't know when the last time was that I had a day off . . . from the things I have to do, I mean. And how come nobody else ever does any of the shopping?

The doctor acknowledged mother's feelings and predicament and talked a bit longer about the feelings expressed by each family member. By this time he was aware of a growing list of items for family work in future sessions. Number one, of course, was the individual and collective feelings of resentment at the unfair treatment that each family member had been feeling subjected to, either at the hands of other family members or on account of George's disease process. George's indignation in this regard appeared particularly acute and demanded rapid intervention. That same feeling expressed by other family members would also need further discussion. Number two, Russell, as the "well" sibling, was certainly hurting, feeling isolated and unnoticed in the flurry of concern and activity that George's condition had stimulated. He was both angry and sad. The family would have to resolve some business there. Number three, mother sounded particularly discouraged, overwhelmed, and exhausted. The doctor sensed a giving-up quality in her manner, and he was not impressed that she was receiving much emotional support from the others. She was going to need help, suggesting item number four: based on the parents' interaction during this initial interview, the doctor felt that their relationship was painfully strained. He hypothesized the presence of marital difficulties antedating the onset of George's disease. The latter, of course, had hardly helped. Where was the emotional support for either parent? They did not appear to be providing it for one another.

The doctor certainly couldn't proceed simultaneously in all four areas. Since George's pain and anger seemed both acute and available, he decided to start there. The pediatrician mused aloud, wondering if perhaps George had begun to express the outrage that they all were feeling—and hiding, since none of them felt entitled to such emotions. He added that it was high time they allowed themselves and one another to complain and to feel all right about doing so; they had the right. The family agreed that such freedom would feel good and that they were interested in pursuing that goal. The doctor replied that he would begin with George, teaching each of them how to complain and express resentment honestly. However, George was to come alone next time, since the doctor sensed the boy probably had a lot more to say about "things being unfair," and perhaps some of them would be easier to say alone. George readily accepted. The doctor told the rest of the family that he would meet with them all again after one or two sessions alone with George. They were agreeable. The doctor closed the interview by giving George a homework assignment. He was asked to write down at home three things that continued to make him very angry about his tumor and his operation. George agreed to the task.

George arrived as expected for the next visit. He had completed his homework assignment. Entitled "Things I Still Resent About My Illness," the paper read:

1. After my operation, when I was going home, I had no idea that I would have further treatments. Nobody had told my parents or me that they had more treatments planned. So it came as a shock to me when they said that they were going to give me radiation treatments for 6½ weeks. That meant that my hair would fall

out, my head would be burned, my throat would be sore, my blood count would drop, and I wouldn't be able to go to school for another 1¾ months.

2. And . . . after radiation I thought that I was done completely. But then my mom wanted me on this special program called chemotherapy, and it is one pain. I have to miss school sometimes, I get sick on these drugs, and every time I have gone (in 9 months), nothing has showed any sign of anything wrong with the tumor. The brain scans and the spinal always show "nothing." There has never been one thing wrong. And I don't know what specific date that it will be over. Every time I ask somebody they say another year to 5 years. I think I would be more calmed down if I knew exactly when it would end. Then I could wait for that day.

3. I hate returning to school, when I know that I am going to have three times as much homework as I usually do.

George discussed each of these freely, acknowledging that he felt especially betrayed by the lack of preparation for planned medical treatments. He felt that too little advance warning had been given him regarding what would happen, how long it would take, and how it would make him feel. He also readily expressed resentment for what he assumed to be his mother's pushing him into chemotherapy. He felt the failure of anyone to consult him was monstrously unfair, especially in light of the side effects and the necessity for ongoing follow-up studies that were all painful. When the doctor asked him if he had shared some of these angry feelings with his parents, he said:

George: No. They don't want to hear any of this. They just tell me I should be thankful I'm still alive.

Doctor: Who can you share things like this with?

George: (tears welling up) Nobody.

Doctor: That's tough. You must have an awful lot stored up then.

George: (nods yes)

Doctor: Since you're doing it, George, then you might as well do it up right. Tell you what I have in mind. You did an excellent job in writing down some of your anger about being sick. I would like you to do some more writing. I would like you to consider each member of your family separately and write down three things about that person, particularly related to your illness, that make you feel angry. Do you understand?

George indicated that he did and set to work immediately, needing no further encouragement. He wrote steadily, using a separate sheet for each person:

Mom

1. She sometimes doesn't listen to me. When Russell starts fights she won't listen to me. She never lets me tell my side of the story, which she knows is the truth, because Russell always makes up something like, "He came into my room and punched me," when Russell really came into my bedroom and punched me. But my mom believes him.
2. She always calls me a big baby all the time when I start crying because Russell punched me for no good reason at all.

Russell

1. He always comes up to me, asks me if I want to play a game with him. Most of the time I say yes, but sometimes I feel sick and say no. When I say no, he'll say something mean like "Oh, I forgot, you are too lazy to play," or "You aren't supposed to come outside and hurt yourself."
2. He beats up on me when I am beating him at a game such as Ping-Pong or baseball or basketball.
3. He never has anything good to say to anybody and he always talks like everyone else is stupid. He never cleans up his messes, so either I have to or we both get in trouble.

Dad

1. Sometimes when I am going to the hospital and he is driving, he will lose his patience with me and say something like "I hate this whole program" or "How come I always have to drive you?" or "I can't stand doing these things for you" or "Next time, get someone else to drive you."
2. He gets mad at me constantly, even if Russell is the one who did wrong.
3. When Russell does something wrong or makes a mess, he will say, "George, get up here and clean this mess" or "Why do you boys make such a mess?"

His absorption in, and enthusiasm for, the task said that what he was writing was important to him and that he wanted to share it with someone. The doctor was appalled by what he wrote. In George's eyes, his mother didn't listen and was pulling away from him in favor of Russell. Russell used George's lack of stamina from his illness to tease and belittle him. And Mr. Nelson's angry, rejecting statements most certainly had stung. Family relationships were in a bad way. Whether each point was literally accurate made little difference actually. The boy was feeling unheard, denigrated, rejected, and betrayed by different family members in different situations.

Now the interviewer rather wished he had not pursued this direction with George alone, for it was quite apparent that communications of the sort George was writing down would need to be aired and altered in a family setting. However, he had begun, and so he continued. George and he discussed the items George had listed. The doctor was struck with this youngster's exceptionally strong sense of fair play in his orientation to school, family, and life. Things were supposed to be right, just, fair, ethical, and honest. Even more than in the first session, it seemed that George considered his disease to have violated all the rules, dealing a staggering blow to his sense of fairness. It was this blow from which he was reeling most heavily and from which he had not recovered. Nor, apparently, had his family.

Doctor: You know, George, I think some of these things are going to have to be discussed with your family.

George: They won't listen (looking very sad).

Doctor: Would you like them to?

George: Well . . . yes. I guess so.

Doctor: I heard that "I guess" on the end.

George: Well, it's kind of scary to think about saying some of this to them.

Doctor: How come?

George: They would think I was complaining.

Doctor: And so? Do you have a right to complain — after what you've been through?

George: I dunno.

Doctor: Well, I feel strongly that you do. You have a right to be screaming from the rooftops as far as I'm concerned.

George laughed at the image, he said, of hanging from some roof hollering his lungs out, moaning and complaining. His remark triggered an impulse on the doctor's part that he immediately discounted and then found himself continuing to consider for the rest of the session. He then said to George:

Doctor: I think I would like to meet with you one more time alone, George, before your family returns for a session. We'll be taking a short hike, so wear old clothes and some walking shoes.

He did not explain further in spite of George's curious questions. The boy agreed excitedly without being sure what he was taking on.

At the next visit, George came prepared. They piled into the doctor's car and drove for a few minutes. The San Francisco Bay area is studded with hills. One of these was near the office. From its heights one could survey all of San Francisco Bay with its bridges, islands, cities, and the Pacific Ocean beyond. It was a stupendous, lonely spot, a place where one might feel that he looked down on the earth from above. George and the doctor climbed the hill by car and parked near the summit. They walked along a hiking trail to a private spot the doctor knew where he sometimes came by himself. It was deserted. They sat on the rocky edge and talked some more of life's unfairness for George. Then the pediatrician said:

Doctor: OK, George, it's time.

George: For what?

Doctor: I'm going to ask you to do something that sounds silly; however, I want you to take it very seriously. I want you to scream one phrase at the top of your lungs: "It's not fair!" I want you to scream it so that the Golden Gate Bridge out there can hear you.

George: (stared at him in disbelief)

Doctor: Go on.

George: (hesitatingly, and then, his voice scarcely above a mumble) It's not fair.

Doctor: Much louder, George.

George: (settling into his position on the rock, he raised his voice considerably) It's not fair!

Doctor: Good. Now much louder still.

George: It's not fair! (He was shouting at last.)

Doctor: Again.

George: It's not fair! It's not fair! IT'S NOT FAIR . . . IT'S NOT FAIR!

George was screaming and he was crying — and he was smiling. Neither he nor the doctor spoke; George was almost breathless. Gradually both his breathing and his crying quieted, and they each sat quietly, looking out over the bay and toward the bridge. George didn't notice, but the doctor had tears in his eyes also. After sitting for maybe 10 minutes more the physician reached over, touched the boy's shoulder, and said:

Doctor: Let's go back to my office.

George: I'm ready.

Neither said very much on the way back. George didn't say good-bye when they returned to his mother's waiting car at the office. He turned and said, "Thanks." The doctor decided it hadn't been a harebrained idea after all.

This "mountaintop" experience was not duplicated in subsequent work with the Nelson family. In fact continuing work went rapidly downhill after that. The next meeting, scheduled to be with the entire family, in reality became a session with the parents alone. Both George and Russell were away on an overnight scouting trip. The interviewer decided not to cancel the session and met with Mr. and Mrs. Nelson.

Both parents were pleased with some changes in George, particularly following his previous interview. They felt that he was no longer as edgy and irritable. "He seems to have less of a chip on his shoulder" was the way father put it. George had discussed the trip to the hill with both his mother and father. Since George was not present, aside from hearing that he was apparently doing well, the doctor did not want to discuss him further. He turned the discussion toward mother and father and their own coping in the face of all that had happened to the family. Each parent was feeling angry and bitter toward the other, with similar complaints. Mother felt unsupported by father, as though she were carrying most of the family responsibilities on her shoulders alone. Father had the same feeling; to him it seemed that the weight of all decision making and particularly care for George fell to him. He felt unnoticed and unappreciated by his wife in his efforts to keep the family afloat. Both were chronically carping at one another.

Acknowledging the feelings of both parents, the doctor suggested that continuing counseling—some with them alone and some to include the children—was essential if they were to feel better about themselves, one another, and their relationship with the boys. They too, just as George, needed to release some of their "unpleasant" feelings and find ways to communicate feelings more effectively. The parents agreed to this plan.

> *Doctor:* Next time, however, I will want to see all four of you. George has some things that he needs to discuss with the family. After that I think I would want to see the two of you alone.
> *Father:* That will be OK.
> *Doctor:* How about for you, Mrs. Nelson?
> *Mother:* Yes . . . OK. Do you think it will do any good, really?
> *Doctor:* You're feeling hopeless about your situation?

Mother: Oh, I don't know . . . sometimes. Well, no . . . but, sure we can come back.

Mrs. Nelson's reluctance was very unsettling; it was the first inkling the pediatrician had that the family and he had not solidly joined. The second indication he had of that lack of joining appeared around the issue of scheduling the next appointment. Christmas was just ahead, and the family was going out of town for a 2-week vacation. Mother asked if she could call to set up the next appointment when they returned. The doctor agreed. Three weeks passed.

By now he was uncomfortable that he had not heard. Growing restless, he called the family. Mother answered and apologized for not calling. They would not be able to continue sessions right at the moment. Her husband would be traveling back and forth to southern California for the next month and a half on swimming team business. She and he had decided that they would prefer to initiate sessions in the future as needed. Right now things seemed to be going much better at home, and George was no longer having difficulty with procedures at the hospital. Could she call if problems were to develop later?

Discouraged, the doctor nonetheless agreed. The family did not subsequently call. Periodically he would call them, sometimes talking to one of the parents or to George. The parents were always "satisfied" with how things were going in their own relationship and positive in their views of George's behavior. The pediatrician could not be sure whether that reflected changes in the marriage and improved coping by George or the parents' determination to put off further family counseling. George himself sounded reasonably happy and busy with his life when the doctor talked to him. He was pleased with the fact that the treatment procedures were no longer causing him to come unhinged. Even so, the doctor felt irritatingly unfinished with George and his family.

Eighteen months have passed since those initial sessions. George is still alive and so far without a recurrence. The longer he survives, of course, the more likely his case represents a cure, an uncommon occurrence with his particular tumor type. Yet, as his mother reminded the doctor during their last phone conversation, they still can't know for sure. She added:

Mother: But you know, nothing's really for sure—ever. We've just given up waiting for the other shoe to drop. Life has to be now, my husband says. He's right.

The family had come a long way, the pediatrician thought to himself. Maybe they will be all right. Even though they and he had not systematically worked together to resolve the family's obvious interpersonal stresses, and even though that fact might always seem frustrating for the doctor to accept, perhaps he had been one help for them along their way.

Discussion. Work with George Nelson and his family was certainly not a total failure. Neither could it be considered a rousing success. Endings such as this particularly stimulate questions about the course of the interviews and the approaches used. Could interviews, for instance, have been handled differently to prevent the family's premature withdrawal from continuing sessions? That is hard to know for certain. Surely withdrawal followed hard on the heels of a focus on the parents and their marital relationship. Sessions were allowed as long as the spotlight remained on George. Perhaps the parents viewed open discussions of their own relationship as just too threatening, and they retreated, taking the boys with them. Unfortunately the pediatrician did not sense this during the work itself but only subsequently as the parents obviously were beginning to flee, and then it was too late. So in retrospect a slower pace with less direct attention to marital discord, perhaps continuing work for a while with the sibling subsystem, might have felt more tolerable to Mr. and Mrs. Nelson. George and his brother certainly needed to discuss and resolve some angry feelings and misunderstandings between one another. A gradually increased emphasis could have been developed regarding feelings and misunderstandings first between children, next between a child and a parent, and finally between parents themselves, approaching the most vulnerable area last. Also the parents had been through a tremendous ordeal with their son's illness. Asking them to turn depleted emotional energies toward a consideration of their own chronic dysfunction with one another may simply have seemed like too much at the wrong time. The interviewer could have discussed this very thought with them and in the process might have spent considerably more time acknowledging the dilemmas and feelings of each parent regarding their present life situation with George.

In summary then the parents' termination of interviewing sessions may have communicated their dissatisfaction with the interviewer's intended direction (discussion of marital discord). A slower interviewing pace and an increased acknowledgement of the parents' plight are two alternate strategies that the pediatrician might have considered using.

The terminal event of death

This third period in the chronology of a child's fatal illness arrives when death, not illness, comes to be considered the foreground topic. Its arrival may be precipitous or gradual. Until this point the disease, its complications, its stresses, and its course have occupied the energies of the patient, the family, and the medical staff. In this third period a focus on the patient's illness course is now joined and perhaps replaced by the realization that death is close, and attention to this phenomenon may dwarf all else. During this period families want help, not with living in the face of chronic illness but with living in the presence of death.

Particularly at this juncture, stimulated perhaps by the realization that time is running out, many parents voice aloud their concerns (although they may have been silently worried for months) regarding what their child knows about his dying, what to tell him, how to talk to him, who should talk to him, and so on. They may frequently turn to the doctor for advice regarding dialogues with their dying child. A family interview including parents and perhaps siblings (with the option of including the ill child in subsequent sessions) can be used to help families deal with this aspect of their child's dying.

We have earlier mentioned that it is not a question of whether to talk to children about their condition but rather how. This holds, we feel, whether one is talking about the name of the condition, that is, the diagnosis, or its seriousness and fatal outcome. Kübler-Ross has found in her work with adults that "all terminally ill patients know the seriousness of their condition" regardless of what they have been told.[4] We have observed that the same is true with children and agree with Vernick and his studies of children with leukemia:

> The children invariably knew their diagnosis, either because they were among the few who had been so informed by their physician or parents or because they had figured it out on their own. Some were aware that they had a life-threatening illness related to the blood without knowing the particular diagnosis. Regardless of age, they all appeared to realize the fact that they could die from their illness. The process by which they reached a diagnosis may be highly circuitous but most of them are able to recall the confluence of telltale cues that first led them to identify their illness. Here are a set of typical responses from a child who had been consciously kept in the dark about the diagnosis and prognosis:
>
> "All of a sudden I got my room redecorated, and all new clothes for

school . . . When we came back from the doctor's office, things were all different at home. I started getting lots of things I never could have before. I never could have a big machine gun that shoots BB's, but the next day my father comes home and he has this gun for me . . . Relatives who never used to visit started coming around and bringing me all kinds of things . . . Sometimes, when I would walk into the room, my mother and father would stop talking and look at me."

By the time a child has undergone some of the procedures used to diagnose and later, to treat leukemia, he has already completed most of the puzzle himself. The shock, guilt, anger, fear, and frustration that overcome the parents are transmitted to the child in various ways. He clearly understands that their distress is related to his own situation, and on this basis alone, he is able to conclude that he is in serious trouble. This is when he most needs to have the questions discussed with him openly and honestly.*

Therefore one could in a family interview assure parents first of all that their child in all probability already knows something very serious is happening.

A pediatrician may also assure them that most children want to talk about their dying. In this regard, Vernick cites the work of two French pediatricians, Raimbault and Royer.[6] While carrying out their first interviews with young patients concerning the children's ideas about their fatal illnesses, these authors were struck by the great frequency with which the patients spontaneously approached the death theme. In all the interviews, the children, either directly through questions and comments or indirectly through picture drawing, or by both means, themselves brought up the subject of death. After having discussed such matters with the children, the authors concluded that chronically and seriously ill children readily and realistically can and do wish to speak about their fears, concerns, and ideas regarding death and dying. Specifically they stated, "When the sick child has the possibility to freely express himself with an adult he will approach the subject of death without restraint."[6] These pediatricians, even with very young patients, used straightforward simple communication techniques, finding no need to become involved in complicated symbolic and interpretive techniques.

That children (1) know of and (2) want to talk about their dying does

---

*Vernick, J.: Meaningful communication with the fatally ill child. In Anthony, E., and Koupernick, C., editors: The child in his family: the impact of disease and death, vol. 2, New York, 1973, John Wiley & Sons, Inc., p. 114.

not mean that one counsels the family to assault a child with a frontal attack, such as telling him he is going to die. Families need to understand that most often they will not have to initiate such discussions by "telling" their child anything. They will help a child and facilitate open communication most effectively by listening and responding openly to his questions about life and death. This process is helped, as Kübler-Ross points out, when staff and family can tune into "the language of the dying patient."[5]

For instance: a 6-year-old patient on our pediatric ward at the University of California, terminally ill with leukemia, was soon to be discharged. It was his family's wish that he be allowed to die at home with them. The parents' wishes were being respected. Just at discharge, the child, Terry, began talking of the upcoming spring baseball season. It was clear to all the staff that Terry would not live for more than a few days, certainly not until spring, and they felt somehow that Terry knew that also. Yet the child began to make statements and ask about playing baseball in 3 months' time.

> *Terry:*   I'm going to play baseball when I get home. There's a big season coming up. It starts pretty soon, well not too soon . . . (pause) . . . Will I be able to play baseball, Dr. Carson?

Dr. Carson felt, and rightly so, that he was being put on the spot; he was at a loss for words. Terry, of course, was talking about death. We have earlier referred to the use of open-ended questions and statements to help children express their worries and fears about illness. Just such a remark would have been quite appropriate at this point with Terry. Whoever was on the receiving end of Terry's comments about baseball might have responded: "Tell me how you see the situation, Terry. Do you think you will?"

Such a question would have invited the child to respond with his own version of how he was viewing the immediate future. The doctor would then have been in a position to respond to the child's feelings around his own prediction. Perhaps most important, such a response would have communicated the adult's willingness to continue the discussion and not close it off. Replies such as: "No, I think you will have to stay in bed," or "Of course you will, Terry," are ways of gently cutting off any further discussion. One might just as well say, "Let's not talk about that, Terry." And the moment for facilitating the child's disclosure of a part of his internal world would be lost.

Family interviews can be used as practice sessions for families troubled by their child's questions regarding death, in much the same way as a practice session was utilized and described in the previous chapter. In that situation a child's questions surrounding upcoming surgery necessitated some practice on the family's part. Similarly, with the help of a family interviewer, parents can be encouraged to face in advance those questions that they most dread hearing from a terminally ill child. Parents may also then in the interview setting learn the technique of responding with an open-ended question that sustains and enlarges the communication. Below are some representative questions from a larger list, questions that specific parents have told us they feared their dying child might ask or had actually asked. Next to the question is one reply that we utilized with them to initiate a role-playing experience with us in the interview, before any subsequent actual conversation between parent and child was held.

Statement or question	Possible reply to open the conversation
1. Sometimes I wish I wasn't here	Where would you rather be? Tell me about it.
2. Why me?	Sure seems unfair. What's the unfairest part of all?
3. I don't have much to live for	You sound pretty discouraged. What makes you feel like giving up?
4. Where do I go when I die?	Tell me what you think it will be like.
5. When I die, can I take my dog?	You worried about being alone? I won't leave. . . . Tell me more about your dog; what would you need him for when you die?

Having parents become accustomed to using such responses (not the specific words given here but rather the approach) in practice sessions and allowing them to expand their remarks into a longer simulated interchange with the child have often been quite helpful in preparing families for the actual discussion at a later time.

Abundant evidence, some already cited here, suggests that children want very much to talk about these issues. And yet there are still critics of open conversation with dying children about their conditions. To them we respond with some words by Clement Smith:

> I think we should get away from the idea that, with children, we must somehow soften blows in a special way. Blows cannot always be softened, but by explanation and sharing, their impact may be made somewhat less concentrated and acute.*

---

*Smith, C.: Help for the hopeless, R. I. Med. J. **39:**491, 1956.

The period following death

Less commonly today, but still too often, a physician considers his work done with a child's death or perhaps when the results of the autopsy are returned. It is not; only the work of the dead child is finished at that point, not that of the physician and certainly not that of the family. Family members may each be grieving at a different level, burdened by separate and different issues. The turmoil of surviving siblings may be easy to overlook, since for various reasons they may believe that their feelings must be hidden. They may not wish to burden their obviously upset parents with their own feelings of upset and sadness. They may have feelings of guilt that they somehow caused the death of their brother or sister through "evil" thoughts or wishes. They may even worry about the possibility of catching the same fatal illness. Because such thoughts and feelings are so charged and frightening, they may be carefully screened from view by the child, and his outward appearance may be misleading to the adults around him absorbed in their own grieving.

Almost no one in the family, adult or child, will have completed his mourning coincident with the child's death. Fear, anger, guilt, and above all sadness are usually painfully present and not at all resolved. The family may be feeling ravaged not just by their child's death, but by staggering medical bills, seriously eroded family relationships, physical exhaustion and symptoms, and significantly strained communication patterns. Thus they may need considerable help just taking up the task of living once again. We would urge the pediatrician not to abandon the group at this point. He may specifically find the use of periodic or regular family interviews an efficient means for keeping tabs on emerging and unresolved family difficulties following the death of a child. It is certainly a direct method for evaluating the mourning process in each family member, not just the adults but children as well, and for offering professional support and counsel in the completion of that process.

Emily Dickinson has a final stanza in one of her poems that describes the feelings of survivors at the bedside of one who has just died:

> And we, we placed the hair,
> And drew the head erect;
> And then an awful leisure was,
> Our faith to regulate.*

*Dickinson, E.: Selected poems of Emily Dickinson, New York, 1924, Modern Library.

It is helping the family to "regulate" their "awful leisure" following a child's death that requires the physician's continuing care and presence.

REFERENCES

1. Anthony, S.: The child's discovery of death: a study in child psychology, New York, 1940, Harcourt Brace Jovanovich, Inc.
2. Binger, C., and others: Childhood leukemia, emotional impact on patient and family, N. Engl. J. Med. **280:**414, 1969.
3. Kübler-Ross, E.: The dying patient's point of view. In Brim, O., and others, editors: The dying patient, New York, 1960, Russell Sage Foundation, pp. 156-170.
4. Kübler-Ross, E.: On death and dying, New York, 1969, The Macmillan Co.
5. Kübler-Ross, E.: Personal communication, 1975.
6. Raimbault, G., and Royer, P.: Thematique de la mort chez l'enfant attient de maladie chronique, Arch. Fr. Pediatr. **26:**1041, 1969.
7. Rothenberg, M.: Reactions of those who treat children with cancer, Pediatrics **40:**407, 1967.

CHAPTER 11

Psychosomatic conditions

THE ORTIZ FAMILY

Alice Ortiz, 15 years of age, trailed along disconsolately after her parents. Her father was first into the office, a picture of crisp efficiency with a manner that said, "Let's get down to business." He was short, trim, dressed in a three-piece suit; everything was well-ordered—his hair, neatly trimmed moustache, white shirt, solid tie, handkerchief, dark socks, and black shoes. His facial expression matched his somber wardrobe, and he carried a copy of *The New York Times* (although this was San Francisco) and a book under his right arm. His wife, two steps behind, seemed to be striving for invisibility. She avoided Dr. Silver's eyes as he greeted her, only belatedly extending her hand beyond her bulky coat sleeve after she saw his outstretched; her large coat was bundled around her such that he could see only a portion of her head rising from the commodious collar. She moved quickly to a chair, two available seats away from her husband, and motioned for her daughter, bringing up the rear, to join her on that side of the room. Alice complied; she was in many ways duplicating the entrance of her mother, maintaining a low profile. She too was wrapped in a heavy coat that concealed. The coat did not do its job, however. The doctor could see she was a beautiful young woman, taller than either her father or mother and with striking dark features and good looks. She loosened her coat as she sat and draped it over the back of her chair; mother did not emerge from her cover. All three looked *very* anxious as the session started.

A fourth family member was not present; Alice's 19-year-old sister was away at college. The parents, both born in Guatemala, had come to the United States as young adults and met and married in this country. Mr. Ortiz had a responsible office position with a shipping company on the San Francisco waterfront. Mrs. Ortiz also worked full-time as a laboratory technician in a medical office. Alice's asthma had brought the family in. The pediatrician had earlier been told by the referring physician, an eminent pediatric allergist, that this was one of the few families in which he felt emotional factors were significant contributors to the child's symptomatology; he himself had witnessed attacks triggered by father's heavy-handed and punitive approach to his daughter.

Since this was a teaching hour, a pediatric resident was also present in the room. This was his first day in the Child Study Unit and his first observation of a family interview. Dr. Silver glanced over and winced; the trainee looked as uncomfortable as the family. When both family and trainee were scared equally, that usually meant that Dr. Silver would have to work very hard throughout the session, since the resident would be another responsibility rather than a co-worker who would help with the interview and the family. He quickly lectured himself not to expect so much of a new trainee. After all this was his first day.

Following introductions all around and a few words about taping the session, Dr. Silver opened the hour by asking each family member in turn what he or she understood about the meeting.

Doctor:	How about you, Alice?
Alice:	Well, it's about my asthma. Dr. Williams, my allergist, said we should come.
Doctor:	I see. For what purpose?
Alice:	I don't know. I think he thinks there may be psychological things about my asthma, as well as physical.
Doctor:	And what do you think?
Alice:	I'm not sure really. I'm wondering if we're going to be talking about medical stuff or . . . (glancing at her father) something else.
Doctor:	So you're feeling confused as to whether today's session is going to be a discussion of medical issues or psychological ones?
Alice:	Yes.
Doctor:	OK. I'll come back to that in a minute. Let me first move to your dad. Mr. Ortiz, what do you understand about this meeting here today?
Father:	My wife asked me to come. Doctor. And Dr. Williams said it would be a good idea. Otherwise I really don't know—I assume that you are an allergy specialist, and you are going to help Alice with her asthma. Will you be giving her allergy tests, that sort of thing?
Doctor:	Oh my, then you have been thinking that I am an allergist?
Father:	Yes.

Doctor: I think I need to explain. I am not an allergist. I am a pediatrician, and I often work with children who are having some particular medical problem — like asthma, for instance. My special focus with them, however, is on the emotional or behavioral parts of that medical problem. And I prefer to work with the whole family, rather than just with the child alone. Alice mentioned a minute ago that Dr. Williams thinks there may be emotional or psychological issues connected with Alice's asthma attacks.

Father: Yes . . .?

Doctor: Tell me how Dr. Williams explained that to you.

Father: He didn't.

Doctor: Oh, then you also must be feeling somewhat confused as to what this meeting is all about, especially since I have now just told you that I am not an allergist.

Father: I certainly am.

Doctor: Maybe we need to talk about terms . . . "psychological things as well as physical" . . . I wonder what Dr. Williams could have meant there? Anybody in the family have any ideas?

Father: (very definitely) No.

Mother: I think what he is referring to . . .

Doctor: Good, Mrs. Ortiz. I was beginning to worry that I hadn't yet gotten over to you . . .

Mother: I think he means that Alice can get an attack just from getting upset.

Doctor: And have you noticed that?

Mother: Yes, often.

Doctor: Tell Alice specifically what you have noticed.

Mother, still looking very frightened, then shared her observations with Alice that her asthma would often seemingly occur when the girl became stressed, anxious, or upset. Alice halfheartedly agreed and then countered that there were just so many things she was allergic to. Her father quickly entered the conversation at this point, affirming her statement with a listing of all her specific allergens and a description of his own recently surfaced allergies and the prolonged diagnostic evaluation in which he himself was currently participating.

It was not a particularly heartening beginning. Father thought Dr. Silver was an allergist; Alice, the identified patient, was showing considerable reluctance in broaching psychological issues; her mother, while tentatively suggesting the presence of psychological factors, was looking scared to death as she did so. No one had visibly relaxed since the start of the hour; the resident was still nervous and wide-eyed. The interviewer wasn't particularly comfortable himself. Hence he decided to retreat to territory that would feel more comfortable for the family and for the resident — territory he could discuss almost mindlessly. It would give him time to organize his thoughts and plan how in the world he would proceed.

> *Doctor:* Alice, it would help me to learn more about your medical condition. Tell me more about your asthma.

She did, and the conversation settled into a discussion of frequency of attacks, medications used, emergency room visits, duration of attacks, at what age she first developed symptoms, and so forth. She and the other family members talked freely during this portion of the interview, and the anxious pall seemed to lift from the room. Even the resident uncrossed his legs. While Mr. Ortiz and Dr. Silver were discussing something about the use of aminophylline, the interviewer glanced at Alice and noticed that she was very close to tears. He said nothing but completed his conversation with her father. The atmosphere was less strained; however, the doctor was getting impatient. He did not want to pursue the subject of bronchodilators for the rest of the session. Clearly the family on their own would not enlarge the discussion to include the subject of feelings and emotions. The pediatrician felt the need to move somehow into the area of family relationships with the Ortizs, but how, in a way they would tolerate? He decided to use Alice's visible tears as a bridge.

> *Doctor:* Alice, I'm wondering what you're feeling inside right now as we've been discussing all of this.
> *Alice:* (very quietly) I don't know.
> *Doctor:* I ask that for a specific reason. Just a few moments ago, as your father was talking, I noticed that you were very upset, quite close to tears.
> *Alice:* Just a cold, I guess (blowing her nose).
> *Doctor:* Somehow, it seemed more than that.
> *Alice:* (Silent for a long time, she finally begins to sob quietly.)

Dr. Silver glanced over at the resident. He had crossed his legs again. Mr. Ortiz was sitting ramrod straight in his chair, unchanged. Mrs. Ortiz had started sobbing in rhythm with her daughter. Clearly something very important was happening; the interviewer chose to remain silent and let the situation proceed. Within a short period of time, Mrs. Ortiz rose from her chair, crying openly and apologizing for her tears.

> *Mother:* Oh, Doctor, I am sorry . . . so sorry. Excuse me please.

She headed for the door. The doctor rose, put one hand on her arm and the other on the doorknob, and gently asked her to stay.

> *Mother:* Oh, I just shouldn't be crying.

The interviewer reassured her that in this room it was all right to cry. Then guiding her back to her seat he asked her to talk about her tears. She indicated that she couldn't bear for her daughter to be upset—darting a look at her husband that he did not return—that when Alice got upset, she did too. The doctor acknowledged that the two of them must be very close and asked if she knew the origin of Alice's tears at this moment.

> *Mother:* No, I don't understand.
> *Doctor:* Would you ask her now—ask her what her tears are about, see if she will put her tears into words.
> *Mother:* What's wrong, darling?
> *Alice:* Just . . . scared, I guess.
> *Mother:* Scared about what?
> *Alice:* (shakes her head indicating that she does not know)

A long silence fell.

> *Doctor:* I bet you have a few ideas, though.
> *Alice:* (nods her head yes.)
> *Doctor:* But it's very hard to talk about?
> *Alice:* (vigorously) Yes.
> *Doctor:* Well, I can see that it's really hard for you to talk right now. I have some ideas too about what's happening on your insides. So don't talk—I'll share my ideas, and you can just let me know whether what I say fits or not. You can just nod yes or no.
> *Alice:* (nods in agreement)
> *Doctor:* If I'm Alice, I am feeling scared because this whole situation is frightening. Here I am with my family sitting in front of two strange doctors: I don't know them. It's hard to talk about important and private things with strangers. That's one reason I am feeling scared. Does that fit?
> *Alice:* Yes.

Doctor:	And there's more?
Alice:	Yes.
Doctor:	Another reason, if I'm Alice, for feeling scared is I'm worried that people won't understand what I'm feeling or trying to say.
Alice:	(again nods that he is correct)
Doctor:	Those were my ideas. I wonder if you have some others, Alice, of your own.

After a long pause, she indicates that she does. There is an even longer silence, and finally, squaring her shoulders while continuing to look at her hands, she softly states:

Alice:	I cannot talk with my father.
Doctor:	(allowing a silence to intervene) You sound very sad as you say that.
Alice:	Very.
Doctor:	Tell me, is there a part of you that would like to be able to talk to your father, a part of you that would like for the two of you to be closer?
Alice:	(nods agreement)
Doctor:	Could you tell him that directly, right now.

Alice looked at her father and did just that. He was listening intently. And the doctor was thinking so far, so good. They had successfully made the transition from medical matters to feeling matters.

Alice said that she very much wanted to be closer to her father, but that communication never seemed to work well between them, that he seemed always angry and dissatisfied with her. Since it was so hard to tell from Mr. Ortiz's implacable face what impact this turn in the interview was having on him, the doctor then said:

Doctor:	Mr. Ortiz, you are obviously listening very hard. What do you see in your daughter's face right at this moment?
Father:	Anguish. I see anguish.
Doctor:	And what does that do to *your* insides?
Father:	I don't know what you mean.
Doctor:	What are you feeling inside?

After some searching and discussion, Mr. Ortiz acknowledged that his daughter's feelings triggered in him a feeling of helplessness. He just didn't know what to do. He then began to defend his customary behavior with her, saying that it wasn't his intention to create distance between them, but he was just so worried about her asthma that her attacks often threw him into a panic, the manifestation of which would be his launching into a "third degree" in which he would question her relentlessly about her behavior during the day. He would probe for anything that might give a clue as to how she allowed an offending allergen into her environment. She would have to list for him the food she had eaten, the places she had been, the activities in which she had engaged, and so on. Ultimately he would explode with an "Ahhhhh, so that was it! How many times have I told you . . . " She would then be severely reprimanded for being irresponsible about her own condition. By this time, of course, she would be intimidated into tears. They would end the interchange with mutual bitterness and alienation. In an effort to support him in his good intentions, the doctor acknowledged that it seemed to be his feelings of helplessness and also concern for his daughter's health that prompted him to be so often upset with her. Mr. Ortiz agreed, and his daughter seemed to hear as well.

Dr. Silver asked father and daughter if they were interested in learning to communicate in other ways and work at drawing closer together. Both were interested; Mrs. Ortiz also signified her willingness to participate in additional sessions. After they made plans for a subsequent interview, Dr. Silver terminated the hour. From a tentative beginning, the interview had progressed well, he thought. The resident was impressed and asked if the interviewer had in some way "planted" the family to demonstrate the effectiveness of a family approach. Dr. Silver took that as a compliment. He discussed the hour and his strategies and direction, and since the resident now seemed willing to enter the fray, he and Dr. Silver made plans for how they would more jointly share interviewing responsibilities when the family returned in 1 week's time.

The family never returned. They cancelled their next two interviews and then indicated that they did not wish to continue at all.

What happened? What went wrong? How was it that the resident and the interviewer felt so positive about the session and sensed the family felt likewise? The family's willingness to pursue the communication of feelings in subsequent sessions had obviously been misread. Why? What had happened that the interviewers seemed to win the battle and then lose the war?

The reader may have his own answers to the above questions. In retrospect we too have found some explanations for the family's disappearance after just one session. Our own explanations are related to possible omissions and/or oversights by the interviewers in three categories: (1) achievement of the goals for an initial family interview, (2) respect for the cultural background of a family, and (3) utilization of some general considerations about families with a psychosomatic member.

A brief discussion of each seems in order.

ACHIEVEMENT OF THE GOALS FOR AN INITIAL FAMILY INTERVIEW

Achievement of goals has already been discussed in Chapter 6. Briefly reviewed, the four interviewer goals is an initial session are:

1. To establish that he will be in charge of the interview
2. To develop a beginning formulation of the problem and a tentative treatment plan
3. To make the interview a "touching" experience for every family member
4. To ensure the family's return

With specific regard to the Ortiz family interview, there was never any doubt that the interviewer was in charge of the process. Hence goal number one fell into place. Likewise goal number two was achieved: a beginning formulation of the problem was made, namely that the expression of feelings was blocked in this family, and a tentative treatment plan was started, that of assisting the family in "unblocking" their expression of feeling with one another. However goal number four, ensuring the family's return, fell flatter than a pancake and was probably related to a simultaneous failure with goal number three, making the interview a "touching" experience for every family member. Quite likely Alice was touched in the interview. Her feelings were heard, acknowledged, and discussed. However, not much attention was paid to Mrs. Ortiz, and it is unclear whether or not the brief interchange around her own tears was sufficient acknowledgement of her distress. Probably more time should have been spent with her in the hour. Regarding Mr. Ortiz, considerable time was spent with him, eliciting and acknowledging his feelings, in a direct attempt to "touch" him. From the interviewer's vantage point, the "touching" seemed to take place. In retrospect sufficient "touching" probably did not occur with Mr. Ortiz. This is demonstrated by the fact that it was Mr. Ortiz who refused to return or to allow the family's participation in subsequent interviews. We must say "probably," however, because it was Mrs. Ortiz who communicated this message to the interviewers. Repeated attempts to talk directly to Mr. Ortiz were unsuccessful.

For Mr. Ortiz to have felt touched in the session, the interviewer not only needed to search out the man's feelings with regard to his daughter, her condition, and his own allergies, he also needed to pay attention to Mr. Ortiz's feelings surrounding the whole family interviewing process itself. That brings us to a discussion of the second category of oversights by the interviewers.

RESPECT FOR THE CULTURAL BACKGROUND OF A FAMILY

Mr. Ortiz communicated in many ways the importance that he placed on being a responsible individual in charge of his family. His dress and his manner suggested it, let alone his nationality and cultural background. Everything about him said clearly, "I consider myself the head of this family." For such a man, too rapid an entry into family business by an outsider — even a kindly observer — could easily be experienced as an intrusion and a derogatory statement about father's ability to manage his family group successfully. An interviewer, pursuing his own goal of establishing that he will be in charge of an interview, may unwittingly suggest to such a father that paternal control is being usurped. In our experience in working with families having a cultural heritage outside that of white, middle-class America, this has often seemed to be the case. Just coming in for a family interview itself, regardless of what is discussed, has been very threatening for some fathers of European, Asian, or Latino background. It is as though the very occurrence of a family interview with an outsider is an indictment of fatherly capabilities, even though it is not viewed or intended as such by the interviewer.

This being the case, considerably more attention to, and support for, Mr. Ortiz's position of leadership in the family needed to take place, especially before facilitating the family's discussion of feelings toward one another.

UTILIZATION OF SOME GENERAL CONSIDERATIONS ABOUT FAMILIES WITH A PSYCHOSOMATIC MEMBER

In our experience psychosomatic symptoms in a family member are often the feelings of that person being expressed in disguise. As one of our staff has noted:

> It is a useful generalization to consider that it suits the body's economy to discharge feelings of all kinds. If the expression of feelings is forbidden by family rules of behavior, those feelings will still press for release although by indirect means. I generally expect to find the most "psychosomatic" difficulty in those families which are most intent on teach-

ing their children to suppress the expression of feelings. The parent's motive is usually based on his own dread of some feeling of helplessness. For example, "If I let my child cry, I won't know what to do to stop her." Or, "If my child loses his temper, I will not be able to stand up under his anger." Since there is nothing that can be done directly to prevent someone from *having* an emotion (short of drugs, psycho-surgery, etc.), families that are fearful of being overwhelmed by other people's feelings generally work to discourage *expressing* feelings. Certain body organs seem far more immediately involved in the discharge of feelings that are not being handled directly. As you might expect, the more vulnerable organs are those which are in dynamic equilibrium between the organism and the environment, e.g., the nervous system, the gastro-intestinal tract, and the respiratory tract. Breathing seems an especially sensitive interface between the self and the outside world. In fact, the German word "angst" from which "anxiety" derives, means a narrowness and refers to the feeling of restricted respiration and tightness that accompanies anxiety.*

It is interesting how often metaphors and similes come to mind when one is either working with or experiencing a psychosomatic symptom. It is more than coincidence, we believe, that an individual with a tension headache will generally describe his pain in terms such as, "I feel like I'm going to explode" or "I'm going to blow my top," and that these same statements are widely accepted metaphors for the expression of anger as well. In this and other instances there has seemed to be an uncanny, almost poetic connection between a given psychosomatic symptom and a particular metaphor that is popularly used to describe a certain feeling. To illustrate, we have worked with family members with:

Headaches who were so angry that they were ready "to blow my top"

Chest pains who were feeling "heartache" and/or that they had something they needed to "get off my chest"

Constipation who were feeling "tied up in knots"

Back pain who were feeling like someone in their lives or some situation was "a pain in the neck"

Vomiting who couldn't "stomach" something in their environment

Dysphagia who were finding something "hard to swallow"

Asthma who felt "choked up" and/or "breathlessly excited" about someone or something

Enuresis who clearly stated that they felt "pissed off"

---

*Leveton, A.: Personal communication, 1972.

It seems almost as though such an individual, perceiving that ordinary, direct methods for expression of feelings are blocked, chooses to get his message to the outside in code in a way that outwits the family proscription against revealing or verbalizing feelings. Thus psychosomatic symptoms and the indirect expression of feelings have seemed to us inextricably linked. None of this, of course, is very far removed from some of the early and now classical writings of Breur and Freud on hysteria,[1] in which connections were postulated between the symbolic expression of unacceptable feelings and somatic symptoms.

Since, at least in part, individuals develop psychosomatic symptoms to symbolize and express feelings because the direct expression of certain feelings is considered unacceptable in that individual's family environment, perhaps a too-rapid encouragement by the interviewer for family members to verbalize their emotions will be too frontal, too direct, and too threatening. This may indeed have been the case with the Ortiz family. Challenging family members so quickly and so directly to transcend their accustomed style of avoiding feelings may simply have frightened them off. An alternative would have been to go much slower, proceeding at a pace that the family could better tolerate. After all, what was the rush?

This discomfort with the direct expression of feelings is one important characteristic of a psychosomatogenic family. There are others that we would like to share with the reader, and for this purpose we return to the writing of Salvador Minuchin, most particularly to his work described in a recent publication, *Psychosomatic Families: Anorexia Nervosa in Context*.[4] Authored by Minuchin and his co-workers at the Philadelphia Child Guidance Clinic, Drs. Bernice Rosman, Lester Baker, and Ron Liebman, this book presents the orientation and approaches of that group to psychosomatic families. A brief summary of their writing follows.

A conceptual model of the psychosomatogenic family

Minuchin and his co-workers have for several years been engaged in a study of patients with one of these three psychosomatic conditions: anorexia nervosa, "brittle" diabetes mellitus, and intractable asthma (the last two judged to be psychosomatic if their symptoms are produced and exacerbated by emotional stress). They have found certain characteristics that are consistent across the families and nonspecific with respect to the type of symptom. Consequently, they have proposed that there is a model for a type of family whose organization predisposes or supports somatic symptoms as an expression of emotional distress; further, they feel that the somatic symptom bearer is not merely the recipient or expresser of emotional stress in the family but, in a dysfunctional kind of way, is a reliever of stress. They developed these findings into a conceptual model of the psychosomatogenic family. According to this conceptual model the development of psychosomatic illness in a child is related to three factors: (1) a characteristic mode of family functioning, (2) involvement of the child in parental conflict, and (3) physiological vulnerability.

A characteristic mode of family functioning. The repetitive transactional pattern of a psychosomatogenic family is characterized by enmeshment, overprotectiveness, rigidity, and lack of conflict resolution. In *enmeshment,* the family members are overinvolved with one another and overresponsive. Interpersonal boundaries are diffuse, with the family members intruding on each other's thoughts, feelings, and communications. Subsystem boundaries are also diffuse, which results in a confusion of roles. An individual's autonomy is severely restricted by the family system. The reader may recall earlier reference to Laura French, a patient with anorexia nervosa, who was asked to construct a family sculpture. The patient put together a small, tight, family circle and inserted herself in the middle; the interviewer then demonstrated that they could not take a step without literally falling over one another. Their enmeshment was readily apparent.

Members of an *overprotective* family have a high degree of concern for each other's welfare. Protective responses are constantly elicited and supplied. When there is a sick child, for example, the entire family becomes involved. Parental conflicts are often submerged in the process. The child in turn feels responsible for protecting the family. This dimension was well illustrated by the Ortiz family. Father's heavy-handedness stemmed from his desire to (over) protect his daughter from her condition. It also seems reasonable that some of Alice's reluctance to open up in the session could well have been her own desire to protect the family (even the father whom she feared) from the "prying" of the interviewers.

Rigidly organized families often present themselves as not needing or wanting any change in the family. Preferred transactional patterns are inflexibly maintained. This is a frustrating characteristic for interviewers to face, since a family is almost always asking for help with a particular child's symptoms while simultaneously communicating, "But do not ask us to change anything." This pattern often accounts in large part for the family's resistance to change. It most certainly was one factor in influencing the Ortiz's nonreturn. Their accustomed transactional patterns were preferred over those suggested by the interviewer. Perhaps for this reason also, a slower pace by the interviewer would have challenged the family's rigidity less directly and encouraged them to return.

Finally, *the lack of conflict resolution* in a family means that it has a low threshold for conflict. Some families handle this by simply denying the existence of any conflict. In other families one spouse is a confronter, but the other is an avoider. Others bicker equally; however, they manage to avoid any real confrontation. Regardless, conflictual issues are not negotiated and resolved. The psychosomatically ill child plays a vital part in his family's avoidance of conflict by presenting a focus for concern, and the family system reinforces his symptomatic behavior to preserve its pattern of conflict avoidance. Difficulties with conflict resolution were prominently displayed in the Ortiz family through Alice's reluctance to speak up to her father in the face of his angry overreaction to her symptomatology.

Involvement of the child in parental conflict. Minuchin and others have felt that the previously described characteristics alone are not enough to explain the etiology and/or maintenance of the child's symptom from a family systems point of view. Therefore they have suggested that the key factor supporting the child's symptom is that youngster's involvement in parental conflict in such a way as to detour, avoid, or suppress the conflict. The symptomatic child may be involved in parental conflict in particular ways. Parents unable to deal with each other directly might unite in protective concern over their sick child. A marital conflict might be transformed into a parental conflict over the patient and his or her management. The child might be recruited into taking sides by the parents or might intrude himself as a mediator or helper. In many families that we have seen with an anorectic child, we have been struck with the family's insistence on a portrayal of the perfect marriage in the perfect family, only to find that once the child's symptom of noneating diminishes, profound marital dysfunction of long standing bubbles up to the surface and announces itself.

Physiological vulnerability. Some type of physical predisposition in a child is a necessary (but not sufficient in itself) component for the appearance of a psychosomatic syndrome. For instance, one does not develop diabetes mellitus without some abnormality in the islets of Langerhans. However, not all individuals with diabetes mellitus develop psychosomatically-induced episodes of acidosis; other features of the psychosomatogenic family must be present for attacks to be so triggered. The same holds true of asthma. A physiological hypersensitivity to specific allergens underlies asthmatic symptoms, even those attacks precipitated or exacerbated by emotional stress.

To conclude our retrospective guesses with the Ortiz family, certainly some interviewing mistakes occurred, as noted in the preceding pages. There may have been others as well. We have partly included our summary of work with this family for that very purpose. We find that "failures" or "situations that just don't work out" with family interviews are frustrating but not rare. Even with clear principles in mind, we sometimes feel like bumblers in our work. Interviewing a family is hard to do; families are very complex. The end is not always satisfying either for the family or for the interviewer. It seems only honest that we allow our failures to appear in print as well as our successes. Such situations are to be expected, by the novice and by the experienced interviewer. Neither category excels in omnipotence.

SCHOOL PHOBIA

In no situation have we encountered psychosomatic symptoms with more regularity than in the group of conditions collectively referred to as "school phobia" or "school avoidance." There are numerous excellent reviews of this syndrome.[2,5,6] It is variously defined as "a partial or total disability to go to school that results from an irrational dread of some aspect of the school situation"[3] or more appropriately as, "poor school attendance, based on unwarranted fear of the school *and/or inappropriate anxiety about leaving home.*"[6]* It is differentiated from truancy in which the child does not usually return home and his parents are not usually aware that he is not in school. On the contrary, in situations of school phobia the parents are usually painfully aware of the child's nonattendance. Rather than reviewing all aspects of the syndrome, we would prefer to summarize the fairly consistent picture that has emerged for us in working with the families of children who are refusing to attend school, ostensibly because of some psychosomatic symptoms, for instance, abdominal pain, headaches, or nausea. We acknowledge that one would do children

*Italics added for emphasis.

a disservice by concluding that all cases of school avoidance are psychological in nature and a reflection of family dysfunction. Surely one would need to ascertain that the problem was not one of peptic ulcer, for instance, or caused by a threatening situation in the classroom or on the playground such as physical violence, a regrettably common phenomenon in today's schools. Having made sure of this, one will still be left with the majority of cases of school avoidance attributable to somatic complaints still unexplained. We would like to discuss our approach to these clinical situations.

The family configuration

Utilizing representative geometric symbols one might construct a diagrammatic configuration as shown for the ordinary situation of a child who freely attends school. Mother and father are shown to enjoy some degree of closeness, relatively closer to one another than either is to the child. The child is placed at a reasonable distance from his parents, between them and his school; both parents and school are fairly accessible to him.

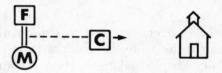

Almost without exception we have detected a different configuration for the family of a child with psychosomatic symptoms who is refusing to attend school. (See diagram on p. 301.) Here father and mother are not close; their distance may be psychological or literal. In either situation they are to a significant degree alienated from one another. It is usually father who has assumed a peripheral position with his family. In addition, the school may often be in a somewhat different place for this configuration. Frequently some factor at school has rendered it a less inviting environment for the child; hence the child sees it as less accessible. There may be peer pressures of some sort, or academic stresses may intervene. The child may be experiencing some conflict with the teaching staff or curriculum. No matter, the end result is that the school is viewed as a more distant and threatening place.

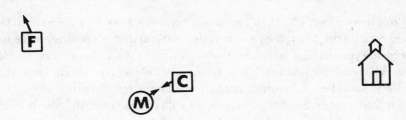

It may take no more forceful precipitant than an upper respiratory infection or a bout of diarrhea to transform the preceding situation into one in which the mother and child become glued together. Each is frightened for his or her own survival should they separate, and each is concerned about the survival of the other should they separate. Mother, unconnected to her husband, is alone. The child, unconnected to his life at school, is alone. They latch on to one another with a vengeance, striving to assuage their own feelings and those of the other simultaneously. At this point the physician is often consulted. Resolution of the crisis requires not only attention to the physical symptom presented, but a return of the family to a configuration at least approaching that in the first diagram on p. 300. Disengagement of the central duo, mother and child, necessitates that one find another connection for each. Ideally for the mother, one needs to help father reenter the family. For the child, one needs to help with a *rapid* return to a school that understands the situation. All of this, of course, requires work with the child, the school, and the *family,* as the following summary indicates.

THE NAKAMURA FAMILY

Fourteen-year-old Nathan Nakamura and his mother were first seen in our general pediatric clinic on November 26. They were both concerned about Nathan's headaches, nasal congestion, skin rash, and "poor" vision. An accompanying note from Nathan's counselor at Franklin Junior High School indicated that the school was also concerned. Nathan had missed 20 days in the last month and a half of school. A new patient workup with appropriate laboratory studies was done by the pediatric resident. She concluded that the patient had mildly decreased visual acuity, a skin rash suggestive of mild psoriasis (this was later confirmed), school phobia, and exogenous obesity. Plans were made for the patient to be seen in the ophthalmology clinic for refraction, and an offer was made to assist in Nathan's steady return to school by a referral to the Child Study Unit for family counseling. Nathan and his mother were not interested, preferring to follow through with getting glasses first to "see what difference this makes." The resident wisely let the family know that the door would remain open for their return if they wished.

On November 28, Mrs. Nakamura called the resident. She had reconsidered and wanted the number to call for an appointment in the Child Study Unit. A pediatrician there said he would be happy to work with Nathan and stressed that he would need to see the entire family for the first visit.

> *Mother:* Well, now, I don't know about that, Doctor. My husband is awfully busy. I thought perhaps that you could see Nathan by himself. Actually with my heart condition I shouldn't be making so many trips myself. I had planned for my sister to bring him in.

The doctor inquired about her heart condition; it did not sound serious enough to prevent her own participation in the visit. So he reiterated that he needed to see the whole family, and that even though Mr. Nakamura was indeed busy, his presence would be essential for the first visit. She agreed to discuss the situation with her husband and to call back the next day regarding confirmation.

Dr. Drew did not hear from her for the next 6 days and attempted to contact her himself. No one answered. The next day, December 5, was their scheduled appointment. They did not call, nor did they show up. He returned the chart to the record room, deciding that he would push no further and that he would probably not hear from the Nakamuras again.

He was wrong.

On January 7, Mrs. Nakamura called, very apologetic. Two days before their scheduled appointment in December, Nathan had voluntarily returned to school, protesting that he would continue regular attendance if his mother would promise that they "did not have to go see that doctor as a family." She agreed. Three days after their missed appointment, Nathan resumed his customary refusal to get up and go to school. Dr. Drew made a new appointment for January 10, again for the whole family.

January 10 arrived; as one might expect, the Nakamura family did not. However, the doctor did receive a call early that morning. Once again Nathan had voluntarily returned to school because of the threat of an impending family interview.

Mother: I just don't know what to do. He promises that he is going to go from now on. And I certainly want to give him every chance to prove himself. I really think he means business this time and that we've got this problem licked. What do you think? Should we cancel today's visit? He seems so willing to follow through now.

Doctor: (with some duplicity) It certainly sounds to me that you've taken care of this problem yourself. That's terrific. Keep up the good work. Why don't we do it this way. I doubt that I am going to need to see you, things are coming along so well. I do have one more opening on January 17 that I will hold open for you, just in case, although it doesn't sound as though you will need to come. I will need you to call me on the 16th to let me know whether you will be using the time or not.

Mother: That would be fine. I certainly want to show Nathan that I have every confidence in him at this point, doing it on his own.

Doctor: Absolutely. Good luck. You can let me know on the 16th. It will probably be the last appointment time that I can hold open for you.

Mother: Thank you so much, Doctor. I will be calling you.

On January 16, Mrs. Nakamura called the Child Study Unit. She didn't even ask to speak to Dr. Drew directly but simply left a message that the family would be coming in the next day.

Finally on January 17, after almost 2 months, the doctor was able to meet Nathan, his mother, and his father. It was an interesting meeting indeed. Mother was perhaps less than 5 feet tall; she alternated her tone between apologizing to the doctor for being 5 minutes late and scowling at Nathan, the cause of their lateness since he had insisted on buying a candy bar on their way to the clinic. As far as the doctor could tell, she did not favor her husband with either of these expressions—in fact she did not look at him. She and Nathan engaged in a mild momentary struggle at the door, Mrs. Nakamura literally pushing Nathan into the office. Nathan, a head taller than she, was easily resisting her efforts and shrugged her hand from his shoulder. Once clear of her, he petulantly entered the office and slammed himself down into a chair, not the one his mother wanted him to occupy. Mr. Nakamura was the last in line. He was very proper, very polite, and very uninvolved in the struggle between his wife and Nathan. He and the doctor shook hands and exchanged pleasantries. His blank smile raised the interviewer's worst fears, and Mrs. Nakamura confirmed them.

Mother: Oh yes, Doctor, this is my husband, Mr. Nakamura. You will have to excuse him. He doesn't speak English, only Japanese.

She must have seen the doctor's face fall, because she hastened to reassure him that *she* would be happy to translate whatever was necessary. Above all the doctor was not interested in Mrs. Nakamura giving his words (and who knows what else) to her husband in a way that Dr. Drew could not possibly check out! Three pediatric residents were joining him that day for the interview. One winked at him, a second covered his mouth with his hand, and the third offered to find a Japanese translator elsewhere in the clinic. The interviewer knew that the individual usually called in such instances was unavailable. He thus said no thanks and decided to try the session on his own.

It was not strictly true that Mr. Nakamura did not speak English. He said "Yes" and "I see" a lot. It is not at all clear whether or not he understood what he was saying. It is quite certain that he did not understand what the doctor was saying. That, coupled with the interviewer's suspicion that Mrs. Nakamura's translations that day were less than literal, particularly fixed the memory of that first interview with the Nakamuras in the doctor's mind. The reader can appreciate that we will not report extended passages of specific dialogue to illustrate the beginning work with these three individuals. Such dialogue would look even more confused on paper than it sounded in actuality. They smiled a great deal, repeated their words often, and checked out messages for understanding over and over. Even so, the residents and Dr. Drew were able to get a somewhat clear understanding of this family's repeating sequence around the issue of school avoidance. These were the events on a typical school morning:

1. Mrs. Nakamura would wake at 6 A.M. and gently rouse Nathan. Nathan kept no alarm clock in his own room.
2. Mrs. Nakamura would then proceed downstairs where she would begin elaborate breakfast preparations. "Nathan likes hot muffins for breakfast." A breakfast bed tray was prepared.
3. At about 6:20 she would release the family dog into Nathan's room. The dog would lick Nathan's face, waking him a second time.

4. By 6:25 both the dog and Nathan would be asleep in bed.

5. Mr. Nakamura, having gotten up at about 6:15, would finish dressing, have a quick breakfast, and be out the door by 7 for his long day at the bank.

6. Nathan would complain that he had a headache and wasn't feeling well.

7. Mrs. Nakamura would feel his forehead and then plead that he try to go to school anyway.

8. They would argue.

9. Mrs. Nakamura would give up and return to the kitchen for her own breakfast, leaving the breakfast tray with Nathan.

10. Nathan and the dog would eat from the breakfast tray in bed.

11. Mrs. Nakamura would notice by about 7:20, after her husband's departure, that the time was getting short. Charging up the stairs, by this time very frustrated that Nathan was not moving, she would begin screaming.

12. Nathan would handle this in a variety of ways. He might lock his bedroom door, or hide under his bed, or, as on one occasion, run past his mother on the stairs, down to the basement, where he secured himself in a closet until 10:30 A.M.

13. Mrs. Nakamura, growing tremendously upset with these maneuvers and with her innumerable trips up and down the stairs, would remember her cardiac condition and finally repair to her bedroom for quinidine and a rest.

14. By midmorning Nathan and his mother would be playing Scrabble, both promising aloud that maybe tomorrow things would go better.

15. Mr. Nakamura would arrive home at 6:30 P.M. to find his wife and son had spent another day home together. By 7:30 he would retire to his desk and a briefcase full of "office work."

By now, of course, the doctors knew that Mr. Nakamura spoke no English. What they did not know until much later was that Nathan spoke very little Japanese. Consequently, mother and father spoke Japanese together and Nathan and his mother conversed in English. Nathan and his father by and large didn't speak together; they couldn't. That didn't stop them from shouting at one another—father in Japanese and Nathan in English. Mother felt that she often had to be the intermediary, that her husband was too demanding to handle Nathan's sensitive nature. Father in turn criticized her perpetual giving-in to the boy and acknowledged that some of his early leave-taking for work was to avoid the predictable, mounting, morning maelstrom.

> *Mother:* What my husband doesn't understand, Doctor, is how helpful Nathan is around the house. Yes, I would rather he were in school also, but he's been such a help to me this past fall. My condition has been acting up, and he's such a good child at helping me with heavy things around the house. My husband is just too busy at work to take care of some of these things at home — I understand that. You'd think he would be grateful for Nathan's help. But . . . what's that? (responding to an interruption from her husband)

The two had a lively, agitated conversation for a few moments. It caused Nathan to shake his head in disgust, at which mother chided him for not showing his father respect. She then turned back to the doctor.

> *Mother:* My husband wanted you to know that one reason he especially wants Nathan in school is that he doesn't want him to be at home where he could be on the street. We don't really like him to be out at all unless one of us is with him. But what my husband doesn't understand is that when Nathan stays home from school, he doesn't leave the house. He and I are home all the time together.

At this point Nathan complained that he never could have any time to himself in the house, that neither parent seemed willing to leave him alone or to trust him.

> *Mother:* Well, Nathan, when you're ready to show us that you're responsible, then we'll believe it, not before.
> *Nathan:* (scowling) See what I mean? They'll never change.
> *Mother:* And what about you, Nathan, what about you?

The reader may feel that this family is beginning to sound familiar, and no wonder. They represent an almost verbatim copy of a family sequence described by Haley and summarized earlier in this text. We refer to Haley's example of a family with a "two-generation problem," one that includes an overintense parent-child dyad that alternately includes and excludes the other parent. Such was the Nakamura family system; they were in a sequence that the family members were repeating over and over. Mother and Nathan were seriously overinvolved; father was drifting in and out of their relationship, but mostly out. In so doing the family was also illustrating the typical configuration that we have come to associate with school phobia, that shown in the diagram below.

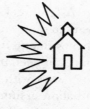

Likewise Minuchin's conceptual model for a psychosomatogenic family was well illustrated. *Enmeshment* was a prominent feature, especially between Mrs. Nakamura and her son. It was further demonstrated by both parents' reluctance to have Nathan away from them on his own. They had few social contacts outside the immediate family and prided themselves on being a "closely-knit family, except for my husband's long working hours, which of course are necessary." With this family the doctor felt the tyrannical implications of the phrase "closely-knit" in a way that he had not before. It also seemed paradoxical but true that this family could visualize themselves as very close, yet without a common language among the three of them. *Overprotection,* particularly that by Mrs. Nakamura toward Nathan, was certainly displayed. Such solicitude was undoubtedly in the reverse direction as well, since Nathan's staying at home enabled him to keep a watchful eye over his mother and her "heart." *Rigidity* was illustrated by the family's repetitive insistence on the same sequence of behavior over and over again. The outline of a typical school morning did not occur just once; it had happened regularly and in the same way for perhaps 30 different school mornings. The family's *difficulty with conflict resolution* was clearly present in all of their behavior with one another. Resolution simply did not occur; a lack of resolution met some need.

The family's sequence, structure, system, and configuration thus seemed clear. The question was how to proceed and help them alter their pattern. The doctor felt that he would have to include the school in any treatment considerations and told the family this. Both parents were delighted that he was willing to contact Franklin Junior High School; however, Nathan resented his intrusion and told him so, declaring that he wouldn't go back, no matter what. They ended the session by making a return appointment for 7 days hence; by that time the doctor would have had time to consult with the school and make some plans for continuing work with the family.

A few weeks prior to seeing the Nakamura family, Dr. Drew had worked quite successfully with a suburban high school in helping one of their students with school phobia return to full-time attendance. The staff had been informed and effective in their efforts to support the doctor's work with that child and her family. He naturally approached this situation assuming that the school would be easily incorporated into therapeutic efforts. He had not reckoned with the likes of an urban, overcrowded, understaffed public junior high school. Just finding the appropriate counselor required four phone calls. He eventually located him, explained the situation, and asked for the counselor's assistance. Protesting his pressed schedule, the man nonetheless agreed. Dr. Drew told him that he anticipated difficulty, that a simple insistence on Nathan's return would not be successful. In his work with the family he would be supporting the family's efforts to get Nathan out the door. In the event of his refusal, would Mr. Davis, the counselor, be willing to arrange for someone from the school to drive to the Nakamuras' home and personally take Nathan to school? Mr. Davis indicated that such a move would be decidedly unusual. However the doctor prevailed, and Mr. Davis himself agreed to use his own car if necessary to drop by Nathan's home and pick him up. Dr. Drew was very grateful and closed by telling him that he was in the process of drawing up a written task sheet for the family. Each family member would be given a copy. Mr. Davis would be sent one as well.

Preparing for the family's next visit then, and feeling that he had enlisted the aid of the school, Dr. Drew made up several copies of the following for distribution to the family, the residents, and Mr. Davis:

Family task: (To begin January 25)
1. Nathan is to return full-time to school immediately.
2. For now, Mrs. Nakamura is to wake Nathan at 6 A.M. by saying:
    "You must get up *now* for school."
    "I expect you to get up and go to school."
    "I have confidence in your ability to get yourself there."
    There is to be no further discussion by Mrs. Nakamura:

No punishments ⎤
No recriminations ⎬ This is to be enforced by
No promises ⎟ Mr. Nakamura
No threats ⎦

3. If Nathan should choose not to attend school, Mrs. Nakamura is to notify:
   a. Dr. Drew
   b. Mr. Davis, who has for now kindly agreed to come to the house and take Nathan to school if necessary.

The task had been designed with several ingredients. First of all, the interviewer wished to communicate to everyone that an *immediate* return to school was expected. He also wanted everyone to be involved in the process and hence designed a task with something for each family member to do: Nathan was to get to school, mother was to wake him, and father was to monitor mother's approaches. He did not really expect that mother would say the precise lines listed. Nonetheless, he wanted to focus on her approach to Nathan and stress that she should not allow herself to be drawn into extended dialogues with him as she had been doing for months. Since the doctor expected that the return process would be stormy and that the task would be sabotaged in some way, he hoped that writing it down would enable him to see at what point and with whom things were not working. He could then address that issue in subsequent family sessions.

On January 24 the family and the doctors met again. The task was presented to them and discussed. To make sure that all understood, the residents and Dr. Drew encouraged the family to role-play a situation in which they carried the task to completion. Surprisingly they complied, and each individual demonstrated that he or she had an understanding of what was being asked. Nathan was as usual sullen and noncooperative; Mr. Nakamura expressed surprise and delight that the solution could be so simple. Mrs. Nakamura kept reiterating, "We'll do whatever you say, Doctor." Events certainly seemed to be proceeding evenly. Regrettably, Dr. Drew did not suggest (paradoxically) that they would fail with the task.

The next morning, the first for implementation of the task, Mrs. Nakamura called. Nathan had not yet gotten out of bed; it was 8:30. The doctor asked for a brief report of what had happened prior to the call. Her husband had not stayed around to supervise her approaches to Nathan. He had gone off to work as usual. She and Nathan had screamed at one another.

Mother: What do I do now, Doctor?
Doctor: Do you have your task sheet available?
Mother: Wait . . . yes, oh, I see; I call Mr. Davis.
Doctor: Right. You know what to do next, Mrs. Nakamura. Thanks for letting me know.

After hanging up, the pediatrician felt vaguely uncomfortable at not knowing what might happen next. He decided to call Mr. Davis to make sure that he was alerted.

School: Mr. Davis? No, I'm sorry; he's not in. He's sick today.

The house of cards that the doctor had so carefully constructed was beginning to crumble. Neither Mr. nor Mrs. Nakamura could be counted on, nor could Mr. Davis, it appeared. Dr. Drew asked to talk with one of Mr. Davis's co-workers or anyone who might be able to help him. After five more phone calls, he was connected to Mr. Davis's supervisor. He explained the situation.

Supervisor: Look, I don't know what this is all about. But Mr. Davis was way out of line when he agreed to come out to the child's home. We don't have enough personnel for that sort of thing. It's against school policy. No, we couldn't possibly send someone else out. You're the doctor—why don't you go over to his house? That would probably have much more meaning anyhow. Do you know how many kids we're responsible for?

Feeling defeated and confused, Dr. Drew decided to do nothing for the moment other than call Mrs. Nakamura. She hastened to tell him that Mr. Davis was ill, and no one else at school seemed to know what to do. He thanked her for the "news" and suggested that the task be shelved until Mr. Davis returned to work.

By the next day the supervisor had apparently reconsidered, because that afternoon Mrs. Nakamura reported that, Mr. Davis still being ill, the school had sent out a graduate student in counseling who was doing her field placement at the school. She had pleaded with Nathan through the locked bathroom door to come out, that she wanted to take him to school. He didn't budge. She positioned herself in front of the bathroom door and stayed there for an hour doing needlepoint, finally leaving when she ran out of yarn and when it became obvious to her that Nathan would not emerge.

On January 29 the family arrived for their scheduled family interview. However, Mr. Nakamura was not with them.

Mother: He just can't keep taking time off from work, Doctor. He won't be able to come anymore until after tax time is over in April.

By now all semblance of the doctor's being in charge of the situation had disappeared. He declared that the task should be scrapped(!), and he and the residents spent the hour working with mother and Nathan on the bitter feelings they were exhibiting toward one another. Dr. Drew was wondering if he could continue with the family without the father's participation, even in Japanese. At the close of the session, however, he did agree to see the two of them again.

They were scheduled to return on February 5. That afternoon, an hour before their appointment, Mrs. Nakamura called. She was frantic, and Nathan was screaming in the background.

Mother: Doctor, I just can't get Nathan to come in for our appointment today. He just refuses. Couldn't we consider putting him in the hospital, please? I'm not sure how much more of this I can stand.

Nathan: (He howls in the background and swears at his mother. He is so loud that the doctor cannot hear her words.)

Doctor: Mrs. Nakamura, I . . .

Mother: What's that, Doctor? I can't hear you; Nathan is so upset. A psychiatric hospital, maybe?

Doctor: (surprising himself that he is getting angry and raising his voice) I will not talk to you under these conditions. Get him quiet. I cannot even hear you.

Mother: What?

Doctor: Unless I can hear you, I am going to hang up.

At this point Mrs. Nakamura left the phone. The doctor heard angry, raised voices in the background; mother was the louder, and then Nathan was quiet. Mother returned to the phone. The doctor congratulated her on her obvious ability in doing what was necessary. She then asked if she could come alone; Nathan just wouldn't agree to continuing sessions.

Doctor: I couldn't possibly do that, Mrs. Nakamura. I am unwilling to work with the family unless you both come.

Mother: Well, how do I get him there, Doctor?

Doctor: That will be up to you. However, in order for me to continue work-

ing with the family, you must both be here. I can see you next on
February 7 at 4. I will expect you at that time.

On February 7, mother and son arrived, the son smiling for the first
time in the doctor's presence. Mother had obviously been successful in
demanding his presence at the session. He had not yet returned to
school. During the course of the interview this rather remarkable interchange took place:

Mother: Nathan, I don't know why I have to keep picking up your room.
You should be able to do that. I've told you over and over again
that your room is your responsibility and that I'm not going to pick
up after you again.

Nathan: Yeah, well, you don't mean it. We both know that. You give in too
easily on everything.

Mother: I just can't stand it looking like a pigsty.

Doctor: Hold it, everyone. Nathan, say that again.

Nathan: What?

Doctor: What you just told your mother.

Nathan: Well, it's true. You give in too easily . . . on everything.

Mother: If that isn't gratitude . . .

Doctor: (interrupting) Nathan, is there a part of you that would like your
mother to say "no" more often?

Nathan: (after a long period of thought) Yes.

Doctor: Tell her that, now.

Nathan: (pause) Mom, I would like you to say "no" more often to me.

Doctor: Say it again.

Nathan: Mom, I *would* like you to say no more often to me.

Doctor: Mrs. Nakamura, were you aware that he felt this way?

Mother: I'm floored. I don't believe it.

Doctor: Are you serious, Nathan?

Nathan: Yes, I am.

Doctor: Then you're going to have to convince your mother. She doesn't
believe you.

Nathan then proceeded to tell his mother that he was uncomfortable
with her giving in on all sorts of issues, that she didn't stand up for herself at all with him, that it was almost like there weren't any rules in the
house, and that somehow that wasn't right. The doctors exchanged
glances. Even with all the turmoil and previous fiascoes with this family,
they were approaching substantive issues between this mother and her
son. Mother heard his request that she set stronger limits and acknowl-

edged that such a shift would be very difficult for her for two specific reasons. First, Nathan was her only child, her pride and joy; saying no to him had always been difficult. Second, she had spent her early years, during World War II, in one of the Japanese relocation camps; she remembered it as a bitter and difficult experience. Her father had died within a year of internment; financially the family had had great difficulty. She resolved that no child of hers would ever suffer or want as she had; her child would have everything asked for and then some. And with time this resolve came to be construed as a determination to avoid the word "no" with Nathan. She glimpsed through her son's words that day the price both she and he had paid for that resolution.

As the hour concluded, both expressed for the first time a genuine willingness to continue in future sessions. Mrs. Nakamura slso shared a letter she had received from school. It was an order for Nathan and his family to appear in court the next day for a truancy hearing. The school had thus decided on some independent action. Dr. Drew asked the family to keep him posted.

At the next session he learned that much indeed had transpired. Nathan and his parents had reported to juvenile hall for the hearing. It had actually been a preliminary event, during which the parents, the child, the school counselor, and the authorities met to discuss future plans. Nathan was shown the room he would occupy in juvenile hall if he was declared truant. This declaration was to be made if he missed one more day of school. Official court procedures were explained to the family. The counselor then offered to drop Nathan off at school for the remainder of the day. He meekly complied.

The next morning Nathan balked. But there was a different sequence this day in the Nakamura household. Father arose first and told both his wife and his son that he would *not* leave the house until Nathan was headed for school. In fact Mr. Nakamura was going to drive him there himself. When Nathan challenged his father's new stance, he was cuffed for his protests. Whereupon he got himself up, dressed, fed, and out the door into his father's waiting car.

There were no more school absences. (In fact in a few months' time, when a city teachers' strike caused pupil attendance in San Francisco to drop to less than half normal, Nathan didn't miss a day. He was later given an award for being one of the few pupils who had not been absent during the strike.)

What had happened to effect such a dramatic and lasting change?

Certainly the fact that mother was beginning to show some strength (for example, getting Nathan to the doctor's office), coupled with Nathan's request for more limits and mother's insight into her own behavior had been hopeful signs just before all of these events took place. However they could hardly account for such a reversal, especially in father's behavior. It would seem that father's different approach was a very significant factor in producing change in the family's accustomed pattern. The physicians had hoped for his active involvement in Nathan's return to school in the beginning family work with the Nakamuras. However, it looked as though the school had succeeded where the doctor had failed. They had certainly stimulated him into a more active and responsible parenting role by setting up a choice with consequences, one of which was juvenile hall. When that was accomplished, whether through pediatricians or through the school, Nathan returned to classes. As to what it was in the school's approach that successfully moved father, one can only guess. Probably the family's very private business was becoming uncomfortably public for the father when the courts were called in and his Japanese heritage would not allow such a humiliation, at which point he very capably took over the reins of his family and brought the situation under control.

Whether this actually explains his change and decision to act one cannot know for sure. In any case the family system changed sufficiently that a return to school was possible. Everyone in the family, including Nathan, expressed relief that their dilemma had resolved itself, at least in terms of school avoidance. Both mother and son asked to continue family counseling to pursue changing aspects of their relationship. Mr. Nakamura kept himself unavailable for future sessions. Since it seemed unlikely that mother and father would make any significant changes in their marital relationship, the doctors focused on helping mother establish a wider circle of social relationships in her community so that she could tolerate letting go of Nathan, allowing him to pursue his own growth, without herself feeling stranded and isolated. They encouraged her to get a part-time job, which she did and enjoyed. Nathan became interested in some after-school activities and began to spend less and less time at home. This was acceptable to mother and father because they felt that he was in some sort of supervised program and not just "out on the streets."

The crisis period with this family covered 3 months, beginning with their first visit to the pediatric clinic in late November for a medical evaluation and ending with Nathan's steady return to school in early February. During that period, a total of five family interviews took place, two with the entire family and three with mother and son. Subsequent work with the family after the crisis resolved continued for another 3 months, with mother and son being seen weekly for family sessions. The principal issue dealt with was their ability to tolerate separation from one another. Both felt comfortable enough with their situation to terminate family sessions in May, before the end of the school year. Subsequent follow-up with the family has extended over 3 years. There have been no recurrences. Mrs. Nakamura now works full-time. Nathan is planning to go to college. Mr. Nakamura is still very busy at the bank.

CONCLUSION

In psychosomatic conditions, just as mentioned in the chapter on common behavioral problems, it is less the specific complaint that matters than the family system. That is what the interviewer needs to elucidate and alter. Children with psychosomatic complaints are very common in pediatric practice. Youngsters with recurrent abdominal pain, chronic headaches, enuresis, ulcerative colitis, tics, encopresis, and anorexia nervosa are but a few of these patients. In our practice a successful outcome with these children had depended on an alteration of the family's system, communication pattern, structure, and repetitive sequence of behavior. Our previously stated maxim has still obtained: figure out the family system, its meaning and purpose, and one will usually figure out the problem and very often its resolution.

REFERENCES

1. Breur, J., and Freud, S.: Studies in hysteria. Translated from the German and edited by J. Strachey, New York, 1957, Basic Books, Inc., Publishers.
2. Eisenberg, L.: School phobia: a study in the communication of anxiety, Am. J. Psychiatry **114:**712, 1958.
3. Johnson, A., and others: School phobia, Am. J. Orthopsychiatry **11:**702, 1941.
4. Minuchin, S., and others: Psychosomatic families: anorexia nervosa in context, Cambridge, Mass., 1978, Harvard University Press.
5. Nader, P., and others: School phobia, Pediatr. Clin. North Am. **22:**605, 1975.
6. Schmitt, B.: School phobia—the great imitator—a pediatrician's viewpoint, Pediatrics **48:**433, 1971.

CHAPTER 12

Developmental disorders

The term "developmental disorder" is considered by some a euphemism for mental retardation. We believe that the term has a broader base and can include various disorders of physical and/or mental and/or psychological development. Strictly speaking then, one might include under the term those disease entities associated with obvious deviations in physical development of the body, such as short stature, precocious puberty, rickets, and various types of congenital anomalies. One might also include entities associated with deviations in central nervous system development and function, such as delayed language development, specific learning disabilities, clumsy child syndrome, mental retardation, deafness, blindness, Down's syndrome, and meningomyelocele. Finally one might include under developmental disorders those conditions associated with combined deviations in psychological and central nervous system development, such as infantile autism and childhood schizophrenia.

Many of these developmental disorders are, or can become, chronic conditions, and chronic conditions have already been described (Chapter 8). Much of what was described in that section is also applicable in clinical work with the families of children with developmental difficulties. However, we have chosen a separate section for our discussion of developmental disorders to illustrate in detail the use of family work in two common clinical situations often associated with developmental conditions: (1) disorders of central nervous system development and (2) disorders with genetic implications.

DISORDERS OF CENTRAL NERVOUS SYSTEM DEVELOPMENT

Alex Tura's father was on the phone: "Educationally handicapped, Doctor, that's what the teacher said, educationally handicapped! Now I don't know exactly what that means, but I do know what she means when she says that maybe Alex should go to a special school. The nerve of that woman — and to deliver that sort of news over the telephone. No conference, no nothing. We just don't know what to do. This is Alex's second year in first grade, and he hasn't been doing too well . . . but they certainly haven't suggested up until now that he didn't belong in the school. She said something about a lot of tests being given, that Alex did very poorly on some sort of "frosting" test — so badly on it, and I guess there were some others as well, that they felt they might not be able to have him stay there. Well, we won't allow that decision to be made just because of one or two tests and by one teacher. We want Alex to have a complete evaluation somewhere else. This is all just nonsense. What is a "frosting" test, do you know? Maybe my wife and I should meet with the principal. What do you think?"

While Mr. Tura is a stranger to the reader, his situation and his desperation will both be familiar to most pediatric clinicians. Parents are frequently being told these days that their child is not "learning as he should," and they can become understandably frantic upon hearing this news. Such parents often turn to the child's doctor for further direction. Since we consider learning handicaps to be, very often, developmental disabilities that pose a tremendous threat to the ongoing health of a child and the child's family, we feel that the pediatric clinician is a logical resource for parents in such a predicament. The pediatrician must, however, be an informed resource, one who understands the reasons for learning difficulty in children, one who is knowledgeable about the community resources available for treatment, and one who is able to work with an interdisciplinary diagnostic evaluation team, utilizing the expertise of professionals outside the field of pediatric medicine.

We have in previous publications[1,2] summarized our work in this area and the evaluation process that we recommend for a child referred with the chief complaint of "school learning difficulty." In addition to close collaboration with the staff of the child's school, complete pediatric history and physical examination, neurologic evaluation, psychological evaluation, hearing, speech, and language assessment, and educational evaluation, we also recommend and routinely include a diagnostic family interview at some point in the assessment process. Lagging academic progress in school is not just a problem for the child experiencing the difficulty but often a family calamity as well. A family interview can be a useful device for evaluating firsthand the impact of a child's school failure on the family. It will also enable the examiner to assess the impact of the family's behavior on the child and his continuing learning difficulty. The gathering of such data allows for the formulation of a comprehensible diagnostic picture regarding the components of a particular youngster's learning difficulties, and it facilitates the formulation of a treatment plan, which often needs to be medical *and* educational *and* psychological in nature. It was thus with the Tura family. Information provided through one diagnostic family interview helped supply many missing pieces necessary to complete the puzzle in order to develop plans for appropriate management of Alex, age 8, and his learning difficulties.

The Tura family

In his initial phone call Mr. Tura had requested a complete evaluation. The pediatrician considered that an appropriate request. First material was gathered from Alex's school, then he had a history and physical examination. Neurological, psychological, and educational evaluations were performed. These studies showed clearly that Alex was a boy of above average intelligence with a specific learning disability of neurodevelopmental origin. His particular difficulties were clustered in the area of visual perception. Spatial relationships and visual sequencing were especially confusing for him. Fine-motor coordination, particularly with paper and pencil work, was another area of educational liability. His previous poor showing on the "frosting" test at school—the Frostig Test of Visual Perception—was certainly borne out by his performance on other measures of visual-motor skill. Alex's specific learning disabilities were fairly limited to this area. In language and auditory skills he was doing nicely, and he was in good shape intellectually. He would certainly require special educational assistance, but he was a youngster who could remain in a public school environment, and with judicious educational remediation he would be expected to do well.

This information, while known by the pediatrician, had not yet been shared with Alex or his family. It would be, of course. However, there was still one diagnostic assessment to be completed before that sharing, an interview with Alex, his parents, and an older brother, Rudy, age 10.

The session began in a somewhat unorthodox manner. As the pediatrician stood greeting the family at his office door, Mr. Tura turned to his family and said:

Father: Now I would like all of you to have a seat and wait for just a few minutes. I have some things I want to discuss with the doctor privately before we all meet together.

Mother: Of course, dear . . .

Doctor: Well, we, that is, I . . .

Father: Go on. It will be just a few minutes.

Without hesitation, everyone in the family meekly turned and headed for available chairs in the waiting room. Mr. Tura maneuvered himself and the pediatrician into the office and pulled the door closed. The pediatrician found time to wonder what in the world was going on, and that was about all. Too bad, because Mr. Tura continued by saying:

Father: I thought there were some things that I ought to tell you ahead of time. We don't need to discuss them with the rest of the family — it would just upset them, but it will help round out the picture for you.

In so short a time the interviewer had already stumbled into strategic trouble — trouble, that is, if he hoped to maintain control of the family interview situation and allow each person to express him/herself openly and honestly. He had just had his interview participant(s) chosen for him, and he was about to have the discussion topics in the family interview assigned, reviewed, and categorized — those discussable and those not to be shared. Furthermore, he was being drawn, whether he liked it or not, into an alliance with one family member, a risky position. For in simply hearing Mr. Tura's remarks, whether or not he agreed to honor father's request for confidentiality, the pediatrician was seriously jeopardizing his relationship with the other family members in the waiting area, who were excluded from the "private" conversation. They were certainly outside wondering: "What are those two talking about . . . and what are we being left out of . . . what are they saying about us . . . why can't we hear whatever it is . . . what will the doctor know now that we don't know . . . how can we possibly feel comfortable in the interview yet to come . . . and who's really in charge around here — the doctor or my father (husband)?"

It is not unusual in the course of family interviewing work for an interviewer to be asked "for a few words alone with you, Doctor, before the rest of the family comes in." The individual requesting private time may have none of Mr. Tura's audacity, but a tactful, polite request can be equally dangerous for the same reasons. Private conversations with the interviewer can alienate other family members, seriously hamper the interviewer's ultimate control over the interview process, and make him privy to secrets that place him in an untenable position with other family members. Such secrets are often attempts on the individual's part to prejudice the interviewer, confirm that one family member is "the patient," limit discussion (for instance, "Please don't bring up the subject of my husband's drinking; it's just too uncomfortable a topic for him to handle right now . . . and not in front of the children."), or otherwise control the interview itself. By and large such private conversations when requested by individual family members serve mainly to decrease the doctor's effectiveness and diminish his freedom in conducting a diagnostic session.

Such a situation is a dilemma for the interviewer. Often the individual requesting time alone with the doctor suggests by his manner that the request is for disclosure of important information—and it often is. The interviewer's curiosity is aroused. To deny the request is also to invite the alienation of this very important person, usually the most controlling member of the family.

There are a number of ways to extricate oneself from this compromising position. First one can use the request to initiate discussion in the family interview itself. In the case previously mentioned, this would require split-second reflexes on the interviewer's part:

> *Father:* Now I would like all of you to have a seat and wait for just a few minutes. I have some things I want to discuss with the doctor privately before we all meet together.
>
> *Doctor:* Mr. Tura. It is important for me to meet first with the whole family. Come on in to my office—everyone—and perhaps you and the family can discuss the purpose of your meeting alone with me further. They look very surprised by what you just said. So perhaps some further understanding and agreement among the four of you is important before a decision is made. I'll just listen.

Or one can simply refuse the request, no explanations given:

> *Doctor:* Mr. Tura, I prefer that we all meet together, initially at any rate.

Or one may refuse by disclosing one's dilemma:

> *Doctor:* That puts me in a bind, Mr. Tura. I am, of course, interested in what you have to tell me. Yet I worry that I will then be placed in a

compromising position somehow with the rest of your family. That being the case, I prefer not to meet with you alone.

Obviously none of these strategies were used by Turas' pediatrician. Once he and Mr. Tura were alone in the office, he chose instead to say:

Doctor: Before you begin, Mr. Tura, let me set some ground rules. I am most willing to hear what you have to say. I am unwilling to share secrets with you that I then cannot openly discuss with the rest of the family should I feel it essential to do so. Therefore whatever we talk about, I reserve the final say as to whether it gets discussed with the rest of the family. I feel you need to know that *before* you tell me anything. Do you understand?

Father: Well, of course, Doctor.

Doctor: That may mean that there are things you had planned to tell me that now you will not want to share. And those things then you will have to keep to yourself. That is your decision.

In this way the doctor left an out for himself and was not boxed into hearing confidences that he must subsequently pretend he had not learned. It was a perfectly appropriate strategy, with one tactical error: he delivered this message only to Mr. Tura; the rest of the family waiting outside did not hear that secret disclosures would be off limits. Consequently their anxiety remained unassuaged. Mr. Tura continued:

Father: I don't quite know the purpose of this — what do you call it? — family conference that we are going to have. But I thought you ought to know that both my wife and Rudy, my older boy, are under a great deal of stress. Perhaps Florence explained the other day, I don't know, did she? No? Well, she has been having some serious physical problems for some time — kidney problems with two major surgeries in the past 5 years and terrible complications with each one. She just isn't strong, and her nerves can't take too much. Now she and I don't always see eye-to-eye on this school problem with Alex. Since her own problems began she's just become so . . . isolated and withdrawn . . . I can't really convince her of the seriousness of his problem. Now all of this has, of course, been getting to me, too, and I have just begun therapy with a psychiatrist — I felt that you should know that. My wife, who probably needs therapy more than any of us, won't have anything to do with it; I have asked her and asked her, but no. Rudy, of course, is a terribly sensitive child. He knows instantly when things are tense around the house, and they are tense most of the time right now. I don't think he can tolerate too much more . . . he gets so upset himself. Doesn't let on to anyone, but I can tell. I can always tell. He begins to look very worried, and he develops these stomachaches and diarrhea. My wife doesn't realize how sensitive he is. I'm sure she doesn't realize what pressure she's putting on him, but . . .

Of course, father was controlling, utilizing all of the tactics previously predicted: striving to establish an alliance with the doctor, suggesting that he, Mr. Tura, was the healthy, responsible, open parent, and portraying his wife as a patient, ominously near some sort of breaking point but stubbornly refusing professional help. He was also suggesting that the doctor stay away from stressful topics in the interview or risk having "two mental cases" come to full flower before his eyes. Belatedly the pediatrician came to his senses and said:

Doctor: Mr. Tura, I can appreciate your concerns as both husband and parent. It is clear that you want the best for both your wife and your children. What you are telling me is very important. I would, however, prefer that it be discussed with the whole family present. I am uncomfortable at our talking in here and at their sitting, worrying and wondering, out there. I am going to have them join us.

Father: Of course, Doctor. We are very open as a family—I told my wife that I was going to have this little chat with you ahead of time; she was in perfect agreement. We can and do discuss everything together.

Doctor: (the contradiction of father's last statement is not lost on him) Good.

The pediatrician then asked the rest of the family into his office, greeting each individual as he/she entered. Their seating arrangement was striking. Mother sat alone, as did Alex. Father and Rudy were in a cluster with Mr. Tura ever solicitous of his older son—arranging his chair, taking his coat, passing him a Kleenex for his runny nose, asking him if his stomach was feeling better, and so forth. Father seemed to have his eyes on everyone, continually taking the measure of his family and how they were doing moment by moment. Of all of them, however, Rudy received the most watching.

Noting this to himself, the interviewer explained aloud, in an effort to recoup with those who had been kept waiting, that he preferred that any discussions should involve the whole family without secrets. Consequently, he had stopped Mr. Tura in his sharing of concerns, feeling that those could appropriately be discussed openly in the family and that other family members had a right to hear about Dad's worries. They were obviously a family that cared about one another and would want to be aware of one another's concerns. The doctor then backed up to introduce the session itself.

Doctor: Before getting to those issues, let me explain what this family session is all about. As part of Alex's evaluation for his learning difficulties, I want to meet at least once with the whole family. Generally in families, particularly in close families such as yours, when something is going on with one family member, all the others are affected by that in some way, perhaps differently for each one. I would like to know some more about that from each of you. How you each get messages across to one another is something else I would like to know more about . . . all different kinds of messages, particularly those having to do with feelings — feelings of happiness, pleasure, sadness, worry, pain, and so forth. Not that there's a right way or a wrong way to handle those messages, rather there are different ways. And I would like to learn more about your ways in this family.

Father: We share our feelings openly with one another, have always felt that was extremely important. Isn't that right, Florence?

Mother: Yes.

Doctor: That's terrific. Let me start this way. Rudy, I'm sitting closest to you, I'll ask you first: How can you tell if your father, for instance, has had a good or bad day at work?

Father: Come on, Rudy, you know the answer to that one, I . . .

Doctor: Just a minute, Mr. Tura. Let Rudy answer this one.

Rudy: Well, with my Daddy . . . well, if he's had a bad day, you sure don't have to guess.

Alex: Yeah, right. Right.

Doctor: What do you mean?

Rudy: He yells. (Both boys agree.)

Father: Now let's be fair, boys.

Rudy: You do, ask mom.

Father: Well now, mother's not feeling well. We mustn't aggravate her right now. Are you sure you're all right, Florence?

Mother: It's nothing, Sam. I'll be all right in a while . . . sometimes, I do have to admit, your voice does get a bit loud. But you boys usually deserve it at those times, I might add. Your father works very hard. The last thing he needs to hear when he comes in the door at 5 is the two of you fighting. It's the last thing any of us needs to hear. I certainly don't, particularly on those days when I'm not even well enough to be up and around. Now Rudy's pretty good about that, but Alex, now . . .

Alex: Geez, what do I do?

Mother: I don't know what it is, but somehow all I have to do is be in bed with my "condition" and you seem to pick a fight with Rudy, Alex. It never fails.

The pediatrician had hoped to make the rounds of every family member, asking how each individual was able to determine the moods and feelings of others. In this family, beginning with just a single question to one member, they were off and running, providing a direct glimpse into many features of their family communication system and structure. Father's need to control, abundantly illustrated in his private preamble to the interview, continued to be displayed by his attempt to take over and answer the doctor's question to Rudy. The boys were able to join with each other in an alliance, at least in their common view of Dad's yelling. However, Mother walked a perilous line alone, striving to agree with her boys and at the same time defend her husband. The end result of the entire interchange was that blame gradually came to rest on Alex as a provocateur, insensitive to his mother's condition and his father's life of hard work. Tentative family roles were thus beginning to emerge: father, the long-suffering controller who was not to be criticized; mother, the sick intermediary, doing a balancing act between children and husband; Alex, the troublemaker; and Rudy, the sensitive, good child.

A decision for interviewers at this point in such an interview is whether to hold to some structure as originally planned or to allow the session to develop its own structure, now strikingly influenced by the family's communication pattern and style. The interviewer choosing to utilize structure might stay with Rudy for a time, exploring (if and) how he could tell when his mother has had a good or bad day; this could be followed by similar comments from Rudy regarding his brother, Alex. The interviewer might then ask Alex to disclose his method for sensing and responding to the feelings and mood of each other family member, and finally the parents could be asked the same questions. To those interviewers for whom the term "good and bad day" seems too bland, one might instead ask each family member to describe more specifically how one can tell when one's wife (husband, child) is upset, worried, sad, angry, or happy. In so doing one would begin to characterize the family's repertoire for expression of feelings and also learn something of the impact of this repertoire on individual family members.

Adhering in this way to a structured set of questions, ensuring that all questions are put to every family member, guarantees that no one will feel slighted, and all family members will be given an opportunity to speak their piece. It also provides a certain amount of order and organization to the proceedings. A disadvantage in pursuing such a course is that rigidity may take over, so that the interview becomes stultifying and an exercise in "talking about" rather than "experiencing." Each interviewer must balance these aspects, arriving at an interview style that is comfortable for him and still gets the job done.

The Tura's pediatrician chose to allow the interview to develop its own form, abandoning (at least for the time being) his neat list of questions and order, since he felt that questions or no, the family was now clearly demonstrating its family system and methods of communicating feelings. Seeing that Alex was in the process of being scapegoated into a "problem," he turned to him:

Doctor: What are you feeling right now, Alex?
Alex: (looking sad) I dunno. I always get blamed. Always.
Father: For some reason, Doctor, most of the time Florence and Alex just don't hit it off anymore. I don't know what it is. Well, I do know — they're so much alike. That's why. Stubborn as mules. If they would just listen to one another more. It really is terribly upsetting, especially for Rudy. He's so sensitive. I can tell right now, for instance, that he's getting uncomfortable with this whole topic. Isn't that right, Rudy? I can tell.
Rudy: Well . . .
Mother: Just let him be, Sam.
Father: Let him be? . . . For what, to develop an ulcer? I don't think you ever understand, Florence, how much this boy takes in and how it affects him. Do you have a bathroom, Doctor?
Doctor: (somewhat taken aback, points to the proper door)
Father: There now, see, Rudy, don't worry. The bathroom is right there when you need it. Just relax. Here, let me rub your stomach, son. That helps.

There was no question that Rudy was being groomed for the role as an invalid, vulnerable child. Father now sat rubbing his son's abdomen.

Father: Your mother and brother just forget sometimes, Rudy. That's all. They don't mean anything by it, I'm sure.

What no one seemed to recognize was that, actually, mother and Alex had done nothing to upset or antagonize Rudy. They had not even spoken to one another or to Rudy during this interchange. Father had simply chided them for not getting along in general. The actual sequence had become lost, somehow, for both doctor and family members. In fact, mother, now intimidated by father's blaming, joined the solicitous ministrations to her older son.

> *Mother:* Here, son, come over here with mother. I didn't mean to upset you. I'm just thoughtless sometimes. I'm not feeling well today either.

Rudy pushed his chair over closer to his mother; she gave him a quick hug. Alex sat by himself looking forlorn and penitent. He received no invitations for caring and attention. Responding to this observation of Alex's isolation, the pediatrician determined to shift the interview in a direction that might more directly approach the important issue of positive validation of the children by their parents.

> *Doctor:* Mr. and Mrs. Tura, I now have a question for each of you. I would like you each to think of some ways in which Alex makes you feel proud. You first, Mr. Tura.
> *Father:* (after a long, painful silence, noticed by everyone) Well, when you do your chores . . . of course, I wish you would do them more often without my having to remind you.

Father's validation was largely obscured by his simultaneous complaint regarding the boy's failure to follow through. The pediatrician attempted once more:

> *Doctor:* I see. Think of something else, some aspect of Alex about which you feel proud and regarding which you don't need to add a negative comment.
> *Father:* Let's see . . .
> *Mother:* (unable to tolerate the embarrassing pause) Alex is very good at taking care of Sparky. That's his dog, and we never have to worry on that score. Alex does a beautiful job there.
> *Father:* That's right. He and Rudy both take care of their animals without any hassle.
> *Mother:* Sometimes, with Alex, it's almost too much with that dog! Sparky comes first and that's all there is to it. The rest of us just have to wait if Sparky needs something. I notice that especially when I'm sick in bed and need him . . . he spends so much time with that dog. He doesn't seem to realize how much I'm depending on him these days.

Now it was mother's turn to discredit her own recognition of Alex's responsible behavior. It was abundantly clear that validation of Alex's emerging capabilities and worth was simply not done easily or clearly by either parent. Far from being a comfortable and accepted skill that they employed, positive acknowledgement of their younger son was generally accompanied by a disqualification or retraction. However, the parents often validated Rudy, although in an injurious manner. Too often it was validation of Rudy's vulnerability, sensitivity, and physical symptoms. Such validation was equally as crippling as *no* validation, training Rudy to become an invalid.

Returning to Alex, if he was not receiving support for his behavior at home, what about school? Well, he certainly couldn't be gaining much validation in that environment since persistent school learning difficulties had prompted his referral in the first place. This unhappy situation was further illustrated when the interviewer turned to Alex and asked him to mention a few aspects of himself about which he knew his parents were proud. Alex fumbled with a few words, became silent, and ultimately said, looking at his father with a weary expression:

Alex: There's nothing that I do that pleases them. Nothing.

The pediatrician noted that both parents looked chagrined and uncomfortable.

Doctor: (to Mr. and Mrs. Tura) What are you experiencing right now?
Father: Well . . . er . . . I'm just realizing that Alex is right. I feel terrible. I never thought about it before . . . and yet . . . thinking about it now, I suppose that actually there is not one area of Alex's life in which he feels successful.
Mother: He certainly doesn't at home with us. We're always complaining about what he doesn't do, the things he forgets. (turning to Alex) Is that true, son . . . does it seem like mostly criticism that you get from your father and me?
Alex: (quietly) Yes.
Mother: Oh . . . I'm so sorry.

Fortunately, neither parent rushed in to discredit the child's feeling or defend his/her own actions. It was a useful moment for producing the desired impact and helping both mother and father to see their son's predicament.

The pediatrician then shifted the course of the interview once again, this time focusing more directly on Alex's learning difficulties and the family's understanding and coping in the face of his continuing failure. Rudy, with all A's requiring a minimum of effort, tended to look down his nose at his brother, calling him stupid, according to Alex.

> *Father:* Come on, Alex — Rudy is very careful of other people's feelings. I'm sure he would never do something like that.
>
> *Alex:* He just doesn't do it when you're around.

Silently the pediatrician tended to agree with Alex, noting that Rudy did not attempt to defend himself at this point. However, the doctor decided to let the issue drop. It was additional evidence of the polarization process underway in the family: one child who was seen as always good, and one who was, if not always bad, then at least usually wrong.

As father had attempted to explain before the interview began, Mr. and Mrs. Tura certainly did not agree on Alex's learning difficulty nor on how to work with him. Father saw his reading failure as a serious problem, stemming from poor study habits and mediocre schools and requiring scrupulous attention and vigilance on the part of both parents. Specifically Mr. Tura saw the need for frequent teacher conferences, close supervision of homework every night, and a strict schedule of study in the home. Mrs. Tura felt that Alex could really do his work if he would just apply himself. She wanted her husband to leave him to his own devices more often regarding schoolwork, so that he could learn for himself what was required. Father predicted certain disaster with such an approach, fearing that Alex would tune out and then drop out before he finished junior high school if they allowed him to handle "the problem" himself. With such discrepant views regarding the origin of and appropriate measures for handling Alex's learning difficulties, it is no surprise that homework sessions became a battleground, often involving everyone in the family except Sparky. Fighting between Mr. and Mrs. Tura could be particularly intense, resulting in strained silences for days afterwards. Mrs. Tura would often take to her bed during such times.

The parents were asked for some information regarding their individual growing-up and especially their experiences in school learning as children. Father was raised by immigrant parents, who, contrary to the American dream, did not successfully climb the ladder to a better life. They insisted that their children succeed where they had failed, however, and from an early age Mr. Tura was given direction, structure, and exhortations to study hard and do well. He did succeed, and he felt that his survival then and now depended on the diligence taught him by his parents. He wanted the same for his own children. Mrs. Tura was a lack-luster student; her parents had felt that education was not terribly essential for a girl and had not pushed her. She wandered through her schooling, never failing but never excelling either. Educational plans beyond high school were interrupted first by her marriage and then finally by her chronically failing health. Two such very different family (of origin) styles had certainly proved difficult for the Turas to integrate as they now attempted to find a common path with their own two boys.

As a final phase of this diagnostic interview, the pediatrician asked each family member to cite one aspect of family behavior that he or she would like to change. Alex volunteered first:

Alex: That's easy. I'd like my Dad to stop smoking.

Parenthetically we have frequently heard this comment voiced by young children regarding one or both parents. At one level it can be heard by parents simply as a child's criticism of a parent's "bad habit." It has usually proved, however, to reflect something deeper than that. It has been first and foremost an expression of caring from the child to the parent, and it also signals that the child has burdened himself with significant worry about the safety and health of that parent. The doctor commented:

Doctor: Alex, I am very touched by your comment. It tells me that you worry about your Dad's health.
Alex: Well, sure.
Doctor: How come?
Alex: What do you mean, how come?
Doctor: I mean, how come you worry about his health?
Alex: Oh . . . you know.
Doctor: I think I do. But I'd like you to tell him out loud.
Father: Oh, he doesn't like the smoke in the house, I know.
Doctor: Wait a minute. I think there's more to it than that. Is there?
Alex: Well . . . yeah.
Doctor: What?
Alex: (embarrassed and looking at father) I care what happens to you.
Father: (genuinely touched) I know you do, son.
Doctor: (after a silent period) How about you, Rudy? What would you like to change in this family?
Rudy: What I would like to change is . . . when Mom and Daddy won't talk in front of us, only after we're in bed.
Mother: What's the problem with that, Rudy?

> *Rudy:* You always say that business . . . "Let's not talk about this in front of the children." And then I hear you at night — hollering — since my room is so close. I feel like you're talking about me . . . especially when you're fighting when you're in there.
>
> *Mother:* Oh, Rudy! (obviously concerned that her son is troubled)
>
> *Rudy:* That's true. Sometimes I feel like *I'm* to blame for your fighting.
>
> *Father:* There, you see. I tell you, this boy is aware. Florence, you need to be more careful.
>
> *Mother:* Sam, Sam, we both need to be more careful.
>
> *Father:* I am careful. I am careful.
>
> *Mother:* Our fighting is no good, no good at all. . .

Again there was a long, silent pause.

> *Doctor:* What would you like to change in the family, Mrs. Tura?
>
> *Mother:* Some of my own actions and reactions . . . I would like to be more open with my feelings. I think Sam . . . er, that is, Alex and I would get along better if I was able to do that better. Sometimes when I'm short with him — and I know I am much of the time . . . it's not that I'm angry with him. Maybe I'm not feeling well or I'm not happy with myself about how I just handled him or something. But he only sees that I'm mad. I wish I could find other ways to express myself.
>
> *Doctor:* Had you ever thought of some family counseling for just that purpose?

At this the pediatrician noted that Mr. Tura began to squirm in his chair.

> *Mother:* Actually I had been considering it recently. . .
>
> *Father:* But do you think you're well enough, Florence? You know I've started therapy myself, and it takes a tremendous amount of energy, I'm finding out.

The doctor was remembering father's earlier complaint that mother would not participate in psychotherapy, though "I have asked her and asked her." Now father appeared to be the unwilling one, a curious stance for one who had tried so hard to involve his wife in treatment. This was obviously a loaded topic, and Alex's evaluation had not yet proceeded to the recommendation stage. That would take place at a subsequent session. The interviewer therefore chose not to pursue this subject further at the moment.

> *Doctor:* Perhaps we can talk more about all that at another time, when we meet to go over the results of Alex's evaluation. Mr. Tura, you

haven't had an opportunity to answer my last question: what would
you like to change in this family?

Father: I would like all of us to express our feelings openly and to be a hap-
pier family.

The pediatrician would have been more encouraged by Mr. Tura's
words if father had not, when the family filed out of the office, sidled up
and said sotto voce:

Father: Doctor, perhaps just before our meeting next time I could have a
few words with you first. The last point . . . there are some . . .

This time the doctor was ready.

Doctor: No, I won't be doing that next time, Mr. Tura. I will need to see you
all together. I too share your concern that the family learn to express feelings openly; consequently, I insist that we all meet together so that such an open sharing can occur. I think our next session is
scheduled for Wednesday, am I right? Fine, see you then.

Discussion. Prior to this interview, as mentioned, the pediatrician
knew that Alex Tura had a specific learning disability with particular
problems in the area of visual-motor function. He now knew much
more. He now had a family context in which to place Alex and his learning difficulties. Among other things he had learned:

1. Alex's father was a man continually struggling to control situa-
    tions, people, and events. In this struggle Mr. Tura was adroit at
    using predictions of doom ("Let him be? . . . for what, to develop
    an ulcer?"), secrets ("Perhaps just before our meeting next time, I
    could have a few words with you first."), blame ("If they would just
    listen to one another more."), generalities ("Of course, Doctor.
    We are very open as a family."), and pseudosolicitude ("But do
    you think you're well enough, Florence? You know I've started
    therapy myself, and it takes a tremendous amount of energy. . .").
2. Alex's mother was a woman who retreated into and made a career
    of her "condition." She too controlled others, her own illness be-
    ing the tool she used for this purpose ("I notice that especially
    when I'm sick in bed and need him . . . he spends so much time
    with that dog. He doesn't seem to realize how much I'm depend-
    ing on him on those days.").
3. The family was actively polarizing the two boys into one good

child and one bad child ("Now Rudy's pretty good about that, but Alex . . .").

4. In addition, Rudy was being programmed to view himself and to behave as exceedingly vulnerable, sensitive, and fragile. He was being encouraged by his father to develop illness as a retreat and as a control manipulation ("There now, see, Rudy, don't worry. The bathroom is right there when you need it. Just relax. Let me rub your stomach, son.").

5. Neither boy was receiving any consistent, clear validation of self-worth or growth toward independence ("Well, when you do your chores . . . of course I wish you would do them more often without my having to remind you.").

6. In fact, communication at several levels in the family was dysfunctional, especially regarding the expression of feelings ("Maybe I'm not feeling well, or I'm not happy with myself about how I just handled him or something. But he only sees that I'm mad. I wish I could find other ways to express myself.").

7. There were strong indications of marital imbalance and discord ("I would like to be more open with my feelings. I think Sam . . . er, that is, Alex and I would get along better if I was able to do that better.).

8. At least one of the boys, Rudy, was feeling partly responsible for his parents' marital stress ("Sometimes I feel like I'm to blame for your fighting.").

9. Finally no one in the family appeared to have an appropriate understanding of the characteristics or dimensions of Alex's learning difficulties. His parents in particular showed widely discrepant styles for approaching and managing Alex for his neurodevelopmental disabilities ("Now she and I don't always see eye-to-eye on this school problem with Alex.").

Is the collection of this sort of information regarding family function necessary in cases such as Alex's? One could argue that the boy had a mild neurodevelopmental specific learning disability and that appropriate special educational assistance should take care of the problem. Yes, special educational help could succeed in assisting this youngster to develop better fine-motor coordination and in teaching him to discriminate correctly between a "d" and a "b," for instance. However, how should his parents be involved in his subsequent learning experiences so they might facilitate his successful learning rather than obstruct it? Would they provide Alex with appropriate validation of self-worth and competence at home while he slowly made gains in school? The answers to these and other questions were extremely important for planning any therapeutic and remedial program for Alex Tura. They could be answered with information learned about the family, its structure, communication patterns, and sequences of behavior. The family interview provided that information; for us such sessions have become an integral part of the diagnostic evaluation of any child with a suspected developmental difficulty. Family influences in developmental disabilities, of which a learning disorder is one variety, are usually a part of the problem and of the solution.

Now the Tura family graphically illustrated its contribution to the "problem" of Alex's learning difficulty as discussed previously. Family involvement would also be necessary for a "solution" in two specific ways in a subsequent family interview. First of all, they would need to receive information regarding the specific characteristics of Alex's learning difficulty. Helping family members to understand that the boy's persistent school failure was not caused by a lack of motivation, poor study habits, or faulty parenting would be the first step in enlisting support for any specific educational remediation around various aspects of visual-motor function. Second, this family was certainly a candidate for ongoing family therapy; family stresses were numerous and fairly serious, ranging from Alex's learning difficulty to Rudy's worrisome symptoms, mother's perpetual illness, father's overcontrolling responsibility for all the family, and marital discord. To alter these stresses would require a significant effort on the family's part, a willingness to embark on a course of family counseling for considerably more than "just a couple of sessions." The family would therefore in a subsequent family interview also require some understanding of its own dysfunctional communication style and the observed impact of such a style on each family member. Recommendations for the possibility of change through future ongoing counseling, along with the interviewer's realistic view that the counseling work would probably be long-term, could be presented at this later time. Helping a family accept a recommendation for ongoing counseling is frequently a pediatrician's job, and most clinicians will agree that at times the task can be frustratingly difficult. Therefore, regarding that issue, we would like to make a temporary aside.

The pediatrician may consider four variables as he sets about helping a family to enter counseling. He must first of all take into account the nature and complexities of the family's problems, for these will dictate not only the specific type of counseling indicated but also within what time frame he must do his work of recommending. If the family's difficulties are mild, or if they are so chronic that "nothing has changed in years," the pediatrician may take several additional sessions exploring the areas of family difficulty before specifically recommending ongoing counseling. The advantage in such a leisurely pace is that the physician is able to build a trusting relationship with the family so that they come to have faith in his observations, his skills, and his eventual recommendation. However, a leisurely pace is not always possible, either because of the acute nature of the presenting family problem (threatened suicide, runaway, delinquency, and so on) or because of the limitations on the pediatrician's time. The latter is then the second variable to consider: how much time the doctor is able to offer in guiding the group toward a therapeutic setting. He must structure his approach accordingly.

Disregard for these aspects of time and timing is often responsible for failed follow-through on a family's part. Families in distress are usually frightened, angry, and confused. Such a group will seldom accept an outsider's directive, offered rapidly and without preparation in the following manner:

> *Doctor:* The tests are all negative; Marilyn's stomachaches are functional. I recommend psychotherapy. I usually send my patients with such problems to Dr. Allen. Here is his address and phone number. Would you give him a call?

No physician should be so pushed for time that the 30 seconds necessary to utter these words is all that he will allow for facilitating a family's move into psychotherapy. The task will always take longer. To what end? Well, aside from inattention to the first two variables of time (that is, the time frame dictated by the family's problem and the time frame the doctor allots for himself), the physician quoted above has also passed over the third variable to consider in facilitating a referral for counseling. This variable concerns the "psychological mindedness" of the family group, their relative openness versus their resistance, their ability and readiness to acknowledge not only their distress but the need to do something about it. Getting a feel for the family's defenses and defensiveness is essential in planning how one will help them move toward further help. Again such a process takes interviewing time.

A fourth variable that will influence the effectiveness of a referral for counseling has to do with the specific resource being recommended. If, for instance, the pediatrician feels that the problem is one that he himself wants to manage, the referral process can be somewhat simpler. His evaluation, already established relationship, and diagnostic observations can usually work to his advantage, so the family comes to feel that a transition from assessment to treatment with the same individual is the logical outcome of the initial visit to the doctor. A referral to another resource may require patient listening on the pediatrician's part regarding, for instance, the family's anxiety at having to start with someone new and unknown. The physician will also need to provide recognition of the family's reluctance and discomfort surrounding the referral and continuing support for a hopeful view (that is, that the family's situation can improve through active participation in ongoing counseling).

These four variables: the time imposed by the family's particular presenting problem, the time available to the physician to effect a referral, the family's readiness or lack of readiness to accept the recommendation, and the features of the actual resource being recommended, will distill into a physician's specific approach with a given family. We have, of course, all experienced clinical situations in which one of the variables, or several combined, has proved an insurmountable obstacle, when a successful referral simply can't happen. Those times are inevitable. One might, for instance, comfortably predict failure for a physician faced with the following situation: A family member is openly threatening suicide. The doctor has approximately 8 minutes to spend with the group. There is abundant evidence that no one in the family can abide looking at his own behavior.

Fortunately such gloomy combined circumstances are not the rule. Even the Turas accepted the pediatrician's referral for ongoing family therapy. Three more 30-minute sessions were held with that family before a specific recommendation for ongoing family work was made. The family problems were of long standing; no acute crises demanded immediate action (variable number one). The pediatrician also had the time to offer follow-up visits (variable number two). And although it appeared superficially that the family possessed a certain readiness to consider psychological factors (one member of the family had already begun individual psychotherapy), the idea of ongoing family or marital sessions was clearly an anxious one for them; they were resistant (variable number three). Briefly summarized, the three additional sessions were spent highlighting the continuing areas of family conflict, particularly between parents and child and between the two children. The family seemed most comfortable with parent-child issues, and discussions were consequently limited to this area. During this period very little work was directed toward specifically emphasizing the marital difficulties, although, to be sure, they were glaringly apparent.

At a point in the fourth session when both parents were agreeing that communication was often frustrating and ineffective with their boys, especially Alex, the pediatrician said:

Doctor: Is this something that you would like to change?

Father: Oh my, would we ever, Doctor! I'm sure my wife would agree (still speaking for his wife).

Mother: (nods her head in assent)

Doctor: Then I am wondering how you would feel about the possibility of ongoing family sessions, specifically geared toward improving your communication with the children and theirs with you?

Mother: Would it help?

Doctor: You have some doubts, it sounds like?

Mother: Well . . .

Doctor: I hear your doubtfulness. And it is also clear that the current situation is not working particularly well.

Father: You can say that again. Florence and Alex, if they could . . .

Doctor: (hurrying to silence Mr. Tura in his blaming of other family members) I would want you to be involved as well, Mr. Tura. You are an extremely important part of the family, and I do not feel that any sort of counseling would be successful without your very important perspective on the family.

Father: I see. And the boys. You mean they would come too?

Doctor: Absolutely. Especially since it is communication between you, the parents, and your children that you want to change. Of course, you and your wife sometimes might have some things that you would like to discuss privately, in which case the children could stay home for that session, but that could be arranged as the situation arose.

Mother: Would we come to see *you*, Doctor?

Doctor: I would like very much to continue seeing you. However, I can also arrange for you to see a counselor closer to home, if you would prefer. I am aware of some excellent resources in your area.

Father: Oh no, I think coming here makes the most sense. You know us now.

Mother and the two children agreed.

The referral was thus accepted. There still remained other particulars of the recommendation to be discussed. The pediatrician told the family, for instance, that he would want to see them weekly for 1 hour each visit. He also wanted the family to know that he felt the work on communication was going to require at least several months of work on the family's part and that he and they could evaluate the duration of counseling more clearly as the work actually got underway. There were also other specifics of appointment time, fee, and so on that need not be detailed here. The referral itself was successful because the doctor attended to the four variables previously mentioned, taking the time to clarify the presence and nature of a specific problem, not only in his eyes but in the family's as well. He was then able to offer specific assistance to the family regarding that particular problem, and a contract for treatment was established.

In fairness to the reader who feels that recommendations for counseling seldom go so smoothly, we should state that the Tura family did participate in sessions as long as the pediatrician focused only on parent-child issues. When in the ninth family interview the doctor began to address marital difficulties more directly, the family abruptly terminated sessions, because "it was getting too expensive." Since to this point there had been no difficulties surrounding the financial aspects of the counseling (and in fact financial arrangements had been discussed), we can only assume that the pediatrician had presumed on his relationship with the family and unwittingly entered an area in which he was not yet welcome. Here, just as during the initial period of referral, proper timing was essential. Yet as the Tura family demonstrated, sometimes the properness of timing in counseling can be evaluated only in retrospect.

Concluding this discussion regarding how one might effect a successful referral for ongoing family counseling, we will now return to the original interview with the Tura family, conducted during the course of Alex's evaluation for learning difficulties.

Contrary to most clinical examples presented throughout this text, the pediatrician interviewing Alex's family made relatively few direct interventions. His omission was intentional. The Tura family had not come initially asking for changes in their style of family function. As they understood the interview, they were participating in a diagnostic effort to elucidate the characteristics of their son's learning difficulties. The pediatrician recognized and honored their perspective in this initial setting. Consequently, he collected family data but did not necessarily act on the information elicited. That would come later after the family had agreed that they wanted assistance. Our trainees have sometimes reported difficulty restraining themselves in this situation. Just seeing dysfunctional behavior, particularly after learning some strategies for altering that behavior, can be for some interviewers an invitation to "wade in and straighten this mess out." But such a move can also be experienced by the family as offensive, intrusive, and ill-timed. Hence a diagnostic family interview such as that summarized calls for continuing attention and monitoring by the interviewer as to how far he will push and how directly he will intervene concerning issues appearing in the session.

The diagnostic family interview with the Turas serves our purposes well in revealing the presence of important family stresses, those associated with, and those above and beyond, a child's stated learning difficulty. It is also a good example of a "sloppy" session in certain respects. As such it conveys much of the flavor of typical interviews. By "sloppy" we refer to the fact that topics sometimes tumbled over one another, issues were not necessarily followed to any conclusion, and sometimes the interviewer seemed to have little form or structure to what he was doing. His questions were occasionally out of sequence, arbitrary, or too abruptly altering of the previous tone. Well, family interviews are like that, especially family interviews held for the purpose of pursuing specific diagnostic information regarding a host of issues, as in the elaboration of a child's learning disability.

As the preceding illustrates, family interviews can be utilized for diagnostic purposes in gathering important information about the families of children with developmental disabilities. We have also suggested that family interviews can be used to share with the family the results of a diagnostic assessment. It is one thing to explain to a family that their child has some difficulty with eye-hand coordination and quite another to share with a family that their child is mentally retarded. Can family interviews effectively serve this purpose? We feel that they can.

Delivering news of this sort to parents amounts to declaring a chronic condition of the most devastating variety in their child. Such an interview should be closely structured around those guidelines that we have presented previously (Chapter 8) for the delivery of bad diagnostic news. By all means one must (1) respect the event, furnishing the time, energy, and support that the family will require of the interviewer. One would also do well to (2) keep medical facts to a minimum, (3) pay careful attention to the feelings shown and expressed by individual family members, (4) withstand the family's silence and grief, and (5) resist the temptation to run away from the distressing scene. The reader may remember that one other rule has generally been included in our summaries of this list from Chapter 8: one needs to share the diagnosis quickly. The "hows" of this last rule can be most perplexing for clinicians who are faced with the actuality of telling parents that their child is retarded. How does one go about such a formidable task? Even with adequate attention to all the other rules above, how is one to share this diagnosis—and how quickly? Excerpts from work with the family of Maria Gomez will illustrate some of the "hows" of family interviewing when helping a family hear for the first time the diagnosis of developmental retardation in one of their children.

The Gomez family

Mrs. Gomez had originally brought her daughter to the pediatrician for a hearing test and a checkup. Maria, age 3½ years, was developing language extremely slowly, so slowly that mother had at times worried there was something wrong with the child's hearing or her tongue ("Could she be tongue-tied, Doctor?"). Mr. Gomez had chided his wife for being overanxious; he knew Maria heard perfectly. He had noticed how much she liked to sit in front of the television, rocking rhythmically to the music of commercials. She certainly had to be hearing the music, he said. Her tongue looked normal to him, and besides her speech was coming along; she was making more and more sounds all the time. Granted her speech, beyond mama, da, and wa, was not often understandable, but pronunciation would improve with time, he maintained. Maybe Mrs. Gomez should go back to her part-time job, he suggested; she just seemed to worry all the time when she was around Maria. Mother, however, could not shake the idea that "something isn't right." It was that continuing concern that prompted her to seek out an evaluation with the pediatrician.

After taking a history and spending some time with Maria, the pediatrician shared Mrs. Gomez's concern. At age 3½, the child had very little expressive speech beyond some unintelligible single syllables. Her large motor skills were lagging; she still tended to take stairs one at a time, would not even attempt riding a tricycle, and could not button, nor was she successful in putting on any of her own clothes. Toilet training had never gotten off the ground. She *did* seem able to hear, the pediatrician felt. He feared the problem would not be that well circumscribed, for he observed to himself that Maria was evidencing serious developmental delays across a wide range of abilities. He suggested to Mrs. Gomez that a diagnostic evaluation was indicated to give a clearer picture of Maria's developmental progress; it would include not just a hearing test but also an evaluation of her language development and some measures of her muscle coordination, thinking abilities, and general development. Several laboratory tests would also be performed. Mrs. Gomez readily accepted the suggestion of this evaluation, adding:

Mother: But my husband will think it's all a waste of time.

Doctor: I'm glad you mentioned your husband, Mrs. Gomez. Because that reminds me, I will certainly want to discuss this evaluation with you *both.* So I would like to arrange an appointment when you and Mr. Gomez can be here. In fact, you have two other children, as I remember. George . . . ah yes, that's right. He's 7 years old now? And Tracy is 2? I would like them to come also. I will want to go over the evaluation with the whole family.

Mother: Well, I don't know about my husband. . .

Doctor: He must be there. It is essential. Would you like me to call him?

Mother: Oh . . . no. I'll . . . I'll talk to him and see.

Doctor: Good. If you do find you want me to speak to him, give me a call. As Maria's father he is a very important person to include in this whole process.

This was one situation, and there are such times, when the doctor's positive expectations regarding father's participation were to no avail. He struggled long and hard subsequently to include Mr. Gomez in the evaluation, most particularly in a diagnostic family interview. But father was perpetually unavailable, sick, held up at work, or tied up with other activities. The evaluation dragged on, uncompleted. As a compromise, rather than losing father altogether, the doctor agreed to combine the diagnostic family interview and summary discussion of evaluation results into one interview, which Mr. Gomez agreed to attend with his wife and the children.

The doctor did not have good news to share with the Gomez family. Maria had had a severely traumatic and hypoxic birth. Complete physical, neurological, laboratory, psychological, and developmental evaluations had yielded no more specific explanation for the fact that Maria was mentally retarded. At $3\frac{1}{2}$ years she was functioning in almost all categories of development as an early 2-year-old. Motor skills, language development, and social development were all at this 2-year level. I.Q. scores were in the low 60's, entirely consistent with the child's behavior and demonstrated developmental pattern. The family could hardly be expected to accept this information with equanimity. It was a devastating diagnosis: idiopathic developmental retardation, possibly secondary to central nervous system damage at birth.

After greetings, introductions, and a brief interchange particularly with the children, the doctor began:

> *Doctor:*   I am glad the whole family was able to come in today. I wanted to be able to talk with all of you about Maria's development — your concerns and the various tests that she has had with us. Mr. Gomez, your wife has already shared with me her questions and worries about Maria. I would like your perspective on the situation as well. How do you see Maria's growth and her development?

While making this overture to Mr. Gomez, the doctor noted that Maria remained inactive and solidly nestled in her mother's lap, sucking two fingers. Tracy, age 2, curious and unrestrained, had wandered over to the toy shelf and was busily exploring what was on it. George, 7 years old, sat dutifully next to his father. The two males formed a unit on one side of the room; Mother and Maria formed another unit on the opposite side. Tracy drifted back and forth between the two groups, alternating trips to them with return visits to the toy shelf. Of the five individuals, only she appeared to be enjoying herself.

> *Doctor:*   (in an attempt to alter the family configuration, interrupting Mr. Gomez before he responds) Hold it just a minute. Mrs. Gomez, see if you can interest Maria in joining Tracy and in playing with some of the toys over there.
>
> *Mother:*   Oh, that's all right, Doctor. I think she's a little tired this morning. You'd probably rather stay here, eh, Maria?

Maria's only response was nonverbal. She buried her face in her mother's shoulder and did not budge. She was beginning to look glued to her mother. The pediatrician had not missed Mrs. Gomez's coded message to Maria, which clearly suggested: "Do not leave my lap, Maria." That brief interaction alone between mother and daughter verified that there was more than one issue to be approached with this family. Many of Maria's difficulties were developmental in nature, undoubtedly stemming from some malfunction in the child's own neurodevelopmental equipment. She was also having difficulty in the process of separation and individuation from her mother. Whether this difficulty was a reflection of her developmental retardation or represented a separate issue was in some ways irrelevant. Since her mother was directly encouraging the child's reluctance to separate, the problem was, around this issue, undeniably interactional, whatever other developmental problems existed.

The pediatrician was about to realize that he had unwittingly played directly into the father's hands:

Father: Actually, that's a large part of the problem right there, Doctor. I keep telling my wife that Maria would be all right if she just wouldn't baby her so much. Why don't you just let her play with Tracy, hon?

Mother: She doesn't want to, do you, Maria? You never seem to understand, Frank, that she's uncomfortable in new situations. And it takes her a while to feel relaxed. Why can't you realize that?

First serious developmental difficulties, then interactional problems between mother and child, and now marital dysfunction entered the picture. The pediatrician would have to set some priorities and organize the session or the interview could soon be out of control. He did.

Doctor: That's an excellent point, Mrs. Gomez. Of course she's uneasy in this situation so far. Why don't you move your chair over closer to Tracy and the toys so that Maria will continue to feel comfortable near you as you gradually ease her off your lap and onto the floor with her sister.

Mother complied and father continued.

Father: You see, my wife, she worries too much; she . . .

Doctor: And you, do have any worries about Maria?

Father: Well, not like my wife, but sure, I wish she was talking more. I guess we all wish that.

Doctor: Tell me what you have noticed about her speech development.

Father went on to explain that he too was worried that Maria was developing speech slowly. He noticed the problem especially since George had been very quick with his language development, and Tracy was already using more words than Maria.

Doctor: You are a careful observer of your children. I've been noticing also here today that Tracy is talking much more than her older sister.

Father: That's right. And I tell my wife, if she wouldn't baby Maria so much, then Maria would have to begin to talk more.

Mother: (rolls her eyes toward the ceiling and says nothing)

Doctor:	I think you've heard that one before, Mrs. Gomez.
Father:	(embarrassed, laughs)
Mother:	I sure have. I try to tell him that if I baby her, it's because in many ways she seems like the baby of the family. But he won't listen.
Doctor:	It's a bone of contention between you two, I can see.

George, silent up to this point, vigorously nodded agreement to the pediatrician's last statement.

Doctor:	That's a bother for you, George?
George:	They always start to fight on this one!

George's remark caused everyone to laugh, partly with embarrassment, partly with relief. The pediatrician was grateful for the shift in intensity to a lighter level.

Doctor:	Let me return for a minute, Mr. Gomez, to your observations of your daughter's development. I hear clearly that you and your wife don't necessarily agree on the reasons behind Maria's slow speech development, but it sounds as though you both do agree that her speech development *is* slow.
Father:	Yes, I guess you would have to say that.
Doctor:	Now, in what other ways have you worried that Maria was perhaps a little behind?
Father:	Well, I know that her teeth are really slow in coming in, but I don't think that means anything. And they're beginning to come through now.
Doctor:	Uh-huh. (silence)
Father:	She's not really all that hot about using her tricycle that we got her for Christmas. And when I put her on it, she just screams. So I gave up on that one.
Doctor:	I see.
Father:	My wife complains that she doesn't even try to dress herself. But that's another one of those . . . if she wouldn't do it for her, maybe Maria would pick it up.
Doctor:	Have you yourself tried that approach with Maria?
Father:	Yes, I did. I tried to teach her about putting her pajamas on. . .
Mother:	Tell him what happened, Frank. (turning to the doctor) It didn't work. He's too impatient. He gets mad, and she starts screaming.
Doctor:	Now you're back to that bone of contention I mentioned earlier.

The pediatrician noticed that by this time Maria had slid off her mother's lap and gravitated toward Tracy and the toys. The difference in the play activity of the two children was striking, even to a casual observer. Maria seemed confused by and/or uninterested in most objects, using them for the wrong purpose or handling them clumsily, putting many of them in her mouth. Tracy was appropriately using the toy telephones, drinking out of teacups, and successfully managing a small train set. Maria would watch her sister and often attempt the same activity; her play seemed to lack the creativity and originality of Tracy's. While Maria was effective as a mimic, it was only mimicry. The doctor determined to use this information to bring the interview closer to a discussion of Maria's evaluation results.

> *Doctor:* Mrs. Gomez, you've done an excellent job in encouraging Maria to play with her sister. You were right—she simply needed to feel comfortable before moving away from you. Is that the way it often is?
>
> *Mother:* (with a sigh) Yeah. She really sticks close.
>
> *Doctor:* I need to talk with you about that a little more. However, as we are talking for the next few minutes, I would like all of you to keep your eyes on the two girls and their play, just pay attention to how they seem to be playing—either together or individually.

The parents and George agreed to do this, and the pediatrician continued to discuss with Mrs. Gomez the fact that Maria "sticks close."

> *Doctor:* Sticking close—that must sometimes be confining for you?
>
> *Mother:* (guarded) Well, yes.
>
> *Doctor:* When do you find time for yourself?

A trace of sadness flashed across mother's face as she acknowledged that Maria afforded her very little time for her own needs. She felt pretty locked in to being one member of a constant duo at this point. With the pediatrician's encouragement she even acknowledged not liking the situation, wishing that somehow she could find more time both for herself and for her husband. It was a useful comment for her husband to hear. As this issue came to a close, at least for the time being, the doctor returned to his previous request of the family:

> *Doctor:* OK. Let's go back to Maria and Tracy. You folks are good observers of children. At what level while they are playing—if I asked you to mention an age level—at what level would you say each is operating? You first, Mr. Gomez.
>
> *Father:* You mean Maria?
>
> *Doctor:* I mean each girl.

Father: Well, I would say that Trace is playing pretty much as I would expect for a 2-year-old; if anything she's maybe a little ahead of her age. But probably 2 . . . 2½ years old, I would guess.

Doctor: And Maria?

Father: She's just about where Tracy is—maybe not even quite as far along, but well—they've been doing most of the same things there on the floor. So I would have to say that Maria is at about a 2-year level also.

Doctor: Does that match at all with what you notice at home?

Father: Oh yeah, the two of them copy one another all the time. Maria likes to play with her sister more than any of the older kids on the street.

Mother and George were then asked for their appraisal of the level of play and activity for each child. They agreed with father that the two girls, both in the office and at home, acted more like twins than siblings with a year-and-a-half difference in their chronological ages.

The pediatrician decided that the way had now been prepared for some discussion of the evaluation results.

Doctor: You all are right on the button. The studies that we have done with Maria, and I want to go over them with you, show exactly the same thing. In almost all respects, Maria is performing and behaving at a 2-year developmental level, rather than her age level of 3½ years.

There was profound silence in the room. After a time the mother looked up and said wearily:

Mother: I knew it. I knew something was wrong.

Father: What does it mean, Doctor?

Doctor: Tell me what you understand about what I have just said.

Father: Well, that is . . . you are saying that Maria is slow, that there's some problem with her development. But what do you mean by that? What kind of a problem and in what kind of development?

Doctor: Slow down, Mr. Gomez. For right now what I am saying is that our tests agree with your own observations. Maria at the present time is mostly at a 2-year-old level in her behavior and in her abilities.

Father: Yeah, right, but what abilities are you talking about?

At this point the pediatrician was able to present some specific examples of Maria's performance on developmental and psychological tests, demonstrating that with various aspects of motor coordination, speech and language development, and social interaction, Maria was succeeding at the 2-year level and rather consistently failing on items beyond that age level. Both parents were listening intently; George was respectfully silent. The two girls continued to play on the floor.

For some families at this point, it is enough to have heard that their child is significantly behind in many aspects of developmental growth. The term "mental retardation" is not spoken aloud nor discussed with the doctor. The point has been made without the explicit use of the term. We do not feel that parents should be assaulted with the term under the banner of "honesty." If the family is loath to utter the phrase, particularly in the initial stages of hearing that their child is developmentally slow, their reticence should be respected. There is abundant time in the future for a discussion of terms and/or other issues. However, with other families, the doctor's initial declaration forces a question from them. It was so with the Gomez family.

Mother: Does this mean, Doctor, that Maria is mentally retarded?

Doctor: Tell me what you mean and understand by that term.

Mother: I don't know, really. I guess mostly what I know is from having seen children on television who look different and they are called what is it . . . mongolism?

Doctor: No, I need you to hear me clearly. Maria does not have that condition. What else do you know about mental retardation?

Mother: (beginning to look stunned) I don't know.

Doctor: How about you, Mr. Gomez?

Father: Mostly I think that it has to do with people who are vegetables, who can't learn, and who have to be in institutions.

Mother: (nodding her head in agreement)

Doctor: Do you see Maria as someone like that?

Father: Absolutely not.

Doctor: I agree. She is not. That is one reason that I am so uncomfortable with the term "mental retardation." Parents so often have terrible . . . and incorrect ideas about what the term means. Maria does not have mongolism; she can learn but it will be slow, and she is certainly not a vegetable. What I need you to understand is that she *is* developing slowly in a number of areas at the present time. Period. It looks to me as though you are all hearing me on that point, am I right?

They all agreed. Even George nodded assent.

Doctor: OK. Now take some time . . . and some breaths. Tell me what you are each feeling now that you have heard the news.

Mother: (tears in her eyes) I am not surprised. . .
Doctor: But there is pain, just the same?
Mother: (nods yes and quietly breaks down)
Doctor: (after a pause) What about you, Mr. Gomez?
Father: It's. . .just one of those things, I guess.
Doctor: How are you feeling inside?
Father: She'll come along, I'm hoping.
Doctor: This has been hard news for you to hear . . . and accept today.
Father: (quietly) Yeah.
Doctor: I can appreciate that, (pause) George?
George: (his tears beginning as he notices those of his mother) Sad.

And in a very loving gesture George rose and put his arms around each parent in turn.

The interview continued, but we will stop at this point. Our purpose in presenting the Gomez family was to illustrate one approach for "how" to share the diagnosis of (develop)mental retardation with a family in the context of a conjoint family interview, and that particular task had now been accomplished.

Discussion. In Chapter 8 we paraphrased, from the writings of Steinhauer and others,[3] six questions that are in the minds of families forced to face the diagnosis of a chronic condition in a child:

1. What's the matter?
2. What (who) caused it?
3. What can the physician do to help?
4. What can the parents do to help?
5. How long will the condition last?
6. Will the child be completely cured?

The presence of mental retardation in a child of course stimulates these same six questions for a family. We point out that essentially only question number one was handled in the initial interview with the Gomez family. Even that one could not yet be set aside as answered and resolved. For instance, Mr. Gomez was partly hearing what the doctor had to say; however, his last comments also indicated his denial and ambivalence at the news. He and his wife would need (and indeed did require) additional discussion just to accept the fact that their daughter was actually lagging in her developmental progress.

Questions two through six had in no way been tackled. However, they were all there, waiting to surface in the Gomez family, just as they are there in all families in similar situations. Consequently many family sessions and/or couple sessions and/or individual interviews are generally indicated if one is working with families to help them accept the diagnosis of mental retardation in their child. With the Gomez family some of the above questions were threatening to break through into the open at any moment: regarding question number two (who caused it?), Mr. Gomez had clearly been holding his wife responsible for Maria's difficulty. This issue would become more prominent should the issue of Maria's hypoxic birth as a causative factor be raised by either of the parents, since such information could easily intensify the notion of maternal blame. Succeeding interviews demonstrated that Mrs. Gomez blamed herself fully as much as her husband did. Much of her protection and solicitude toward Maria was offered in an effort to handle and relieve her own feelings of self-blame for having "caused the problem." The parents also wanted further tests and treatments by the doctor to "make sure" (question number three: what can the physician do?). They wanted very much to be involved in a program of diet, language stimulation, instructional play, or anything that would accelerate their daughter's progress or ameliorate the basic problem. While there were specific helps that they could and eventually did provide, it was extremely hard for them to accept that a certain and significant amount of Maria's developmental growth could not be externally imposed. Question number four (what can the parents do?) thus revealed itself. They had many questions about the future, such as prognosis, schooling, and their dreaded fear of institutionalization. Those concerns, of course, reflected their understandable preoccupation with questions numbers five and six (how long will the condition last? And will the child be cured?).

Each of the above concerns required discussion and repetition, with a willingness on the pediatrician's part to recognize that, for instance, just because he had reassured them on two separate visits about inappropriateness of current institutionalization for Maria, the subject was not necessarily resolved. He needed to explore with the family what had reactivated the concern this time. Sessions were not frequent. The family visited the pediatrician for a "talk session" about every 2 to 3 months, but over a period of 2½ years. Approximately 8 months after the initial session, they asked for the pediatrician's help in locating a parents' support group for the families of retarded children. The fact that they could see themselves as being able to use what such a group had to offer signaled to the pediatrician that they had come a long way in accepting the reality of developmental problems in their daughter.

DISORDERS WITH GENETIC IMPLICATIONS

So far in this chapter we have illustrated the use of family interviewing at two different time points during the evaluation and treatment of a child with a developmental disorder. We began initially with a demonstration of the technique when used for diagnostic purposes, as the evaluation of the child's condition is in process. We then discussed family interviewing at a later date, when the diagnosis of the developmental condition is shared with the family. For a third clinical illustration of family interviewing in conditions of this kind we will move beyond these two initial time periods to another, when the family has heard the diagnosis, and they are struggling to reckon with it. Shock and denial are replaced by an acknowledgement of the facts. Along with realization for many families comes a preoccupation with Steinhauer's[3] second question: what (who) caused it? It is only a short jump for family members from that question to another: am I (are you, are we) somehow responsible?

There are countless developmental disorders in which the above questions become tremendously troublesome foci for parental thought, rumination, and worry. Parents indict themselves and one another with reasonable and unreasonable issues alike, from medications taken during pregnancy, to dietary indiscretions, to smoking, to illnesses, recent or long ago, to not wanting the baby in the first place, and so forth. Perhaps one of the most painful concerns for parents of developmentally disabled children to face and resolve is the notion that they, the parents, have caused the child's condition because of "bad" genes or chromosomes, an outstanding worry especially when the developmental condition is one actually associated with hereditary factors, genetic dysfunction, or chromosomal abnormality. Parents of children with such a genetically determined disability are regularly urged to seek genetic counseling for their many concerns and questions about the genetic aspects of their child's condition. It is certainly an appropriate step to take and represents one facet of comprehensive and proper medical care for such a child and his family. The prototype of a developmental problem for which genetic counseling is sought is Down's syndrome, a developmental disorder nowadays clearly recognized by most parents, even before they are told, as connected to chromosomal, and therefore genetic, factors.

The Strand family

Yet how does one impart the information essential for appropriate genetic counseling to these parents without also inadvertently aggravating the parents' heightened sense of self-blame for having produced chromosomes that resulted in an affected child? Dr. Burnett, a pediatric resident, was facing such a task with the Strand family. The parents, a young couple in their late 20's, had asked him for genetic counseling assistance. Their only child, Sheila, now 2 months of age, had been suspected in the newborn period of having Down's syndrome, and chromosome studies had confirmed the clinical diagnosis. The parents were told when Sheila was almost 1 month old. Of course they had been tremendously shaken by this news, yet seemed to be coping reasonably well. They were now beginning to face, among other dilemmas, the question of having subsequent children and the possible risks involved. It should be mentioned that chromosome studies had also characterized Sheila's problem as one of straightforward trisomy 21. The Strands, without chromosomal evidence of translocation, with a negative family history, and with maternal age under 35 years, stood approximately 1 chance in 100 of having another child born with the same condition. This information had not yet been shared in detail with the family.

Dr. Burnett studied arduously beforehand to make sure that he had the right genetic information regarding Down's syndrome. He found that this was a condition for which statistical information was readily available and certain. The clarity with which numbers and statistics had been established in Down's syndrome was somewhat reassuring to him; he hoped the family would have a similar reaction. After some introductory remarks he got down to business.

> *Doctor:* Mr. and Mrs. Strand, you asked to meet with me so that we might discuss some of the genetic factors associated with Down's syndrome. I think it might be useful if we were to back up and start from the beginning. Tell me first of all what you understand about what causes Down's syndrome.
>
> *Mother:* Just what you told us when we first talked with you, that there is something wrong with Sheila's—er—chromosomes. She got that from us somehow—we gave her too many or the wrong kind or

something. But I felt perfectly fine all during the pregnancy, I don't understand it.

Father: I worry about all those dental X-rays you had, Jean, before we even knew you were pregnant.

Mother: He had me wear a shield, Harry. What do you think, Doctor? Could X-rays have damaged my chromosomes or genes or whatever? I was only about 6 weeks pregnant at the time. Incidentally you had . . .

Father: The first 12 weeks of the pregnancy are the most important—that much I know. And it's chromosomes that are the important things to consider; genes are different. Yes, I know I had some X-rays too about that time, but not as many as you had with that dentist.

Doctor: Let me explain a little about genes and chromosomes. It may help to clarify things.

From his reading Dr. Burnett had prepared a short description of the causes of Down's syndrome. He was eager to use it so that the parents would have a correct understanding of current medical knowledge surrounding the condition, "if only they will stop blaming one another long enough for me to say what I have to say," the doctor added to himself. Aloud he continued:

Doctor: While the underlying causes of Down's syndrome are still unknown, an extra chromosome is always present. Chromosomes are very tiny structures that contain the hereditary factors—genes. Every cell in the body has a complete set of chromosomes. In a normal human, a complete set of chromosomes equals 23 pairs. In each of the 23 pairs, one chromosome comes from the mother and one comes from the father, to make a total of 46 chromosomes. In Down's syndrome, the baby has an extra chromosome in one of the pairs, making a total of 47 chromosomes. This extra chromosome is responsible for Down's syndrome and Sheila's condition.

Mother: The extra chromosome—it must come from the mother, am I right? I remember that you said before that mothers who are over 40 have a greater risk of having a baby with Down's syndrome. And you certainly never hear anything about its being dangerous for fathers over 40 to have babies. It's always "older mothers" . . .

Doctor: Sometimes it is the mother. But the extra chromosome can come from either parent. Let me draw some diagrams for you. Now there are X chromosomes and Y chromosomes, but for the time being we don't need to bother with the Y chromosome. That's the male sex chromosome and the female doesn't have any. The problem in Down's syndrome isn't on the Y chromosome anyway. It's on the twenty-first X chromosome.

The doctor drew the following diagram:

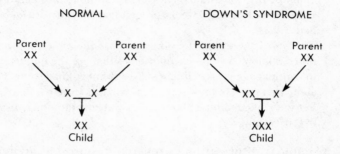

Doctor: Now the egg from which the baby develops normally receives one chromosome of each pair from the mother and one from the father. Since each cell has 23 pairs, a baby receives 23 chromosomes from each parent. Therefore a normal baby has a total of 46 chromosomes in every cell in the body, as does each parent. In the case of Down's syndrome a mistake occurs. The egg from which the baby develops receives two chromosomes of the twenty-first pair from one of the parents and one chromosome 21 from the other parent, giving the baby an extra chromosome. Therefore a baby with Down's syndrome has a total of 47 chromosomes in every cell in the body, not 46, the normal number.

Dr. Burnett had finished. It had gone reasonably well, he concluded. They had stopped talking to one another, and they appeared to be listening intently to his words. He had been careful to phrase his words in understandable English, rather than medical jargon, yet the formulation had been medically correct. So far, so good. Now he had one more brief summary planned for the Strands. He knew they were worried about having another affected baby, and he felt that they deserved some statistics on that issue.

Doctor: Do you have any questions about what I have said so far?

Neither parent spoke. They were beginning to look dazed.

Doctor: OK. Let me go on. I know you are worried about having other children. Let me reassure you on that one. Only in rare cases is Down's syndrome inherited, and in your case it is not; the chromosome studies we did showed us that. In your situation a woman younger than 35 years old has 1 chance in 100 of having another child with Down's syndrome. By age 45, as you remembered my telling you, the mother's chance of having a child with Down's syndrome is 1 in 50. But you're a long way from that. Now, while the chances are always in favor of having a normal child, no parent can ever be absolutely certain. A test is available to determine whether or not an unborn child will have Down's syndrome. This test, called amniocentesis, would involve a chromosome examination of the fetus, the unborn baby developing in the womb. The developing fetus grows inside a fluid-filled sac. With a needle some fluid can be removed from this sac. The amniotic fluid contains cells shed by the fetus. These cells can be grown and examined in a chromosome examination to find out whether or not the fetus is affected with Down's syndrome. Amniocentesis could be performed safely at 15 weeks of pregnancy. If the fetus were to have Down's syndrome, you the parents would choose either to continue or terminate the pregnancy.

By this time, Dr. Burnett felt even better. He had covered a very difficult topic and included all the essential factors that he had hoped to discuss. This time when he offered the parents an opportunity for questions, father managed a lackluster inquiry about whether medical insurance would cover a procedure such as amniocentesis. Mrs. Strand had nothing to say beyond a polite thank you to the doctor for his time and information.

On the way home, neither spouse had much to say to the other. This was curious, because they had heard potentially good news. Future successful pregnancies and normal subsequent children were to be anticipated, and amniocentesis seemed a most reassuring technique to have waiting in the wings. Why then were they both feeling so disagreeable, dissatisfied, and unsettled? The doctor had told them what they needed to know. Hadn't he?

Discussion. In our view the Strands' discomfort was a result of the fact that they had been *told* accurate information by the pediatrician, but they themselves had not been *heard.* Dr. Burnett had unwittingly demonstrated one of the most common errors made by physicians in family interviewing work—one mentioned in Chapter 2. He had focused on content and information to the exclusion of process and behavior in the interview. In his desire to transmit the correct and necessary facts, he had relegated the family's interactional behavior in the office to "background status," something to be circumvented in order to accomplish his single-minded task. It was an unfortunate decision on Dr. Burnett's part. Both parents were terribly preoccupied with questions of blame, particularly genetic blame, regarding their daughter's condition. Father was both suggesting that mother was the carrier of defective genes and working hard to absolve himself of any contributing role. His wife was similarly concerned. The mother's pain was if anything more intense around the issue, because she appeared to fear that her husband's innuendos were accurate, and that she was the donor of the extra chromosome. The pediatrician neither declared the obvious presence of this most stressful issue between them nor acknowledged the parents' considerable pain surrounding it. Rather he ignored the topic, and the couple left the session with their uncomfortable feelings of self-blame and other-blame intact. In fact the family's program to make mother the culprit was possibly even intensified by the work of the pediatrician. He had indeed talked about risks relating to advanced maternal age, a facet of the problem that Mrs. Strand had previously on her own taken to mean: mothers, not fathers, are to blame for Down's syndrome.

Genetic counseling of this kind, as with family interviewing in general, requires a successful balancing act by the interviewer, with attention to the dispersal of necessary information *and* with equal attention to the feelings, behavior, and process displayed by the family in the session. Skewing the interview too heavily in either direction can produce difficulties. A preoccupation with facts, tables, risks, ratios, and statistics leads to the sort of difficulties experienced by the Strands. An exclusive emphasis on feelings, emotions, and behavior with no information offered produces not only incomplete and inadequate medical care but also a feeling by the family that, while they have had some kind of "therapy," they have received none of the necessary facts around which to plan their present or their future. This balancing between content and process in genetic counseling interviews is particularly delicate. The family's process and behavior certainly requires attention and intervention. In genetic counseling, however, there is also a body of information that the family must hear and understand. They must know the facts about future risks in subsequent pregnancies, about the possibility of the condition appearing later in currently normal siblings, about the risk to future generations of the family, about the advisability of sterilization, and so forth. Consequently, the content in such interviews can never really be put aside. It is very important data. Because it is so important, and because so often physicians are comfortable discussing information and uncomfortable acknowledging feelings, genetic counseling interviews are particularly prone to become data discussions with insufficient regard for the feelings and behavior of those involved, as the Strand family discovered.

In this regard we would like to say a few words about the use of diagrams by physicians in interviews. Diagrams such as the one used by Dr. Burnett are often employed by a physician to clarify, whether he is helping a family to understand the specifics of a child's interventricular septal defect, the rudiments of kidney function, or the anatomical location of the appendix. It is wise to remember that sometimes what the physician sees and draws as clarity, the family may experience as informational overkill. We have been particularly impressed with this discrepancy in observing trainees attempt the explanation of hereditary transmission of specific diseases. All too often it has been an excruciating experience for us to watch an earnest student physician tallying on paper the X's and Y's of a particular chromosomal condition, never realizing that the family has gotten lost. Too polite to hurt the doctor's feelings and too embarrassed to express their inability to follow the lecture, the family patiently waits for the doctor to finish. For them and for the doctor as well it has been an exercise in pseudoclarity. Consequently, when a trainee reaches for a pencil to start drawing chromosomal patterns for families, we have experienced an urge to reach simultaneously for an antacid.

And yet we would not like to leave the reader with the impression that genetic counseling interviews need be invitations to dyspepsia. One can do reasonably well if one provides for both information exchange and discussion of feelings in the interview.

Had Dr. Burnett received some supervision along these lines prior to his encounter with the Strand family, the interview might have gone somewhat differently. For example:

Doctor: Mr. and Mrs. Strand, you asked to meet with me so that we might discuss some of the genetic factors associated with Down's syndrome. I think it might be useful if we were to back up and start from the beginning. Tell me first of all what you understand about what causes Down's syndrome.

Mother: Just what you told us when we first talked with you, that there is something wrong with Sheila's—er—chromosomes. She got that from us somehow—we gave her too many or the wrong kind or

something. But I felt perfectly fine all during pregnancy, I don't
understand it.

Father: I worry about all those dental X-rays you had, Jean, before we even
knew you were pregnant.

Doctor: I am hearing that a big problem for each of you right now is . . .
what or *who* is responsible for this whole business?

Mother: Well, of course—she's our child, after all. We had to cause it
somehow.

Doctor: You're feeling very responsible.

Mother: (nods yes)

Doctor: That's a very heavy feeling to be carrying around. How do you
even bear it?

Mother: Sometimes I think I can't. (very sad)

Doctor: I don't blame you. Mr. Strand, were you aware of this particular
worry pressing down on your wife?

Father: She talks about it all the time. Sure.

Doctor: How is it for you?

Father: Well, like I say, the only thing I can come up with are those dental
X-rays she had at the beginning.

Doctor: No, no. I wasn't explicit enough. What I meant was how is it for you
to see your wife in so much distress, feeling that she is somehow at
fault for Sheila's difficulty?

Father: (long pause) . . . very hard.

Doctor: How are you able to comfort her at those times?

Father: I'm not, really. There's nothing I can say, it seems like.

Doctor: And how does that make you feel?

Father: Pretty . . . helpless.

Doctor: What an awful spot for each of you. One is feeling responsible,
and the other is feeling helpless.

Both parents admitted that the feelings that the doctor had acknowledged and labeled were correct. He had begun to direct them away from
a blaming and defending stance with one another.

Doctor: I think both of those feelings need a lot more discussion. It is clear
to me that you, Mrs. Strand, are *not* responsible for Sheila's condition. And it is equally clear to me, Mr. Strand, that you do *not* need
to continue feeling helpless. Yet my saying that does not change
things, I realize.

Mother: (emphatic) Nope.

Doctor: From the sound of that, you will not easily allow blame to be lifted
from your shoulders.

Mother: (nods her head in agreement)

Doctor: As I say, it is an issue that needs much more talking through. However, I am also aware that you wanted to talk about some specific questions regarding future pregnancies. And I do not want the time to get away from us. Would you prefer that we continue talking as we are about your feelings, or do you want to shift for the moment so that your specific questions get answered? We are going to need to talk about both — your questions and your feelings.

Mother: Well, I do want to know about having other babies.

Father: Yeah, me too.

Doctor: All right. I'm not forgetting about your feelings, I want you to know. (pause) What specifically do you want to know about having babies?

Mother: Well, should we even consider it or what? I certainly would never want to have this happen again.

Doctor: Let me say that only in rare cases is Down's syndrome inherited. And I can reassure you that in your case it is not so. The chromosome studies we did showed that . . .

The doctor at this point could continue with his short previously described informational discourse regarding the risks and safeguards in future pregnancies for the Strand family. His return to a discussion and airing of parental feelings might be achieved subsequently by a simple statement on his part to that effect. For instance:

Doctor: If what I've told you about future pregnancies now seems understandable, I would like to return to that earlier issue — one of you feeling helpless and the other feeling responsible. Mrs. Strand, I would like you to tell your husband one way in which he might help you to feel even slightly less responsible. I say even slightly because — he can't take that feeling away, I realize that, but how could he help?

Mother: (tears) . . . Well, he could stop talking about those damn X-rays for one thing.

Doctor: Tell him that directly.

And so forth. The point is made: there can be room for both informational and interactional feeling issues in an interview of this sort. Such room, however, must be organized, developed, and encouraged by the interviewer.

REFERENCES

1. Gofman, H., and Allmond, B.: Learning and language disorders in children: part I, the pre-school child, Curr. Probl. Pediatr. **1:**10, 1971.
2. Gofman, H., and Allmond, B.: Learning and language disorders in children: part II, the school-age child, Curr. Probl. Pediatr. **1:**11, 1971.
3. Steinhauer, P., and others: Psychological aspects of chronic illness, Pediatr. Clin. North Am. **21:**825, 1974.

CHAPTER 13

The single-parent family

Interviews throughout this book have been referred to intentionally as family interviews, no matter whether the participants included an entire family, the parents with selected children, or the parents alone. This was done to emphasize our belief that family interviews are determined not so much by who is in the room as by what is inside the interviewer's head. If the interviewer is thinking in terms of systems, homeostasis, relationships, interactional issues, structure, communication, sequences of behavior, and so on, even though he is face to face with less than a complete family, perhaps even only one individual, then his set, his orientation, and his interventions will be based on a model of the family as the patient-client, and in that context he will be doing family interviewing, family therapy. To be sure, there are times when, for family therapy to be effective, either the entire family or specific family members must attend. However, there are many other times when this is not the case; as long as the interviewer maintains a family orientation in his handling of the interview, he may effectively alter family functioning and relationships without the presence of every family member.

While we have utilized clinical examples with less than complete family participation to illustrate this point, until now we have chosen intact families to demonstrate the use of family interviewing in a clinical pediatric setting. That is, we have purposely selected families populated by two parents living under the same roof, both available for participation in interviews. This was done to verify that:

1. Fathers are important; they have too long been overlooked in comprehensive pediatric care. Those delivering health care to children need to expand their view beyond the traditional mother-child duo in the office to one that includes parents and child — a trio.

2. Pediatricians who understand the importance of the father in a child's health care will be successful in encouraging fathers to attend office visits. Fathers *will* participate. They are usually essential and unique contributors in family interviews and in family interactions.

All well and good. However, we are not so fossilized as to have missed the changes that have occurred in the structure of many traditional two-parent American families. The following conversation with a child attending our clinic makes the point:

Doctor: Now, George, when you come to the clinic tomorrow, we are going to be meeting with you and your family. Is your father going to be able to make it?

George: Which father do you mean?

Doctor: The one who is married to your mother.

George: Do you mean my stepmother or my birth-mother?

Doctor: I'm not quite sure, George. Which one are you living with?

George: This week I'm staying with my aunt.

Doctor: But your mother, the one who came with you this morning . . .

George: That was my father's friend, Josie.

Doctor: And is that your stepmother?

George: She was, but she moved out. She brought me in today because my dad and Laurie went up to the Sierras for the weekend.

Doctor: I don't understand — do you call your mother Laurie?

George: No, my mother's name is Ellen. Laurie, I haven't met her; she's going to be moving in with Dad . . . after Ron moves out.

Doctor: Do I know Ron?

George: I don't know. He's tall, has a moustache . . .

Doctor: I guess not. Is he related to you?

George: I'm not sure.

Now George may even understand the term "significant other," but just figuring out whose is whose at the moment may be beyond him, and if George is having trouble sorting out the cast, then the interviewer is certain to have difficulty. We recall one family interview in which we asked a child's mother to invite the rest of her daughter's family for a diagnostic family interview on the pediatric ward. When they arrived the group included: the 9-year-old patient, her mother and mother's second husband, their 22-month-old daughter, and two other children of the mother's first marriage, the patient's brothers. There were also: the patient's father and his second wife, their two children, and one child from the father's first marriage, again the patient's brother. This collection of 11 individuals made the interview even more confusing by their seating arrangement and behavior in the session. The patient's mother and father, long divorced and now each married to new spouses, chose to sit together; they obviously enjoyed a continuing close relationship. Their current spouses likewise gravitated to one another, seemingly very familiar, and the patient spent the entire session sitting on *their* laps, to a large degree disregarding both natural parents. The other children were hopelessly entangled among one another, and just calling an individual by the correct name loomed large as a task for the interviewer.

Undertaking the interview of such a large group is in some ways an invitation to pandemonium, but not necessarily unjustified or irresponsible. In the previous example it was exactly the essential lack of boundaries demonstrated so dramatically between the two families that was responsible for considerable stress in the hospitalized child and the large collection of people around her. And that feature required restructuring and alteration through subsequent family sessions.

This family represents one end of the spectrum, a situation in which there seem to be too many people. It is not particularly unusual. Altered views in the United States about marriage, divorce, separation, living arrangements, and the permanence of relationships have significantly increased the number of children who are in the process of becoming accustomed to a changing array of adult figures in their lives, some clearly labeled in traditional terms: mother, father, stepfather, stepmother, or parent, while others are somewhat less traditionally defined: "aunt," "uncle," friend, roommate, lover, or just, Ron.

If modern views about marriage, separation, and divorce have produced a significant number of environments with numerous parent and adult figures for children, then they may also be said to have produced a veritable deluge of environments with few parent and adult figures for children. We thus turn to the opposite extreme, the child who through parental separation, divorce, or death is living predominantly with one parent and seeing his other parent less often, at regular or irregular intervals or not at all. In our experience this other end of the spectrum is currently the more common. Somewhere between one fourth and one third of our family interviews are now held with such one-parent families.

Do these interviews call for different approaches or strategies to be used? Theoretically we would say no. All of the aforementioned principles underlying family interviewing and family therapy hold whether one is dealing with an intact family or a family in which one parent is no longer available.

We do consider one-parent families somewhat more difficult to work with, however, mainly because there is one less adult to contribute his or her own perspective regarding family behavior, and when one family member is absent the temptation is very great for someone in the family to speak for him and about him, often distorting the facts. In addition, if that member is permanently absent, there is no way for the interviewer to correct these distortions. This fact requires considerable diligence on the interviewer's part to interrupt and stop the "talking about" behavior before it becomes established in interviews.

Another feature of some specific one-parent families renders the interviewer's job more difficult. We refer to those families composed of two individuals only: one parent and one child, without other siblings and without other adults. Such a combination has given rise to our admonition that "duos are deadly." The typical situation is that of a mother living alone with her preteenage daughter. The two of them can coalesce in a grand manner, frustrating the therapist's best efforts to introduce unwanted change into the family's existing system. Consider Paula, age 9, and her mother, Mrs. Frazier. Paula had been refusing to go to school in the morning; she and her mother also slept together in the same bed. They had done so for some time. The doctor felt that each should sleep alone and in the course of an interview said:

> *Doctor:* I think we need to get back to a discussion of the sleeping arrangements at home.
> *Mother:* That's not really a problem, Doctor. Do you think so, honey?
> *Paula:* (shakes her head no)
> *Mother:* Actually we help each other get to sleep. Sometimes my legs are aching so much, and no one can rub legs like Paula. She's magic! And her room is way down the hall, not very well heated, and there's a streetlight outside her window. It makes sleeping in there very difficult. What don't you like about that room, Paula? Tell the doctor.
> *Paula:* The light—it shines in, right in my eyes. And the TV—that's in Momma's bedroom. We like to watch it in bed together . . . and snuggle when it's cold.

Their relationship with one another does indeed sound too attached and in need of some rearrangement. What might have helped the interviewer at this point would have been the presence of a father, a man who could interrupt with:

Father: Look here, I think this girl ought to be sleeping in her own bed. You give in to her entirely too much, Hazel.

But there was no father. Even the presence of a sibling might have helped if that child had offered:

Brother: I don't see why she gets to be in there, and you won't let me! She gets to do everything!

But there was no brother, either. There were only mother and daughter, each committed to maintaining the status quo and easily able to form a tight alliance against any possible intrusion by the well-meaning interviewer who hoped to change their behavior.

It should also be mentioned that undeniably the pediatrician was running into trouble largely because he was imposing his judgment on the family, pinpointing a "problem" where none existed in the family's eyes. He was pursuing a problem important only to him and in so doing was bound to meet resistance from the family members.

Even in situations not so predetermined by the doctor's misdirection, it often appears relatively simple for a family of just two to maintain a cohesive, united front vis-à-vis the interviewer. We have consistently observed that this is much harder for them to do if even just one additional family member is present, raising the total to three. In a family with more than two individuals alliances are less permanent and fixed. There always seems to be someone who is for the moment "on the outside" of a two-person coalition—someone who is therefore unwittingly able to provide the interviewer with some information, remark, or behavior that offers an entrance into the family system. For this reason we much prefer to work with a family unit of three or more individuals. Sometimes if the nuclear family has consisted of only two people, we have circumvented the problem by inviting a grandparent or other relative to join the sessions. At other times we have settled for the fact that two family members it shall be, recognizing that the work may be slow and potentially more frustrating than we had anticipated.

Another characteristic of one-parent families often adds to the difficulties encountered by a family interviewer. These families have a way of being beset by profound real-life problems, economic, occupational, geographic, and so on. One adult is generally being asked to take on a job that heretofore traditionally has been assumed to require the shared energies of two parents. The disruptions to family functioning engendered by that fact alone can sometimes be tremendous. In a sense the single parent with a child has often, in the course of becoming single, had many of his resources halved while being asked to personally assume total responsibility for twice as much as previously required. Such a state of affairs can often precipitate considerable practical dilemmas as well as painful psychological stress. Some of these dilemmas and stresses will depend for resolution on actual changes in the family's external world, in addition to any rearrangements of their style of relating, communicating, or behaving with one another through counseling. This dimension — that frequently some of the realistic problems faced by the single-parent family are beyond the control of the family and beyond the control of the interviewer — is uncomfortable, forcing an interviewer to acknowledge his own limits and those of the family, thus contributing to one's growing feeling that "single-parent families are hard."

Does this mean that working with single-parent families is to be avoided by the fledgling family interviewer? By no means. In our own clinical situation, working with such families could not be avoided even if one wished to: they are simply too numerous in our patient population. And while family interventions may at times be difficult with one-parent families, we find the work is not impossible nor is it necessarily unrewarding or unsuccessful. There are in fact two specific family systems commonly presented to us in a pediatric setting by single-parent families that we have often found amenable to change through judicious family interviewing: (1) the "helpless" family and (2) the "glued-together" family.

THE "HELPLESS" FAMILY

If a pediatrician faced by a family observes his own responses shifting first from sympathy and regard into sadness and feeling overwhelmed and then finally toward irritation and impatience, probably the family is one of the "helpless" variety to which we refer. In San Francisco such a group may typically consist of a young mother and one or possibly two small children, the children generally of preschool age. Father may or may not have been on the scene at one time. At present he is not available, nor does he contribute to the family's welfare. Mother is often unemployed or working only episodically. She and her child(ren) live in very modest circumstances, and life is clearly too hard and too complicated for them. The family feels quite alone against the rest of the world. Friends are few, and if any extended family are nearby, they tend to be critical rather than supportive. As the family's story unfolds, one feels considerable empathy for this collection of waifs attempting to make their way in life against incredible odds. To be sure, there are the very real complexities for the family of finding bread to put on the table and then securing the table itself. In addition there is often another dimension to the family's plight. In the course of the well-child examination mother discloses that she is not only buffaloed by the landlord, the job market, and the disconnection of her telephone, she is equally stumped by how to manage her child and the child's behavior. She seems to lack practical know-how for mothering. She may not explicitly ask for help in this area, yet it is clear that she needs it.

Nutrition, limit setting, appropriate expectations, proper medical and dental care, sleep requirements, learning, social relationships with peers, and so on are either unrecognized as important issues in child rearing or handled by mother with random bursts of energy, usually ineffectually. Since the family's functioning is seldom based on any sort of predictable organization, the family in reality often appears to consist of all children, and while one individual is somewhat older than the other(s), it is a toss-up which of the two or three is in charge of most family operations.

Onto this sinking ship steps the health care worker, very quick to locate the major leaks and set about repairs, convinced of his "rightness" and assured that the family will be forever grateful for his assistance. While patching a major hole in the bow (for instance, helping the mother to get her telephone reinstalled so she can return to her former job, which required the use of her home telephone), he is chagrined to learn that a new defect has spouted elsewhere in the hull, thanks to deliberate hatchet action by the child (for example, a steadfast refusal to eat anything but cold cereal with water, not even milk). The rescuer-repairman rushes to that area of the ship, attends to the problem (for instance, mother's willingness to knuckle under to her 2-year-old's demands), then returns to his previous repair (the telephone) only to find that mother has reopened the original leak by her own action (refusing to let the lineman in the apartment after the doctor's careful negotiations himself with the telephone company). Such frantic, scurrying activity, around countless other issues, continues until either gradually or suddenly the health care worker realizes: "This ship *is* sinking . . . and furthermore my own feet are under water!" At this point he abandons ship, taking his rescue fantasies with him. What he does not learn until somewhat later is that this very ship has listed into and out of several other ports (health clinics), still precariously but very much afloat, both before and after his own experiences with the vessel. The health care worker had of course fallen into the trap of "doing for" rather than helping the family members to help themselves.

A helpless family such as we have described logically calls forth one's best rescue efforts. There are times when direct assistance regarding resources and information may be indicated and may do much to alleviate a family's distress and dilemmas. At other times a family manipulates the doctor through helplessness, stimulating his most heroic efforts and then providing, through holding on to their own frustrating behavior, a demonstration of how and why the doctor's counsel won't work. It is in those instances, when the doctor feels used and manipulated, that his feelings may well shift from empathy to irritation, from concern to frustration and rejection.

It may not be possible initially to differentiate a single-parent family that will effectively use helpful direction from one that will exploit the physician's helpfulness, undermine his suggestions, and continue to remain stuck. However, the two categories sort themselves out in short order as the physician makes beginning interventions. Generally one of three routes is chosen by the family:

1. The family listens, accepts, and welcomes the doctor's direction, utilizing the help provided as a model for approaching and improving other areas of family stress. For instance, a mother complained that her child was a poor eater, that she just didn't know how to encourage her daughter to eat, nor was she sure what foods the child should be encouraged to eat. The doctor gave the mother some specific information regarding appropriate nutrition for a 2½-year-old and helped her to recognize that a sizable element of the child's balkiness was mother's tendency to switch foods at the first whimper of disinterest from the child. Mother understood that her own persistence in the situation had been a missing element. She altered her own behavior in this regard. After some temporary testing by the child, mealtime hassles were reduced. Mother then independently applied the same change in her own behavior to handling bedtime for the child, a chaotic affair. That problem behavior also subsided quickly.

2. The family listens, accepts, and welcomes the doctor's suggestions. They act on his advice and resolve the specific problem at hand. At the next visit they present problem number two and patiently await the doctor's suggestion. Eventually that problem is resolved with direct counsel by the physician. Subsequently problem number three, then four, then five, and so on are put before the pediatrician, who has by this time become labeled in everyone's mind as the family's troubleshooter and seer. The family itself has become no less "helpless" than when they first appeared in the office. Indeed there is no need for them to develop their own resources; their resource is sitting in the office talking to them. Unknown to them, however, he may be starting to feel drained and as though the family's well-being continues to rest on his shoulders alone. This situation (which the doctor has unwittingly encouraged by his actions) is tolerable only to a point, after which the family may find themselves seeking a new doctor, their sense of helplessness unabated.

3. The family listens to the doctor, but they do not accept his direction, either through direct means, challenging the suggestions and offering repetitive "yes, but . . ." behavior, or indirectly, by simply not following through in their lives with the suggestions offered.

A family that travels route number one is, of course, everyone's favorite. It is a pediatrician's dream that families will use his direction to help themselves, applying principles that he has introduced to numerous other life situations. It is families like these for whom directive counseling and advice were designed in the first place.

Families who follow routes number two or three require something different. In these situations directive "helping" either intensifies the family's basic core of helplessness or doesn't work. In either case such "helping" isn't helpful, since it merely supports the basic problem.

These families may benefit more from strategies designed to increase their sense of responsibility rather than lessen it. Perhaps this can best be illustrated by a glimpse of one family presenting the same problem first to a doctor committed to helping through advice and subsequently to a more understanding physician who determines to assist the family by mobilizing their frustration into action, thus giving them the opportunity to use their own strengths.

Mother: She just refuses to stay with the babysitter anymore. She starts screaming in the morning as soon as I take her over. I even tried walking away anyhow, but do you know, I could hear her—hysterical—when I was a block away. If she doesn't settle down, I'm going to have to give up my job. I can't leave a child who's that upset. What do you think I should do?

Doctor: Oh, I think you must keep your job. That's crucial right now.

Mother: I agree, but I can't leave Allison when she's like that.

Doctor: Have you tried staying with her for a few minutes after you both arrive at the babysitter's house?

Mother: Yes, but that doesn't work. She just clings to me all the more.

Doctor: I wonder if maybe it's not time to consider a change of babysitter. You've had some problems before with this particular woman, as I remember.

Mother: Yes, but her rates are the most reasonable that I've found.

Doctor: Your mother was keeping her for a while. Could you consider trying that again?

Mother: My mother spoils her something awful . . . and then gives it to me when I pick Allison up about what a rotten job I'm doing.

Doctor: Have you considered nursery school for Allison?

Mother: Yes, but Allison doesn't seem to like being in a large group of children. That's why this woman was so ideal. There are only two other children besides Allison. I don't know what I'm going to do. Oh, and also, I think I may have to move soon . . .

Doctor: How come?

This doctor has a number of ready, even sensible suggestions. He has not realized, however, that his suggestions will always be matched by an equal number, plus one, of "yes, buts" by the mother. She will need some acknowledgement of her own difficulties before she can move toward hearing any advice. Helpful advice prior to this will only increase mother's dependence on the doctor.

Another physician tries his hand. He does not fall into accepting mother's demand for advice.

Mother: She just refuses to stay with the babysitter anymore. She starts screaming in the morning as soon as I take her over. I even tried walking away anyhow, but do you know, I could hear her—hysterical—when I was a block away. If she doesn't settle down, I'm going to have to give up my job. I can't leave a child who's that upset. What do you think I should do?

Doctor: Tell me your own ideas.

Mother: Like I said, I'll have to quit work. That's all.

Doctor: Is that what you want to do?

Mother: Well . . . no, I don't.

Doctor: Then don't do that.

Mother: Well, what else can I do? You haven't heard her, Doctor. She's incredible.

Doctor: You're right. I haven't heard her. And since you have, you're really the only one in a position to decide what must be done. You've got a real problem on your hands.

Mother: Some help! I don't need you to tell me that.

Doctor: I'm sure you don't. So what *are* you going to do?

Mother: I don't know. She's just going to have to settle down. I'm not giving up my job.

Doctor: Good idea. How will you help her do that?

Mother: I don't know. Maybe I'd better have a talk with the babysitter first. I don't really know what's been going on there recently. Would it do any good to talk to her, do you think?

Doctor: What would you talk to her about?

Mother: Oh, never mind. I do have some things I've been wanting to ask her; I'll just do it. I may have to move soon, you know . . .

Doctor: Uh-huh.

In this situation Allison's mother is getting increasingly frustrated and increasingly more decisive. Unable to manipulate the physician through her helplessness and complaining, she receives from him recognition of her own abilities and thus mobilizes herself into some course of action and begins, at least in this one episode, to take charge of her own life and to learn problem solving. A continuing decrease in this mother's helplessness will depend on similar approaches used by the physician as additional life problems are brought to him by Allison's mother for "his" solution.

THE "GLUED-TOGETHER" FAMILY

We have encountered a number of single-parent families, usually a mother-child combination, in which relationships appear to be stifling growth. The closeness may have begun as an appropriate drawing together following the event that precipitated the loss of the second parent, whether it was separation or death. It is understandable that the two surviving members of such a family may turn to one another for support and nurturance, and a close bond may indeed be formed, serving a useful temporary function as a source of strength for the two individuals who feel that they have shared a common difficult life experience and fate. Sometimes, it appears, this augmented closeness can become something more than a temporary coping mechanism. Mother and child gradually become more and more interdependent, clinging to each other and preferring intensified contact with one another to the formation of new relationships with age peers or with others outside the now very small family. The result is a family of two that increasingly isolates itself from the outside world, developing an intrafamily closeness and intimacy that can be problematic both for mother and for child. The child is not given opportunities to separate and grow toward independence, and the mother sees little need for expanding her own horizons into adult companionships.

The Lane family

Mrs. Lane had no idea that this stifling togetherness was contributing to some of the difficulties she was having with her 9-year-old daughter, Ann. She knew only that she had been having an increasing problem getting her youngster to attend school regularly, and the pediatrician, after giving Ann a clean bill of health, had suggested that the two of them return to his office in 3 days for an hour's conversation about the problem. She agreed but hoped, she said, that the interview would not really take that long; she had other things to do. This was the week before finals, and Mrs. Lane was a full-time student. If finals week went well, she would have her bachelor's degree after literally years of work, during which she had raised Ann singlehandedly, held down one and sometimes two jobs at a time, and accumulated enough university units to have come very close now to her degree. The doctor congratulated her on her soon-to-be-reached goal and said that he would keep in mind that time for her was really short.

The actual interview opened in an interesting way. First of all, Mrs. Lane was late. Apparently her car had broken down en route. She and Ann had simply left it parked by the side of the road and come the rest of the way via public transportation. Mother looked tired, hurried, and exasperated. Ann was holding on to her mother's right thigh; the other arm was around her mother's waist.

Mother: Don't do that, Ann. I'm hot. Stand up, stand up. Don't hang.

Ann grumpily moved, but only a few inches away from her mother. She did not return the pediatrician's greeting and did not look at him.

Mother: Doctor, I'm so sorry, but could I use your bathroom? In all the upset with the car and so forth, there just wasn't time to take care of
things like that, although I had allowed plenty of time when we
left.

Doctor: Sure. (indicates the bathroom)

Mother: (moving toward the door) Now you wait right here, Ann. Momma
will be right back.

Ann shook her head no and moved right along with her mother, never
allowing the physical distance between them to exceed 3 inches. Mother
looked somewhat exasperated and tried with her own hands to peel Ann
off her body but to no avail. The child persisted in clinging. At the door
itself mother conceded defeat and said:

Mother: Oh, all right. You can come in, too, but I want to be able to be by
myself once we're in there. Do you understand?

Ann's response was to engineer both her mother and herself inside and
close the bathroom door.

The pediatrician preferred not to imagine exactly how certain functions were being performed behind the closed door but simply waited
for mother and daughter to emerge, which they eventually did — together, of course. Mother sat down, and Ann joined her in the same chair. In
fact she settled into her mother's lap. Mother made no moves to discourage Ann and accepted the maneuver as though she were most accustomed to it.

Mrs. Lane went on to describe her concerns about Ann. They were
simply extensions of actions that the pediatrician had already observed
in the office. Ann whined about going off to school in the morning and
sometimes feigned stomachaches. The stomachaches always disappeared
by 9:30 A.M. after mother had called in sick at work, resentfully deciding that she would have to stay home with Ann for the day. Ann balked
in the same way when it came to sleeping alone at night, and Mrs. Lane
had handled that just as inconsistently, sometimes allowing Ann to sleep
with her, sometimes joining Ann in the girl's bed, and sometimes refusing to give in to Ann's demands. The last usually resulted in a sleepless
night for both of them, and Mrs. Lane, feeling that she had to reserve
some energy for her university studies to say nothing of her job responsibilities, tended less and less to take any sort of stand with Ann. In the
middle of this disclosure to the pediatrician she twice interrupted herself
with a somewhat forced, unconvincing aside to Ann.

> *Mother:* Ann, you're awfully heavy on my lap. Wouldn't you like to sit over there?
>
> *Ann:* No
>
> *Mother:* Please . . .
>
> *Ann:* No.
>
> *Mother:* All right for you! (using a teasing tone and giving her daughter a friendly squeeze, then rolling her eyes up in a gesture of exasperation)

Watching the two of them so tightly intertwined, the pediatrician noted a literal change in his own breathing pattern. His chest felt constricted and tight. It was this sensation more than anything else that now prompted him to act. Following Mrs. Lane's second such conversation with Ann, demonstrating that neither had any intention of altering the physical configuration of the family, the pediatrician took matters into his own hands. Rising from his chair, he moved over to the couple and lifted Ann off her mother's body and into an available chair.

> *Doctor:* Ann, I need you to sit there during this talk.
>
> *Ann:* I don't like sitting here. I want to sit there (pointing to her mother's lap).
>
> *Doctor:* I need you to sit where you are.

Surprisingly, Ann made no effort to test the doctor's stern tone that carried no ambivalence or invitation to test; although it was clear that she was not happy in her new spot, she stayed put. The doctor continued:

> *Doctor:* (to mother) How does that feel?
>
> *Mother:* (sigh) Oh, much better. She's really a lapful at 9 years of age. I was having trouble breathing.
>
> *Doctor:* So was I, watching the two of you.
>
> *Mother:* Ann tends to be somewhat shy around strangers.
>
> *Doctor:* What about at home?
>
> *Mother:* We're very close.
>
> *Doctor:* What does that mean?

Mother described their life together at home. The initial incident with the bathroom in the doctor's office was not an isolated happening. Ann often demanded to accompany her mother into the bathroom at home. There was also the previously described problem with maintaining separate sleeping arrangements at night. Going off to school wasn't going well either. Even studying had become a joint endeavor. Mother did her schoolwork at the kitchen table; at those times Ann refused to be in an-

other part of the house, even if she herself had completed her homework. Instead she would busy herself with some activity at the table, insisting on remaining until her mother left the room. There was a hint of
exasperation in mother's voice as she related all of this, enough that the
pediatrician decided to risk asking:

Doctor: Tell me, Mrs. Lane, when do you ever find time for yourself — private time for just you alone?

Mother: To tell you the truth, I haven't had time to myself since Ann's father cleared out 4 years ago. I don't really see that I have much
choice. I haven't had money for babysitters, and besides as I said,
Ann is so shy around strangers, she just refused to stay with people
the few times I tried cooperative babysitters. It just never worked
out. Sometimes I think to myself, and this is embarassing to say . . .
Oh, if I could only go to the bathroom alone, what I wouldn't give
for that!

Doctor: Do you feel that you have a right to some privacy . . . for yourself?

Mother: (looking somewhat taken aback) I've never really considered much
about my "rights" at all . . . in anything. I've been so busy for so
long that I have just sort of assumed that this is the way life is going
to be.

Doctor: Is this the way you want it to be?

Mother: Well . . . no, not exactly, but I don't see that I have any choice.

Doctor: I'm not so sure.

Mother: If you're suggesting that I start hiring babysitters, forget it. That's
just too expensive. I can't afford it.

Doctor: That doesn't sound like a good idea. However, if you were to begin
to arrange some time for you alone in your life, where would you
start?

Mother: Well, I don't know. I see what you're driving at . . . and you know
I've never thought of it in terms like this.

Doctor: It is very clear to me that you are a woman who puts a premium on
responsible mothering, and . . .

Mother: Well, of course. I want to do the best for Ann, and I have been worried about her.

Doctor: OK — I would like you to tell her directly right now what your worries have been about her.

Mother: Oh, she knows.

Doctor: I am sure you have discussed it before. Do it once more, this time in
front of me.

Mother: Well, OK, Ann, are you listening to me? How can I say it? I'm worried . . . I'm worried about . . . your ego.

Ann:	(looks blankly at her mother and says nothing)
Doctor:	(to mother) Find out if she understands.
Mother:	Do you know what I mean?
Ann:	No.

Mother went on to explain that she feared that Ann lacked self-confidence and was so shy around people because she didn't respect herself and her own abilities very much. She didn't seem to have much faith in herself. Ann indicated that she understood her mother's last words.

Doctor:	And how are you teaching Ann to have respect for herself?

Mother indicated with frustration that she just didn't know how to get that across; it seemed to be a very difficult lesson for Ann to learn.

Doctor:	I wonder if you can teach her what you haven't learned for yourself?
Mother:	What do you mean?
Doctor:	Would you agree that you tend to put your own needs aside generally in favor of Ann's?
Mother:	Well, of course. Any mother ought . . .
Doctor:	(interrupting) Wait . . . if you are not demonstrating that you respect your own needs — for privacy and time alone, for instance . . .
Mother:	Yes?
Doctor:	Then Ann will not respect those needs in you, nor will she be learning any good models for developing the ability to see her own needs as important. Are you following me?
Mother:	Yes, I am.
Doctor:	You do put your own needs aside with Ann. That is clear . . . Nonetheless, I am often hearing a resentful edge in your voice when you do so, at least here in the office. Am I hearing correctly?
Mother:	(after some hesitation) You're right, Doctor. There is. I try . . . I try to do so much for her, and it never seems to be enough. There just isn't enough of me to go around.
Doctor:	Uh-huh. Then perhaps in order for you to be able to give more freely to your daughter — especially a sense of strength in herself, you must first nourish and respect some of your own needs, so that you have something of that to offer . . . something beside resentment, that is, so that Ann does not become in your eyes simply one large insatiable demand.
Mother:	That's it! That is often the case, especially with school and the job. I just can't do it all.

Doctor: So back to my earlier question, if you were to insert into your life some time for you, a time for you to be alone and meet some of your own individual needs, where would you begin?

Mother: (after considerable silent thought) I think if I could have time to myself for studying in the evenings, that would help, especially now, during finals.

Mrs. Lane, with the pediatrician's directive questions and acknowledgement, next planned the specific changes that would be required for her to have evenings devoted to solitary studying uninterrupted by Ann's presence and activity. Mother decided (with the pediatrician's support) that she, not Ann, would continue to work at the kitchen table. It represented the best work space with the best light. Ann would be required to stay out of the kitchen from 6:30 P.M. until mother had completed her studies for that evening. Since Ann had a desk and work space in her own bedroom, this would present no hardship. Mother said that until now she had not realized that she had absolutely no place that was hers, rather than theirs, in their entire apartment.

Mother: And what I am saying is that I guess I might like the kitchen to be my private space on weeknights from 6:30 until about 9.

Ann: No . . . I can't study by myself in my room.

Mother: Well . . . would you rather be . . .

Doctor: Wait a minute. Are you giving Ann the choice? Or is this one time you decide? Are you asking her or are you telling her?

Mother: It's my decision, I guess.

Doctor: You guess?

Mother: Oh, dear.

Doctor: If this time it is going to be your choice, then you need to tell her that directly, now.

Mother: The doctor's right. I am going to do what is good for me for once, Ann.

Ann: (sulks and is quiet)

Doctor: So is this one way in which this whole thing could not work out for you — that you would continue to put your own needs and wants aside and let Ann decide?

Mother: Yes, it's almost automatic with me, Doctor.

Doctor: Right. Tell me some other ways in which the two of you could make this proposed change not work out.

Mother: Well, I'm sure Ann could insist on being in the kitchen with me, no matter what I want.

Doctor: OK. And how could you handle that?

> *Mother:* If need be . . . I would just have to pick her up and carry her out of the room.
>
> *Doctor:* And would you be able to do that?
>
> *Mother:* (laughs as though she enjoys the thought of that) Yes, I really think I could. It would certainly take her by surprise.
>
> *Doctor:* And you . . . would you surprise yourself by your own strength and ability?
>
> *Mother:* Probably.
>
> *Doctor:* What else could sabotage your new plan?
>
> *Mother:* . . . I don't know.
>
> *Doctor:* Think of something *you* could do to undermine it.
>
> *Mother:* (embarrassed) I guess I could decide it's not important enough after a day or so to make a hassle out of.
>
> *Doctor:* That's right.
>
> *Mother:* No . . . no, that won't happen. I want to change things so they will be good for me, too.
>
> *Doctor:* Then it will be up to you.

When the session ended a few minutes later, mother left with a smile and Ann left pouting and refusing to even look in the pediatrician's direction. He noted with interest that mother and child were physically quite separate as they went out the door.

At a return visit in 2 weeks, the mother reported that she had implemented her plan successfully and that her studying for finals had been the most enjoyable that she had done in several years. Ann had actually been quite reasonable once they were home and had never challenged her mother's new rule. In fact mother had felt so confident about her new success that she had initiated an additional rule, enhancing her "self-boundary" even further. She had declared the bathroom off limits when she was using it. Ann had been testing this one strenuously with banging on the bathroom door. Mother was handling this behavior at the moment by simply locking the door and refusing to be intimidated. She was thus providing a role of strength from which Ann could model her own behavior.

Unfortunately, a third visit was prevented by the family's suddenly being called back semipermanently to Washington because of a family emergency, serious illness in Mrs. Lane's sister. Had sessions not been interrupted, the pediatrician would have continued during additional interviews in this direction, amplifying and supporting the development of appropriate boundaries between this mother and her child, allowing each to grow toward individuation and independence. Their beginning moves in this direction had been most encouraging. However, the degree of their mutual dependency was significant and could not be expected to disappear after only two sessions. Considerable ongoing work would be required, and it is regrettable that the work was interrupted. A note accompanying mother's payment 6 weeks after the second visit expressed Mrs. Lane's continuing success in the two areas that she had begun to alter, privacy in the evenings and privacy in the bathroom. She also expressed a wish for continuing professional help and asked for the name of a pediatrician "who doesn't just give shots. I want one who listens and then talks." The referral was made to one of our former trainees practicing pediatrics nearby in Seattle.

It seems fitting that we conclude our writing with this family. Mrs. Lane and her daughter, Ann, were each demonstrating serious and potentially handicapping difficulties along their individual and collective roads of growth toward independence. Their difficulties in this area were reflected in their communication, their family system, their family structure, and their repetitive sequences of behavior, as previously described. Utilizing a family view and interventions based on a family approach as proposed by this text, the doctor was able to facilitate a family change, providing a beginning experience for each family member in gaining slightly more independence, individuation, and autonomy. In short the doctor facilitated a small growth step in this family. To our minds, he was practicing very competent pediatrics, for facilitating growth is perhaps the basic responsibility of a pediatric clinician. The clinical example attests one final time to our belief that attention to a child's (and adult's) behavior frequently requires attention to his growth toward independence. Helping individuals grow toward this independence and individuation — the pediatrician's job — may often be assisted by the physician's close attention to the family as the treatment unit.

Index